T-Cell Lymphoma

Editor

ERIC D. JACOBSEN

HEMATOLOGY/ONCOLOGY CLINICS OF NORTH AMERICA

www.hemonc.theclinics.com

Consulting Editors
GEORGE P. CANELLOS
H. FRANKLIN BUNN

April 2017 • Volume 31 • Number 2

ELSEVIER

1600 John F. Kennedy Boulevard • Suite 1800 • Philadelphia, Pennsylvania, 19103-2899

http://www.theclinics.com

HEMATOLOGY/ONCOLOGY CLINICS OF NORTH AMERICA Volume 31, Number 2
April 2017 ISSN 0889-8588, ISBN 13: 978-0-323-52410-0

Editor: Stacy Eastman
Developmental Editor: Kristen Helm

Hematology/Oncology Clinics (ISSN 0889-8588) is published bimonthly by Elsevier Inc., 360 Park Avenue South, New York, NY 10010-1710. Months of issue are February, April, June, August, October, and December. Business and Editorial Offices: 1600 John F. Kennedy Blvd., Ste. 1800, Philadelphia, PA 19103−2899. Customer Service Office: 3251 Riverport Lane, Maryland Heights, MO 63043. Periodicals postage paid at New York, NY and at additional mailing offices. Subscription prices are $397.00 per year (domestic individuals), $742.00 per year (domestic institutions), $100.00 per year (domestic students/residents), $453.00 per year (Canadian individuals), $919.00 per year (Canadian institutions) $536.00 per year (international individuals), $919.00 per year (international institutions), and $255.00 per year (international and Canadian students/residents). International air speed delivery is included in all *Clinics* subscription prices. All prices are subject to change without notice. **POSTMASTER:** Send address changes to *Hematology/Oncology Clinics of North America*, Elsevier Health Sciences Division, Subscription Customer Service, 3251 Riverport Lane, Maryland Heights, MO 63043. Customer Service (orders, claims, online, change of address): Elsevier Health Sciences Division, Subscription **Customer Service, 3251 Riverport Lane, Maryland Heights, MO 63043. Tel: 1-800-654-2452 (U.S. and Canada); 314-447-8871 (outside U.S. and Canada). Fax: 314-447-8029. E-mail: journalscustomerservice-usa@elsevier.com (for print support)**; **journalsonlinesupport-usa@elsevier.com (for online support)**.

Reprints. For copies of 100 or more, of articles in this publication, please contact the Commercial Reprints Department, Elsevier Inc., 360 Park Avenue South, New York, New York 10010-1710; Tel.: 212-633-3874, Fax: 212-633-3820, E-mail: reprints@elsevier.com.

Hematology/Oncology Clinics of North America is covered in *MEDLINE/PubMed (Index Medicus), EMBASE/Excerpta Medica, and BIOSIS.*

Contributors

CONSULTING EDITORS

GEORGE P. CANELLOS, MD
William Rosenberg Professor of Medicine, Department of Medical Oncology, Dana-Farber Cancer Institute, Boston, Massachusetts

H. FRANKLIN BUNN, MD
Professor of Medicine, Division of Hematology, Brigham and Women's Hospital, Harvard Medical School, Boston, Massachusetts

EDITOR

ERIC D. JACOBSEN, MD
Department of Medical Oncology, Dana-Farber Cancer Institute, Assistant Professor in Medicine, Harvard Medical School, Boston, Massachusetts

AUTHORS

MUSA AL-ZAHRANI, MBBS, MD
Division of Hematology, Faculty of Medicine, Gordon and Leslie Diamond Health Care Centre, University of British Columbia, Vancouver, British Columbia, Canada; Faculty of Medicine, King Saud University, Riyadh, Saudi Arabia

ALESSANDRO BROCCOLI, MD
Institute of Hematology "L. and A. Seràgnoli," University of Bologna, Bologna, Italy

DAI CHIHARA, MD, PhD
Department of Lymphoma/Myeloma, The University of Texas MD Anderson Cancer Center, Houston, Texas; Department of Internal Medicine, The University of New Mexico, Albuquerque, New Mexico

CLAIRE DEARDEN, BSc, MBBS, MD, FRCP, FRCPath
Department of Haemato-Oncology, The Royal Marsden Biomedical Research Centre, London, United Kingdom; Department of Haemato-Oncology, The Royal Marsden NHS Foundation Trust, Sutton, Surrey, United Kingdom

TEJASWINI M. DHAWALE, MD
Assistant Professor of Medicine, University of Washington School of Medicine, Seattle Cancer Care Alliance, Seattle, Washington

CHRISTOPHER DITTUS, DO, MPH
Assistant Professor of Medicine, Division of Hematology and Oncology, University of North Carolina at Chapel Hill, Chapel Hill, North Carolina

MICHELLE A. FANALE, MD
Department of Lymphoma/Myeloma, The University of Texas MD Anderson Cancer Center, Houston, Texas

FRANCINE M. FOSS, MD
Hematology and Bone Marrow Transplantation, Yale University School of Medicine, New Haven, Connecticut

MICHAEL GIRARDI, MD
Department of Dermatology, Yale University School of Medicine, New Haven, Connecticut

STEVEN HORWITZ, MD
Associate Attending, Department of Medicine, Memorial Sloan Kettering Cancer Center, Associate Professor, Weill-Cornell Medical College, New York, New York

NICOLE R. LEBOEUF, MD, MPH
Assistant Professor, Department of Dermatology, Clinical Director, The Center for Cutaneous Oncology, Dana Farber Cancer Institute, Brigham and Women's Hospital, Harvard Medical School, Boston, Massachusetts

SHINICHI MAKITA, MD, PhD
Department of Hematology, National Cancer Center Hospital, Tokyo, Japan

ENRICA MARCHI, MD, PhD
Hematology-Oncology Fellow, Center for Lymphoid Malignancies, Columbia University Medical Center, New York, New York

NEHA MEHTA-SHAH, MD
Fellow, Department of Medicine, Memorial Sloan Kettering Cancer Center, New York, New York

OWEN A. O'CONNOR, MD, PhD
Professor of Medicine and Experimental Therapeutics, Director, Center for Lymphoid Malignancies, Columbia University Medical Center, New York, New York

JOHN T. O'MALLEY, MD, PhD
Clinical Instructor, Department of Dermatology, The Center for Cutaneous Oncology, Dana Farber Cancer Institute, Brigham and Women's Hospital, Harvard Medical School, Boston, Massachusetts

ALEXANDER G. RAUFI, MD
Hematology-Oncology Fellow, Center for Lymphoid Malignancies, Columbia University Medical Center, New York, New York

MAXWELL B. SAUDER, MD, FRCPC
Cutaneous Oncology Fellow, Department of Dermatology, The Center for Cutaneous Oncology, Dana Farber Cancer Institute, Brigham and Women's Hospital, Harvard Medical School, Boston, Massachusetts

KERRY J. SAVAGE, MD, MSc
Medical Oncologist, Department of Medical Oncology, British Columbia Cancer Agency, Vancouver, British Columbia, Canada

ANDREI R. SHUSTOV, MD
Associate Professor of Medicine, University of Washington School of Medicine, Seattle
Cancer Care Alliance, Seattle, Washington

J. MARK SLOAN, MD
Assistant Professor of Medicine, Division of Hematology and Oncology, Boston University
Medical Center, Boston, Massachusetts

AMIT SUD, MBChB, MRes, MRCP
Department of Haemato-Oncology, The Royal Marsden Biomedical Research Centre,
London, United Kingdom; Department of Haemato-Oncology, The Royal Marsden NHS
Foundation Trust, Sutton, Surrey, United Kingdom

KENSEI TOBINAI, MD, PhD
Department of Hematology, National Cancer Center Hospital, Tokyo, Japan

PIER LUIGI ZINZANI, MD, PhD
Professor, Institute of Hematology "L. and A. Seràgnoli," University of Bologna, Bologna,
Italy

Contents

Peripheral T-cell lymphoma, not otherwise specified (PTCL-NOS), corresponds with a heterogeneous group of mature T-cell lymphomas. Recent gene expression profiling studies have identified at least two molecular subgroups (GATA3 and TBX2). Standard treatment and outcomes remain poor. High-dose chemotherapy with autologous stem cell transplantation is incorporated into primary therapy for young fit patients but remains ineffective for most and has not been tested in a randomized study. Several novel agents have been approved for use in relapsed/refractory PTCLs, and although response rates are modest for most, durable remissions have been reported. Selecting rationale combinations and incorporating predictive biomarkers will be important moving forward to improve outcomes in patients with PTCL.

Anaplastic large cell lymphoma (ALCL) is one of the most common peripheral T-cell lymphomas, and the incidence is higher in blacks than non-Hispanic whites. ALK-positive and ALK-negative ALCL are distinct subtypes that have different characteristics and clinical outcomes. Breast implant–associated ALCL is a rare lymphoma that has a good survival outcome, and a recent study showed that total capsulectomy is essential for treatment. Brentuximab vedotin (BV) is a standard treatment for relapsed/refractory ALCL. The response rate is high at 80–90%; however, once the disease progresses in patients on BV, survival outcome is very poor, with a median overall survival of less than two months.

Angioimmunoblastic T-cell lymphoma is a follicular T-helper–derived neoplasm displaying a peculiar morphologic appearance and biological complexity. New mutations have been described that contribute to elucidating the underlying pathogenetic events. The disease behaves aggressively and typically affects elderly patients. The outcomes reported with anthracycline-containing regimens are poor; therefore autologous transplantation in first remission should be offered whenever possible. Newer approaches are urgently needed for relapsed and refractory patients. Newly approved agents show activity in pretreated patients but response durations are short. Innovative induction strategies (CHOP + biologic agent) should be designed to enhance response quality, facilitate transplantation, and prolong survival.

Extranodal natural killer/T-cell lymphoma, nasal type (ENKL), is a rare subtype of non-Hodgkin lymphoma, and its treatment outcome was previously poor. Novel treatment strategies have improved the outcomes of ENKL remarkably in the last decade. Nowadays, patients with localized nasal ENKL are recommended treatment with concurrent chemoradiotherapy, and their 5-year overall survival rate is approximately 70%. In patients with advanced or relapsed/refractory disease, the efficacy of L-asparaginase–containing therapy has been confirmed. However, there still remain unmet needs in the treatment of ENKL. Continued efforts should be made to further improvements in the treatment of ENKL.

Adult T-cell leukemia/lymphoma (ATLL) is a rare T-cell disorder that is etiologically linked to chronic infection with human T-cell lymphotropic virus type 1. ATLL is divided into four subtypes: acute, lymphomatous, chronic, and smoldering. The acute and lymphomatous variants are often described clinically as the aggressive types of ATLL. Treatment strategies traditionally have focused on antiviral therapy with zidovudine and interferon-alpha and combination chemotherapy. Novel therapeutic approaches include the use of monoclonal antibodies, anti-CCR4 therapy, immunomodulatory therapy, and anti-TAX vaccines. Future research must focus on multi-institutional clinical trial participation because of the rarity of this deadly hematologic malignancy.

T-cell prolymphocytic leukemia (T-PLL) is a rare and aggressive T-cell malignancy. T-PLL can be distinguished from other lymphoid diseases by the evaluation and integration of clinical features, morphology, immunophenotyping, cytogenetics, and molecular features. The current therapeutic approach relies on immunotherapy followed by a hematopoietic stem cell transplant in selected cases. Clinical outcomes are generally poor, although insights from genomic and molecular studies may increase our understanding of this disease, with the promise of additional effective therapeutic options.

Peripheral T-cell lymphomas represent 10% to 15% of non-Hodgkin lymphomas and comprise more than 20 different entities. Treatment of very rare T-cell lymphomas can be challenging because there are no large or randomized studies to guide clinical decision making and treatment paradigms are often based on small series or imperfect data. Although a strict algorithm cannot be written with certainty, through the literature that exists and clinical experience, themes and principles of approaches do emerge that when coupled with clinical judgment allow reasonable and logical decisions.

Francine M. Foss and Michael Girardi

Mycosis fungoides and the Sezary syndrome (SS) are rare lymphomas of $CD4^+$ helper T cells. There is stagewise progression from patch/plaques to thicker tumor lesions/diffuse erythroderma. Blood involvement is a characteristic of SS. Outcomes are related to the extent of skin, blood, lymph node, and visceral organ involvement. Patients with limited patch and plaque disease are treated with skin-directed therapies. More advanced/refractory disease is treated with skin-directed therapies and oral or systemic immunomodulatory agents. Single-agent chemotherapies are used against tumors, refractory plaques, and lymph node and visceral involvement. Allogeneic stem cell transplantation is a potentially curative strategy for advanced/resistant disease.

Maxwell B. Sauder, John T. O'Malley, and Nicole R. LeBoeuf

Primary cutaneous $CD30^+$ lymphoproliferative disorders encompass lymphomatoid papulosis (LyP), primary cutaneous anaplastic large cell lymphoma (pcALCL), and indeterminate cases. LyP is a benign disorder characterized by recurrent crops of red or violaceous papulonodules. Patients with LyP are at an increased risk of a secondary malignancy. pcALCL is characterized by a solitary red to violaceous nodule or tumor larger than 20 mm. LyP is benign, is limited to the skin, and self-resolves, with a 5-year survival rate of 100%; pcALCL is limited to the skin and responsive to directed therapies, with a 5-year survival rate of over 95%. Aggressive chemotherapeutic regimens should be avoided.

Tejaswini M. Dhawale and Andrei R. Shustov

Peripheral T-cell lymphoma and natural killer/T-cell lymphomas (PT/NKCL) make up a diverse subgroup of non-Hodgkin's lymphomas characterized by an aggressive clinical course. The use of hematopoietic stem cell transplantation (HSCT) in the treatment of PT/NKCL remains controversial because of the absence of randomized controlled trials. The best available data suggest that certain subtypes of PT/NKCL may benefit more from the application of HSCT than other subtypes and that this benefit results from their unique clinical characteristics and underlying biology. Ultimately, however, prospective randomized controlled trials are needed to clarify the optimal type and timing of HSCT in patients with PT/NKCL.

Peripheral T-cell lymphomas (PTCL) are a heterogeneous group of mature T-cell malignancies associated with exceptionally poor prognoses. Currently, chemotherapy remains the standard of care, but outcomes are suboptimal, with 5-year survival rates ranging from 15% to 25%. In recent years, several novel agents, including pralatrexate, romidepsin, belinostat, and brentuximab vedotin, have been approved for the treatment of relapsed/refractory PTCL. In addition, numerous other therapies with different mechanisms of action and targets are currently under investigation. This article discusses in detail agents currently available, those currently under investigation, and active combination trials.

HEMATOLOGY/ONCOLOGY CLINICS OF NORTH AMERICA

THE CLINICS ARE AVAILABLE ONLINE!
Access your subscription at:
www.theclinics.com

Preface

Peripheral T-Cell Lymphoma: The Beginning of the End of the Beginning

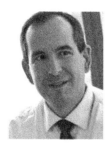

Eric D. Jacobsen, MD
Editor

The peripheral T-cell lymphomas are a group of heterogeneous mature T-cell neoplasms with disparate biology and heterogeneous clinical behavior ranging from very indolent to extremely aggressive. As a group, these lymphomas are rare in North America and Western Europe, accounting for approximately 10% of all cases of non-Hodgkin lymphoma. Certain histologies, most notably adult T-cell lymphoma/leukemia and extranodal NK/T-cell lymphoma, are more common in parts of Asia, Africa, and South America but rarely encountered in other areas of the world. The rarity of these diseases makes them a challenge to study in the lab and in the clinic. Until recently, there were few clinical trials devoted specifically to T-cell lymphomas, and most treatment paradigms were extrapolated from regimens utilized in aggressive B-cell lymphomas, typically with disappointing results. A lack of in vitro and in vivo models further hampered scientific advance and developmental therapeutics.

The last decade has witnessed an increase in drug development for T-cell lymphomas, with four agents (pralatrexate, romidepsin, belinostat, and brentuximab) now approved by the US Food and Drug Administration for the treatment of relapsed or refractory disease. This compares quite favorably, at least in pure numbers if not clinical impact, to the one agent (rituximab) approved for the treatment of diffuse large B-cell lymphoma in the last 20 years. We have also witnessed the advent of randomized trials in T-cell lymphomas—something that was nearly unheard of even a few years ago. Although the approval of these agents and the existence of randomized trials represent a significant step forward, the reality remains that the treatment outcome for most patients with peripheral T-cell lymphoma remains poor, and our understanding of the biology of these diseases is still inadequate. In order to complete clinical trials in a meaningful timeframe, we must lump together varied T-cell histologies that often share limited biological or clinical characteristics. The fact that the most common

Hematol Oncol Clin N Am 31 (2017) xiii–xiv
http://dx.doi.org/10.1016/j.hoc.2017.01.001
0889-8588/17/© 2017 Published by Elsevier Inc.

histology is called *peripheral T-cell lymphoma, not otherwise specified,* speaks volumes to the amount of work that still needs to be done to better understand the pathogenesis of these disorders.

The utility of chemotherapy remains and is likely to remain limited in most subtypes of peripheral T-cell lymphoma. Therefore, further elucidation of the genetics and molecular biology of these disorders will be critical to move the field forward. In this issue of *Hematology/Oncology Clinics of North America*, we present a broad-ranging discussion on the current status of the peripheral T-cell lymphomas. Most articles focus on a specific histology and review current treatment paradigms as well as key emerging data on biological and therapeutic advances. Other articles focus more broadly on experimental therapeutics and stem cell transplantation. Regardless of the focus, each article represents a cutting-edge, up-to-date discussion by a renowned expert in the field.

Peripheral T-cell lymphomas remain one of the great areas of unmet need in hematologic malignancies. Paradoxically, advances in the understanding of the biology of these diseases may make the conduct of clinical trials more challenging. For instance, completing a trial specific to angioimmunoblastic T-cell lymphoma is already daunting, but finding sufficient numbers of patients with angioimmunoblastic T-cell lymphoma who harbor an IDH2 mutation may discourage even the most stalwart clinical investigator. Yet such trials can and should be done. In order to meet this challenge, we must put personal and institutional aspirations aside and collaborate on a global scale to conduct trials based upon rationale targets, not histology or expediency. I hope this issue gives you an appreciation for the challenges we face but, more important, a deeper understanding of how those challenges are slowly but inexorably being confronted.

Eric D. Jacobsen, MD
Department of Medical Oncology
Dana-Farber Cancer Institute
Assistant Professor in Medicine
Harvard Medical School
Mayer 219
450 Brookline Avenue
Boston, MA 02215, USA

E-mail address:
eric_jacobsen@dfci.harvard.edu

Peripheral T-Cell Lymphoma, Not Otherwise Specified

A Review of Current Disease Understanding and Therapeutic Approaches

Musa Al-Zahrani, MBBS, MD[a,b], Kerry J. Savage, MD, MSc[c,*]

KEYWORDS

- Peripheral T-cell lymphoma, not otherwise specified • PTCL-NOS • CHOP

KEY POINTS

- Peripheral T-cell lymphoma, not otherwise specified (PTCL-NOS), is a heterogeneous subtype of peripheral T-cell lymphoma (PTCL).
- Gene expression profiling has identified GATA3 and TBX21 molecular subgroups with biologic and prognostic implications.
- A number of novel therapies show promise in relapsed/refractory PTCLs.

DEFINITION AND CLASSIFICATION

Peripheral T-cell lymphoma, not otherwise specified (PTCL-NOS) corresponds to a heterogeneous group of mature T-cell lymphomas, which does not fit into any of the specifically defined entities. The postulated normal counterpart cells are activated mature T lymphocytes, mostly CD4[+] central memory type of the adaptive immune system.[1] PTCL-NOS was introduced initially in the Revised European American Lymphoma classification in 1994 as PTCL—unspecified[2] and updated to PTCL-NOS in the World Health Organization (WHO) classification.[1,3] More recently, it has been

Disclosure Statement: Dr K.J. Savage has received honoraria and participated in advisory boards for Seattle Genetics, BMS, Merck, Infinity, Abbie and Celgene; consulting for Servier. Dr M. Al-Zahrani has nothing to disclose.
^a Division of Hematology, Department of Hematology, Faculty of Medicine, Gordon and Leslie Diamond Health Care Centre, University of British Columbia, 2775 Laurel Street, 10th Floor, Vancouver, British Columbia V5Z 1M9, Canada; ^b Faculty of Medicine, King Saud University, Riyadh 12372, Saudi Arabia; ^c Department of Medical Oncology, British Columbia Cancer Agency, 600 West 10th Avenue, Vancouver, BC V5Z 4E6, Canada
* Corresponding author. Department of Medical Oncology, British Columbia Cancer Agency, 600 West 10th Avenue, Vancouver, BC V5Z 4E6, Canada
E-mail address: ksavage@bccancer.bc.ca

Hematol Oncol Clin N Am 31 (2017) 189–207
http://dx.doi.org/10.1016/j.hoc.2016.11.009
0889-8588/17/© 2017 Elsevier Inc. All rights reserved.

hemonc.theclinics.com

appreciated that a subset of PTCL-NOS has overlapping features with angioimmuno-blastic lymphoma (AITL). Genetic studies have confirmed the presence of recurrent mutations in AITL, including *TET2*, *IDH2*, *DNMT3A*, *RHOA*, and *CD28* mutations that also occur in PTCL-NOS that manifest a T-follicular helper (TFH) phenotype. For this designation there must be expression of at least 2 TFH-related antigens, including CD279/PD1, CD10, BCL6, CXCL13, ICOS, SAP, and CCR5.[4,5] This common phenotype has led to the introduction of a new umbrella category in the 2016 WHO classification termed 'nodal PTCL with a TFH phenotype,' which encompasses follicular T-cell lymphoma (FTCL), AITL, and other nodal PTCL with a TFH phenotype.[6] Despite these similarities, clinical and pathologic differences remain so both entities are retained in this category. For example, FTCL more often presents with localized disease with fewer systemic symptoms.[6]

PATHOLOGY

The morphologic spectrum of PTCL-NOS is extremely broad. Most commonly, the pattern of lymph node involvement is often diffuse but can be interfollicular or para-cortical with effacement of the normal architecture (**Fig. 1**A).[1] There can be a rich in-flammatory background of normal cells and tumor content can be low.

The cytology is often pleomorphic, with most cases consisting of a mixed population of small and large cells with a high proliferation rate[1] (see **Fig. 1**A). The malignant

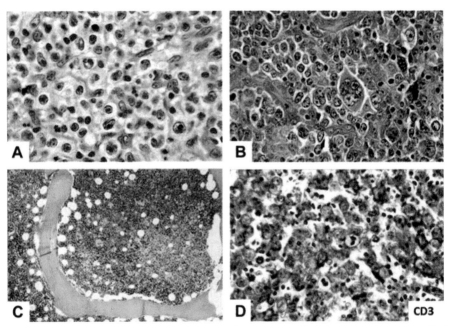

Fig. 1. (*A*) peripheral T-cell lymphoma, not otherwise specified (PTCL-NOS) composed of pleomorphic medium to large cells with clear cytoplasm and nuclear irregularities; both mitotic figures and single-cell necrosis are noted. (*B*) PTCL-NOS composed of pleomorphic large cells with occasional giant cells Reed-Sternberg–like cells with polylobated nuclei. (*C*) PTCL-NOS involving the bone marrow showing an ill-defined pleomorphic infiltrate with a nonparatrabecular localization associated with increased reticulin fibrosis and an admixed reactive inflammatory infiltrate. (*D*) The tumor cells are positive for CD3 with a predominant membranous pattern.

cells are medium or large cells with irregular nuclei, prominent nucleoli and many mitotic figures. Reed-Sternberg–like cells can also be seen (see **Fig. 1**B). High endothelial venules may be increased in some cases and the distinction from AITL may require extensive immunophenotyping.[1]

Phenotypically, PTCL-NOS typically shows expression of the pan T-cell antigens CD3 (see **Fig. 1**D), CD2, CD5, and CD7 with loss of 1 or more of the antigens in up to 80% of cases. It is most commonly derived from non-cytotoxic CD4$^+$ T cells, but rare cases can be CD8$^+$, CD4$^+$ CD8$^+$, or CD4$^-$ CD8$^-$. Expression of cytotoxic markers tends to be associated with CD8 positivity and associated with an inferior outcome (**Table 1**). In most cases (>85%) of PTCL-NOS, the malignant T cells express T-cell receptor-$\alpha\beta$, but rarely, malignant T cells are either of $\gamma\delta$ derivation or negative for both (T-cell receptor silent).[1] Rare Epstein–Barr virus–positive cases can occur and may also be associated with a more aggressive course (see **Table 1**). PTCL-NOS occasionally can display a strong expression of CD30 (**Fig. 2**), which makes the distinction from ALK$^-$ anaplastic large cell lymphoma (ALK$^-$ ALCL) challenging. Some features that are helpful in diagnosing the latter are the presence of hallmark

Table 1
Select studies of biologic prognostic markers in peripheral T-cell lymphoma, not-otherwise specified

Prognostic Marker	First Author	Outcome	Comment
Immunohistochemistry			
EBV (EBER) positive	Dupuis[33]	Unfavorable	MVA marker NS; effect only <60 y
	Went[29]	Unfavorable	MVA marker NS
	Weisenburger[34]	Unfavorable	MVA marker NS; effect only >60 y
Ki-67 $\geq$80%	Went[29]	Unfavorable	MVA marker significant
Cytotoxic marker positive[a]	Asano[32]	Unfavorable	MVA marker significant
CD30 positive	Savage[10]	Unfavorable	MVA marker significant (vs ALK$^-$)
	Piccaluga[4]	Unfavorable	Not evaluated in MVA (vs ALK$^-$)
T-helper receptor profile			
ST2(L) or CCR5 or CXCR3	Tsuchiya[19]	Favorable	Not evaluated in MVA
CCR4	Ishida[18]	Unfavorable	MVA marker significant
% transformed cells >70%	Weisenburger[34]	Unfavorable	MVA marker significant
Gene expression profiling			
Prognostic gene signatures			
Proliferation signature	Cuadros[15]	Unfavorable	MVA signature significant but not Ki-67)
NFKB signature	Martinez-Delgado[12]	Favorable	MVA signature significant
GATA3 signature	Iqbal[9]	Unfavorable	Not evaluated in MVA
$\gamma\delta$ T/NK-cell signature	Iqbal[9]	Unfavorable	Not evaluated in MVA

Abbreviations: ALK$^-$, ALK$^-$ ALCL; EBV, Epstein–Barr virus; MVA, multivariate analysis; NS, nonsignificant.
[a] TIA-1 and granzyme B.

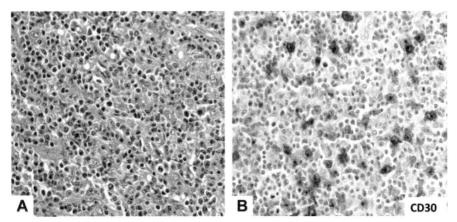

Fig. 2. (*A*) Peripheral T-cell lymphoma, not otherwise specified with a polymorphic cellular composition, with a mixed population of small and large malignant cells admixed with reactive cells, including small lymphocytes, histiocytes, and abundant eosinophils. High endothelial venules are easily seen. The malignant cells are predominantly of medium size with variable clear cytoplasm, irregular nuclei, conspicuous nucleoli, and frequent mitotic figures. (*B*) The CD30 immunostain highlights a minor subset of malignant cells, predominantly the large cells, with strong CD30 expression with a dotlike paranuclear and membranous pattern.

cells, a sinusoidal growth pattern, and coexpression of epithelial membrane antigen. In addition, CD3 is positive more frequently in PTCL-NOS, and EMA and cytotoxic markers are more often positive in ALK⁻ ALCL. (For more information, please see Dai Chihara and Michelle A. Fanale's article, "Management of Anaplastic Large Cell Lymphoma" in this issue.)

MORPHOLOGIC VARIANTS

Three morphologic variants have been described in the WHO 2008 classification, namely, lymphoepithelioid also known as Lennert's type, follicular, and T-zone.[1] The prognostic and clinical significance of these variants is unclear, although it is useful to recognize their presence because their pathology could be confused with other subtypes of lymphoma and with reactive processes.

The lymphoepithelioid variant typically shows diffuse interfollicular growth and is characterized by a prominent reactive infiltrate of epithelioid histiocytes. The neoplastic cells are CD8⁺ in most cases and the inflammatory cells can be admixed with scattered Reed-Sternberg–like cells that are usually Epstein–Barr virus positive. The follicular variant can mimic follicular lymphoma growth forming intrafollicular aggregates with a TFH phenotype and can be associated with a t(5;9) (q33;122) *ITK-SYK* translocation and is now included in the newly defined category of nodal T-cell lymphomas with a TFH phenotype.

The T-zone variant is characterized by a perifollicular growth pattern in the usual T-zone of lymph nodes and the neoplastic cells are small with minimal atypia.

INDOLENT VARIANT OF PERIPHERAL T-CELL LYMPHOMA, NOT OTHERWISE SPECIFIED

Recently, an indolent variant of PTCL-NOS has been recognized that involves the thyroid and can be seen in the setting of autoimmune thyroiditis.[7] The tumor cells are CD3, CD4, and CXCR3 positive, supporting a TH1 derivation. These cases are extremely rare but seem to be associated with an indolent course and may undergo spontaneous regression in the absence of any therapy. In addition, irradiation of the thyroid can lead to clearance of the peripheral blood.[8]

GENE EXPRESSION PROFILING OF PERIPHERAL T-CELL LYMPHOMA, NOT OTHERWISE SPECIFIED

Gene expression profiling (GEP) has been used to gain insights into the biology of PTCL-NOS but also to refine the diagnostic classification. The GEP reflects the malignant T cells and the microenvironment, which can be a major component and it is important to note that application of molecular classifiers ultimately reassigns cases to another PTCL subtype approximately 20% of the time.[9] Importantly, CD30⁺ PTCL-NOS can be distinguished from ALK⁻ ALCL using a molecular classifier[10] and linkage to clinical information supports an inferior prognosis in the former in this and other studies.[10,11]

For more than a decade, a number of studies have attempted to use GEP to identify biologically meaningful and possibly prognostic subgroups in the heterogeneous PTCL-NOS and provide insight into the underlying pathogenesis.[4,9,12–16] Disease rarity and the previous need for frozen tissue biopsies to perform microarray studies has prevented large-scale GEP studies in PTCLs. As described, a subset of PTCL-NOS with TFH features has overlapping features with AITL and this is also supported by GEP studies.[11] However, for the remaining cases, cytologic and phenotypic features are diverse.

A landmark study analyzed the GEP of 372 newly diagnosed pretreatment PTCL tumor samples with a goal of developing molecular classifiers for the main PTCL subtypes, including 150 cases with a pathologic diagnosis of PTCL-NOS.[9] After molecular classification of the PTCL-NOS, 55 cases (37%) were reassigned, including 13 as γδ–PTCL-NOS that were identified using a natural killer cell classifier, but also had high expression of CD3γ and CD3δ messenger RNA and T-cell receptor-γ chain transcripts and, interestingly, had similar outcomes to the extranodal natural killer cell/T-cell lymphoma cases.[9] With the addition of 26 cases of AITL that were reclassified as PTCL-NOS, there were 121 cases in total with bona fide PTCL-NOS. Unsupervised analysis using hierarchical clustering identified 2 major subclusters: one group had high expression of *GATA-binding protein 3 (GATA3)* and target genes (*CCR4, IL18RA, CXCR7, IK*); the other had an higher expression of *T-box 21 (TBX21) (T-bet)* and *EOMES* and known target genes (*CXCR3, IL2RB, CCL3, IFN-γ*). These signatures seemed to correlate with GATA3 and TBX21 protein expression by immunohistochemistry (see **Fig. 3**C, D). A molecular classifier was developed to distinguish *GATA3* from *TBX21* PTCL-NOS cases, but there were still approximately 20% of cases that remained unclassified (**Fig. 3**A).[9] Both *GATA3* and *TBX21* are transcription factors that are master regulators of gene expression profiles in T helper (Th) cells that skew Th polarization into Th2 and Th1 differentiation pathways, respectively, supporting that cell lineage is a key factor in defining PTCL-NOS subgroups. However, the correlation of *GATA3* and *TBX21* subset and Th counterparts is imperfect, and felt to reflect the system plasticity.[17] Importantly, for the subset of cases with outcome information (n = 106) the prognosis was inferior in the *GATA3* group (n = 37) with a 5-year overall survival (OS) of 19% compared with 38% in the *TBX21* group (n = 49) (*P* = .01) with the unclassifiable group (n = 20) somewhat intermediate (see **Fig. 3**B).[11] Interestingly, CCR4 (*GATA3* profile) and CXCR3 (*TBX2* profile) protein expression have been found to be previously associated with unfavorable and favorable prognosis, respectively (see **Table 1**).[18,19] However, a subset of cases within the *TBX21* subgroup with high expression of a cytotoxic gene signature had an inferior

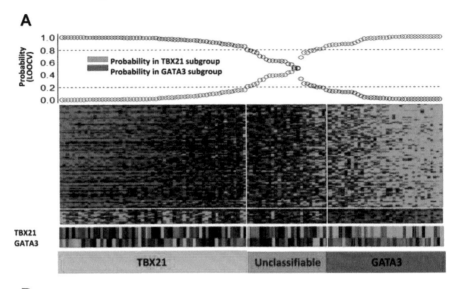

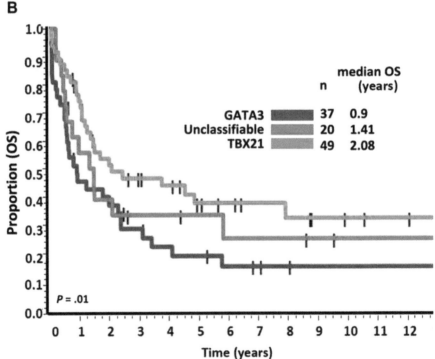

Fig. 3. Two major molecular subgroups within PTCL-NOS with biological and overall survival differences. (*A*) Bayesian predictor for GATA3 and TBX21 subgroups developed using cases derived from hierarchical clustering and leave one out cross validation testing was used for classification. (*B*) Overall survival (OS) of molecularly defined GATA3 and TBX21 subgroups showing differences in outcome (*P* = .01). (*C*) Representative cases in the TBX21 subgroup (H&E) with TBX21 immunostain demonstrating positivity from 40% to 80% of cells whereas positivity in GATA3 was <10%. (*D*) Representative cases in GATA3 subgroup immunostained with GATA3 showing positivity from 50% to 80% of cells, and were negative for TBX21. (*From* Iqbal J, Wright G, Wang C, et al. Gene expression signatures delineate biological and prognostic subgroups in peripheral T-cell lymphoma. Blood 2014;123(19):2919; with permission.)

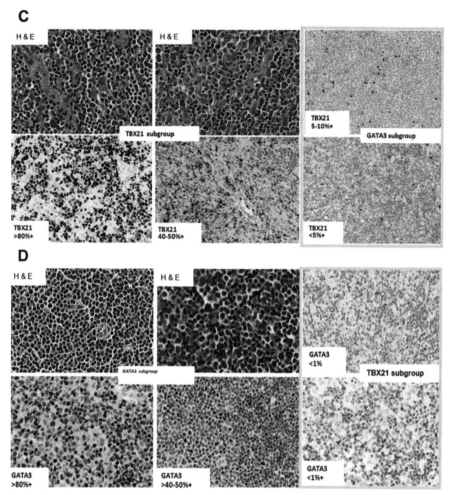

Fig. 3. (*continued*)

outcome, highlighting again the heterogeneity and complexity of classification.[11] Nevertheless, this represents the first study to demonstrate molecularly defined subgroups of PTCL-NOS that seem to be biologically and prognostically meaningful. The *GATA3* group was marginally enriched for mammalian target of rapamycin and *MYC*-related genes and showed significant enrichment of PI3Kinase-induced gene signatures, which may highlight key therapeutic targets. A separate study demonstrated that *GATA3* expression by immunohistochemistry in PTCL-NOS was associated with an inferior survival.[20] These results are intriguing, but represent unadjusted survival analyses and have not yet been validated in a larger patient series or applied in clinical practice. Further, it is unclear whether the unclassified group represents a biological entity or represents low tumor content.

RECURRENT MUTATIONS IN PERIPHERAL T-CELL LYMPHOMA, NOT OTHERWISE SPECIFIED

Next-generation sequencing studies in PTCL-NOS have provided some insight into the underlying genomic landscape in PTCL-NOS, but a large-scale study has not yet been published. The subset of TFH-like PTCL-NOS are characterized by similar mutations described in AITL[21]; however, for the remaining cases the full mutational spectrum still needs to be explored.

A study of targeted sequencing was reported in PTCL-NOS, with samples derived from formalin-fixed paraffin embedded tissue, which included 237 genes chosen for their relevance in other hematologic malignancies. This study demonstrated mutations were most commonly observed in epigenetic mediators (eg, *KMT2D [MLL2]*, *TET2*, *DNMT3A*), but also in genes involved in T-cell receptor signaling pathways (eg, *TNFAIP3*, *APC*, *CHD8*) and tumor suppressor genes (eg, *TP53*, *FOXO1*, *ATM*).[22] Cases with alterations in histone methylation (*MLL2*, *KDM6A* or *MLL*) had an inferior survival ($P = .0198$). It is unknown whether any of these mutations correlate with the efficacy of emerging novel agents, but this will be important to study in the future.

EPIDEMIOLOGY AND CLINICAL FEATURES

PTCL-NOS accounts for about 26% of all PTCLs, which in turn represent approximately 10% to 15% of all non-Hodgkin lymphomas in Western countries.[23] Most patients present with advanced stage disease with a median age of 60 years and there is a slight male predominance. The majority of patients present with widespread nodal disease, and extranodal involvement is common with the skin and gastrointestinal tract being the most affected sites.[1] Bone marrow involvement is more common than in diffuse large B-cell lymphoma (see **Fig. 1**C).

PROGNOSIS

The majority of cases of PTCL-NOS lymphomas behave aggressively and exhibit frequent relapses with poor outcome. The 5-year OS rate is typically in the range of 20% to 30%, although there is considerable variation depending on prognostic variables[23–26] (see **Table 2**). Some models exist that stratify patients into different risk categories to help predict outcome. The International Prognostic Index[27] (age >60, elevated serum lactate dehydrogenase [LDH], stage III or IV disease, Eastern Cooperative Oncology Group Performance Status $\geq$2, and >1 extranodal sites) is primarily used in diffuse large B-cell lymphoma, but it retains its significance in some of the PTCL subtypes, including PTCL-NOS[22] (**Table 3**). It is notable that even the low-risk group has a poor outcome.

The Prognostic Index for T-cell lymphoma was developed specifically for peripheral T-cell lymphoma, unspecified/NOS and incorporates age, elevated LDH, and poor

Table 2 Outcome of PTCL-NOS in select retrospective and prospective studies			
First Author (Study)	**Population**	**PFS/FFS**	**OS**
Savage et al,[31] 2004 (BCCA)	Retrospective	29% (5 y)	35% (5 y)
Vose et al,[23] 2008 ITLP	Retrospective	20% (5 y)	32% (5 y)
Ellin et al,[25] 2014 (Swedish)	Retrospective	21.3% (5 y)	28.1% (5 y)
Schmitz et al,[26] 2010 (German)	Prospective	41% (3 y)	53.9% (3 y)
D'Amore et al,[49] 2012 (Nordic ASCT)	Prospective	38% (5 y)	47% (5 y)

Abbreviations: ASCT, autologous stem cell transplant; BCCA, British Columbia Cancer Agency; FFS, failure-free survival; ITLP, International T-cell Lymphoma Project; OS, overall survival; PTCL-NOS, Peripheral T-cell lymphoma, not otherwise specified.

Table 3							
Survival of patients with PTCL-NOS by prognostic models							
International Prognostic Index[23]				Prognostic Index for PTCL-NOS[28]			
Risk Factors	Cases (%)	5-y OS (%)	5-y FFS (%)	Risk Factors	Cases (%)	5-y OS (%)	5-y FFS (%)
0/1	28	50	36	0	20	50	34
2	35	33	18	1	38	40	22
3	22	16	15	2	29	22	13
4/5	15	11	9	3/4	13	11	8

Abbreviations: FFS, failure-free survival; OS, overall survival; PTCL-NOS, Peripheral T-cell lymphoma, not otherwise specified.

performance status as well as bone marrow involvement[28] (see **Table 3**). In addition, a Ki-67 of 80% or greater also associated with a worse outcome in PTCL-NOS and along with elevated LDH and poor performance status can be integrated into a 3-factor score with widely disparate outcomes (2-year OS of approximately 65% vs 40% vs <15%; P<.0001).[29] Other pathologic[30,31] and molecular features that are associated potentially with outcomes are shown in **Table 1**.[9,10,12,15,16,18,19,29,32–34]

DEFINING THE OPTIMAL PRIMARY THERAPY OF PERIPHERAL T-CELL LYMPHOMA, NOT OTHERWISE SPECIFIED

Cyclophosphamide, doxorubicin, vincristine, prednisone (CHOP) is considered the standard therapy in PTCLs, including PTCL-NOS[35] and, to date, no other regimen has clearly shown to be superior to CHOP. In the International T Cell Lymphoma project, more than 85% of PTCL patients received CHOP or a CHOP-equivalent regimen and the outcomes remain unsatisfactory with a 5-year failure-free survival of only 20% in PTCL-NOS[23] (see **Table 2**).

Further, in this study, the OS of patients with PTCL-NOS receiving an anthracycline-based regimen as part of their primary therapy was similar to those that did not suggesting that anthracyclines may not impact outcome and has led to the exploration of novel non–anthracycline-based regimens in the front-line setting. In contrast, the Mayo Clinic performed a similar analysis and found that PTCL-NOS/AITL patients that received non–anthracycline-based chemotherapy had an inferior outcome.[36] Given the potential biases introduced, in particular, patient fitness, which may dictate the use of a less aggressive regimen, it remains an open question whether anthracyclines are an essential treatment component in the management of PTCL-NOS.

The GOELAMS group (Groupe Ouest Est d'Etude des Leucemies et Autres Maladies du Sang) performed the first randomized, phase III, multicenter study in patients with PTCL comparing a novel dose intensive regimen, VIP (cycles 1, 3, and 5; etoposide, ifosfamide, cisplatin)/rABVD (cycles 2, 4, and 6; adriamycin, bleomycin, vinblastine, dacarbazine) with 8 cycles of CHOP-21. In total, 88 patients with PTCL were randomized, the majority of whom had PTCL-NOS (n = 57; 65%). With a median follow-up of 110 months, the 2-year event-free survival (EFS) was similar for VIP/ABVD and CHOP-21 arms at 45% and 41% (P = .7), respectively. The median OS was 42 months for both arms and the overall response rate (ORR) was 62%, including the 39% complete response (CR) rate. This study is a useful benchmark of outcomes with CHOP chemotherapy in a clinical trial population.[37]

LIMITED STAGE PERIPHERAL T-CELL LYMPHOMA, NOT OTHERWISE SPECIFIED

The majority of patients with PTCL, including PTCL-NOS, present with advanced stage disease. As such, there is very little information describing the outcome and optimal treatment approach in limited stage patients. The impact of radiotherapy in the subset of patients with PTCL-NOS with stage 1 disease was evaluated in the International T-cell Lymphoma Project and there seemed to be a benefit compared with chemotherapy alone ($P = .018$).[38] The Mayo Clinic evaluated 75 patients with limited stage PTCL, 29 of whom had PTCL-NOS with stage 1 and 2 disease. Although it is unclear what proportion had extensive stage 2, B symptoms or bulky disease, the 2-year progression-free survival (PFS) for PTCL-NOS, ALCL, and AITL was approximately 50% and comparison of combined modality therapy and chemotherapy alone yielded similar outcomes.[39] Thus, given the small number of patients in these trials, it remains unknown what the optimal number of cycles of chemotherapy are in limited stage PTCL-NOS and the added benefit of radiotherapy. However, given the poor outcome with CHOP it seems that integration of radiotherapy is a reasonable approach.

CHOP ALTERNATIVES FOR THE PRIMARY THERAPY OF PERIPHERAL T-CELL LYMPHOMA, NOT OTHERWISE SPECIFIED

The addition of etoposide, typically in the form of CHOEP, was explored by the German High-grade non-Hodgkin lymphoma (DSHNHL [Deutsche Studiengruppe Hochmaligne Non-Hodgkin Lymphome]) study group in a retrospective analysis performed on completed prospective studies.[28] Combining PTCL-NOS, AITL, and ALK⁻ ALCL, there was a trend to an improved EFS for select young good risk patients (<60 years of age, normal LDH) incorporating etoposide (3-year EFS 60.7% vs 48.3%; $P = .003$), but the OS was similar. The Swedish Registry Study similarly reported that use of CHOEP was associated with an improvement in PFS ($P = .008$) in multivariate analysis with a trend toward an improved OS ($P = .052$) in PTCL patients less than 60 years of age, excluding ALK⁺ ALCL,[25] but also did not evaluate PTCL-NOS separately. A US retrospective study did not find a benefit in adding etoposide ($P = .80$), again combining all PTCL patients.[24] Taken together, it remains unknown whether the addition of etoposide is truly improving cure rates in PTCL-NOS, but these data have been used as the rationale to include CHOEP as a first-line chemotherapy option in PTCL-NOS in the National Comprehensive Cancer Network and European Society for Medical Oncology guidelines. CHOEP should only be considered in younger patients, given that the toxicity is higher than with CHOP.

It has been postulated that doxorubicin efflux from tumor cells, via the multi drug resistance product P-glycoprotein, is the cause of anthracycline resistance in PTCL.[40] In an attempt to improve outcomes, a new front-line regimen, PEGS, was piloted in a phase II study by the Southwest Oncology Group (SWOG0350), which incorporates cisplatin, etoposide, gemcitabine, and methylprednisolone, all of which are not affected by P-glycoprotein. In total, 33 eligible patients were enrolled, 26 of whom were treatment naïve; however, the efficacy was disappointing with a 2-year PFS of only 12% and a 2-year OS of 31%. For PTCL-NOS, the ORR was only 47% and the CR was 26%.[41] Whether this was due to suboptimal dosing of gemcitabine, a known active drug in PTCLs, or the absence of alkylating agents in this regimen, is unknown. There is an ongoing UK study comparing CHOP to gemcitabine, cisplatin, and methylprednisolone (GEM-P) (NCT01719835) in the upfront setting.

Several other studies have evaluated the addition of a novel agent to CHOP-(like) chemotherapy. Alemtuzumab (Campath-1H) is a monoclonal antibody that binds to CD52, an antigen present on B, T, and natural killer cells and variably expressed in patients with PTCL. Several PTCL studies have shown high CR rates of up to 70% with alemtuzumab when combined with CHOP. However, the profound immunosuppression and increased rate of opportunistic infections, including a 25% risk of cytomegalovirus reactivation, has been problematic.[42–44] The best results were seen in a phase II study evaluating CHOP-alemtuzumab in newly diagnosed PTCLs (n = 24) reported by GITIL (Gruppo Italiano Terapie Innovative nei Linformi), which showed improved toxicity, with cytomegalovirus reactivation only present in 9%. The CR rate in PTCL-NOS was 71% (n = 14) and the projected 2-year PFS for all patients was 48%[34]; however, follow-up was short and several other phase II studies demonstrated no clear benefit of the addition of alemtuzumab.[45] Further, the phase III ACT-2 (Phase III Study of CHOP-14 Plus or Minus Alemtuzumab in Peripheral T-cell Lymphoma of the Elderly) trial was recently reported comparing CHOP-14 with CHOP-14 and alemtuzumab in newly diagnosed patients with PTCL greater than 60 years of age failed to show any advantage in EFS (CHOP-14 + A 26% vs 23%; $P = .254$) or OS (CHOP-14 + A 38% vs 56%; $P = .120$).[46] Although PTCL-NOS was not reported separately (n = 45; 39% of total), it is unlikely that a benefit will be seen in specific subtypes. The ACT1 trial evaluating the impact of alemtuzumab in younger patients with a planned consolidative ASCT has not yet been reported.

A number of other novel agents added to CHOP have been explored, including denileukin diftitox and bortezemib with CR rates in PTCL-NOS of 33% and 32%, respectively. Interestingly, a phase II trial of CHOP with everolimus demonstrated a CR rate of 60% in PTCL-NOS, which may have biologic rationale given the recent GEP findings.[47] Further, the Food and Drug Administration (FDA)–approved histone deacetylase (HDAC) inhibitors (HDACI) romidepsin and belinostat are under investigation in combination with CHOP in the front-line setting and brentuximab vedotin is being studied with CHP in CD30$^+$ PTCLs given promising results in ALCL.

It remains unknown whether dose intensive regimens may improve the outcome in PTCL-NOS, but this forms the basis of the rationale for consolidative autologous stem cell transplantation (ASCT) in first remission. The DSHNHL group compared CHOEP to dose-escalated (high-CHOEP) or a mega-dose (MegaCHOEP) variant, which incorporated stem cell rescue; however, neither approach seemed to improve OS. The MD Anderson Cancer Centre reviewed 135 patients with PTCLs receiving CHOP or an intensive regimen[48] and the 3-year OS was similar (CHOP 62%, dose intensive 56%). A US retrospective study also did not find a difference comparing CHOP with a more dose-intensive regimen (PTCL-NOS; n = 107; 31%). The common challenge for all of these studies is the combining of diverse PTCL subtypes in outcome analyses and there are very few data in specific disease subtypes, including PTCL-NOS.

ROLE OF CONSOLIDATIVE AUTOLOGOUS STEM CELL TRANSPLANTATION IN FIRST REMISSION

In an attempt to improve cure rates, consolidative high-dose chemotherapy and ASCT is a common practice and endorsed in guidelines. However, it is challenging to know which patient to select for this intensified approach and failure of primary chemotherapy continues to be a concern. The data for ASCT come from retrospective series and a few prospective trials that included heterogeneous populations of patients with different PTCL subtypes.

The largest prospective study was reported by the Nordic Group and evaluated 160 patients with PTCL, including 62 patients with PTCL-NOS (39%), who received CHOEP-14 if less than 60 years of age or CHOP-14 if greater than 60 years, for 6 cycles followed by BEAM ASCT if an objective response was demonstrated.[49] The transplant rate was 70% and with a median follow-up of 5 years, the 5-year PFS and OS were 44% and 51%, respectively, for all PTCL patients, and estimates for PTCL-NOS were 38% and 47%, respectively (see **Table 1**).

Reimer and colleagues[50] reported the outcome of 83 PTCL patients enrolled in a phase II study of CHOP for 4 to 6 cycles followed by high-dose chemotherapy/ASCT in responding patients, of whom 32 (39%) had PTCL-NOS. With a median follow-up of 33 months, and transplant rate of 66%, the results were similar to the Nordic study with a 3-year PFS and OS of 36% and 48%, respectively, for all patients; subtype-specific results are unknown. Not surprisingly, the 3-year OS for those who underwent ASCT was much better at 71%. The Centre for International Blood and Bone Marrow Transplant Research (CIBMTR) evaluated the outcome of PTCL patients receiving either allogeneic SCT (allo-SCT) or ASCT in first-line or beyond. For PTCL-NOS patients undergoing ASCT, the 3-year PFS and OS were 33% and 42%, respectively, but results specifically for CR1 PTCL-NOS patients was not reported. Taken together, the results with consolidative ASCT in PTCL-NOS are better than historical retrospective reports (see **Table 1**), but selection bias remains a problem for study interpretation in a clinical trial population; however, a randomized study is not likely feasible. Limited studies suggest that for patients with PTCL in a CR, outcomes with and without consolidative transplantation are similar[24]; however, subtype-specific benefits may exist and, given the high relapse rate of PTCL-NOS, consolidative ASCT remains a reasonable approach in young patients. (Please see Tejaswini M. Dhawale and Andrei R. Shustov's article, "Stem Cell Transplantation in T Cell Lymphoma," in this issue, for more details.)

TRANSPLANT FOR RELAPSED/REFRACTORY PERIPHERAL T-CELL LYMPHOMA

Although there have been no randomized, controlled studies evaluating the role of ASCT specifically in relapsed/refractory PTCLs, multiple small retrospective studies have been reported that typically have combined histologic subtypes and some have evaluated both allo-SCT and ASCT in outcome analyses. Collectively, these studies support that ASCT in relapsed PTCL remains a potentially curative option if chemosensitivity is demonstrated, similar to the practice for diffuse large B-cell lymphoma. Although most note superior salvage rates with ASCT in ALCL, very few have reported outcomes specifically in PTCL-NOS. Song and colleagues[51] evaluated 36 patients with relapsed/refractory PTCL, including 20 patients with PTCL-NOS who underwent ASCT and the 3-year EFS was 23%. The CIBMTR evaluated 241 patients receiving either an ASCT or allo-SCT.[52] Considering only PTCL-NOS patients who underwent ASCT beyond CR1 (n = 28), the 3-year PFS and OS rates were 29% and 42%, respectively.

There are more limited data evaluating allo-SCT but it remains a viable option, particularly in those with refractory disease. A French retrospective study evaluated the outcome of 77 patients with PTCL undergoing allo-SCT, including 27 with PTCL-NOS, most of whom underwent myebloablative conditioning (n = 19) and the 5-year EFS for PTCL-NOS patients was 58% and 63%, respectively, although it is unclear what proportion were transplanted in CR1. Responses were observed after donor lymphocyte infusion, supporting the existence of a graft-versus-lymphoma effect. A recent systematic review and meta-analysis reviewed the efficacy and safety of allo-SCT in PTCLs.[53] The pooled 3-year OS was 49.6% and there was no difference between allo-SCT and ASCT. Rates of acute and chronic graft-versus-host disease were 27% and 30%, respectively, and the treatment-related mortality was 24%. (Please see Tejaswini M. Dhawale and Andrei R. Shustov's article, "Stem Cell Transplantation in T Cell Lymphoma," in this issue, for more details.)

NOVEL THERAPIES IN RELAPSED/REFRACTORY PERIPHERAL T-CELL LYMPHOMA, NOT OTHERWISE SPECIFIED

The outcome of patients that fail front-line therapy is very poor with a median OS of only 6.5 months in PTCL-NOS in the absence of transplantation, highlighting the need for improved therapies.[54] The most significant progress in recent years in the management PTCL has been the evaluation of novel agents specifically in relapsed/refractory PTCLs leading to the FDA approval of 4 agents, 3 of which are approved for use in PTCL-NOS, namely, pralatrexate, romidepsin, and belinostat (**Table 4**).

Pralatrexate is an antifolate drug that was designed to be efficiently internalized by the reduced folate carrier that regulates the internalization of natural folates required for purine and pyrimidine biosynthesis and it was the first FDA-approved drug specifically for relapsed/refractory PTCL. In the PROPEL study (Study of Pralatrexate With Vitamin B12 and Folic Acid in Patients With Relapsed or Refractory Peripheral T-cell Lymphoma), pralatrexate was administered to 111 patients with relapsed/refractory PTCL (30 mg/m^2 weekly for 6 weeks in a 7-week cycle), just more than one-half of whom had PTCL-NOS (n = 59; 53%). The median ORR was 29% for all patients with a CR rate of 11%, which was similar in the subset with PTCL-NOS (ORR 32%; see **Table 4**). For all patients, the median PFS and OS were 3.5 and 14.5 months, respectively, and the median duration of response (DOR) in responders was 10.1 months. The most common side effect was mucositis, occurring in 71%, but grade 3 to 4 events occurred only in 22%.[55]

There is a growing body of evidence of a class effect of HDACI in PTCLs. Romidepsin is a potent class 1 selective HDACI that induces histone acetylation leading to antitumor effect through different mechanisms. FDA approval in 2011 occurred following the report of a phase II trial of romidepsin in 131 patients with relapsed/refractory PTCL (PTCL-NOS, n = 69; 53%). The ORR was 25%, the CR rate 16.6%, the median DOR was 16.6, and the median PFS was 4 months.[56] In PTCL-NOS, the ORR was 29% and rate of CR/CRu was 14%. Grade 3 or 4 drug-related events included infection at 6%, neutropenia at 18%, and thrombocytopenia at 23%.[56] An update of this trial was reported with a longer follow-up and has shown a longer median DOR of 28 months with the median not yet reached in those achieving a CR and no difference observed between PTCL subtypes, although patient numbers in this comparison were small.[57]

Belinostat, a nonselective HDACI, was approved by the FDA in 2014 for relapsed/refractory PTCL. In the pivotal phase II multicenter BELIEF trial (A Multicenter, Open Label Trial of Belinostat in Patients With Relapsed or Refractory Peripheral T-Cell Lymphoma), 129 patients with relapsed/refractory PTCL received belinostat (1000 mg/m^2 on days 1–5 every 21 days) and in the evaluable patients, the observed efficacy was similar to romidepsin (ORR, 25.8%; CR, 10.8%) with an ORR in PTCL-NOS of 23.3% (see **Table 4**). Responses were durable with a median DOR of 13.6 months and a median that was not reached but exceeded 29 months in those who achieved CR.[58] There was less bone marrow toxicity (grade 3–4: anemia, 11%; thrombocytopenia, 7%; and neutropenia, 6%).[58] It is unknown whether recently reported mutations in epigenetic mediators correlate with response to these agents.

Brentuximab vedotin is an antibody drug conjugate that is composed of an anti-CD30 antibody conjugated to monomethyl auristatin E, an antimicrotubule agent that is released inside the cell after the binding of the antibody drug conjugate to CD30. Brentuximab vedotin has striking efficacy in relapsed/refractory ALCL (ORR, 86%; CR, 57%; median PFS, 13.3 months)[59] leading to FDA approval in this setting. Brentuximab vedotin was subsequently evaluated in other CD30$^+$ non-Hodgkin lymphomas, including PTCLs. The results in CD30$^+$ PTCL-NOS were modest, with an

Table 4
Novel therapies in PTCL with a focus if efficacy in PTCL-NOS

Drug	Study	All PTCL (n)	ORR/CR (%)	PTCL All Med PFS (mo)	PTCL All Med DOR, (mo)	PTCL-NOS (n)	ORR/CR (%)	PTCL-NOS PFS (mo)	PTCL-NOS DOR (mo)	FDA Approved PTCL-NOS
Pralatrexate	Phase II	109	29 (11)	3.5	10.1	59	32 (NA)	NA	10.1	Yes
Brentuximab vedotin (CD30+ non-ALCL)	Phase II	34	41 (24)	2.6	7.6	22	33 (14)	1.6	7.6	No
Romidepsin	Phase II	131	25 (15)	4	28	69	29 (14)	NA	16.6	Yes
Belinostat	Phase II	129	26 (11)	1.6	13.6	77	23.3 (NA)	NA	NA	Yes
Duvelisib	Phase II	16	47 (13)	NA	NA	NA	NA	NA	NA	No
Alisertib	Phase II	30	30 (7)	3	3	13	31 (8)	NA	NA	No
Mogamulizumab	Phase II	29	34 (5)	2	NA	16	19 (6)	NA	NA	No
Lenalidomide	Phase II	29	24 (NA)	4	5	14	NA	NA	NA	No
		54	—	2.5	3.6	20	20 (0)	NA	NA	
		10	30 (all CR)	—	—	24	30 (all CR)	NA	NA	
Nivolumab	Phase II	5	40 (NA)	NA	10.6–78.6+	NA	NA	NA	NA	No

Abbreviations: ALCL, anaplastic large cell lymphoma; CR, complete response; DOR, duration of response; Med, median; NA, not applicable; ORR, overall response rate; OS, overall survival; PFS, progression-free survival; PTCL, peripheral T-cell lymphoma; PTCL-NOS, peripheral T-cell lymphoma, not otherwise specified.

ORR of 33%, CR of 14%, and a median PFS of only 1.6 months, which underscores the fact that these are different diseases.[60]

OTHER NOVEL THERAPIES

Duvelisib (International Prognostic Index-145), a dual oral inhibitor of phosphoinositide-3-kinases (PI3K) delta and gamma has shown promise in PTCLs. PI3K-δ and PI3K-γ isoforms have important roles in T-cell function and are pivotal in cell signaling and regulate multiple cellular functions linked to oncogenesis and growth. Duvelisib was evaluated in a phase I trial in 33 patients with relapsed/refractory PTCLs and, for the 16 patients with PTCL, the reported ORR was 47% and CR was 13%.[61]

Alisertib is a reversible inhibitor of aurora A kinase that lead to cell cycle arrest by interfering with centrosome separation in mitosis with encouraging results in the subset of 8 patients with PTCLs in a phase I study with an ORR of 50%.[62] A phase II study from the SWOG group evaluated this drug in 37 patients with relapsed/refractory PTCL and the ORR was 30% (CR of 8%) and was the same in PTCL-NOS (ORR, 31%; CR, 8%).[63] Further, in the first phase III study in this setting, the Lumiere trial randomized 271 patients (n = 118, PTCL-NOS) to either alisertib or investigator's choice systemic therapy (pralatrexate, romidepsin, gemcitabine) and failed to show any difference in ORR (35% [alisertib] vs 46% [comparator]; P = .07) and the median PFS was only 3.5 months in both groups.[64] Results by histologic subtype have not yet been reported.

Mogamulizumab (KW-0761) is a humanized anti-CCR4 (CC chemokine receptor 4) monoclonal antibody that that has shown promise in patients with relapsed/refractory CC4-positive PTCL. CCR4 is a marker for type 2 helper T cells and is expressed by the malignant T cells. Patients with PTCL-NOS with CCR+ tumors have a shorter survival time when compared with those with tumors that are CCR4-.[18] In a multicenter phase II study, mogamulizumab was used in 38 patients with relapsed/refractory CCR4$^+$ PTCL (PTCL-NOS, n = 16) and cutaneous T-cell lymphoma. In the PTCL-NOS patients, 3 responded (19%; 1 CR and 2 partial responses); 6 patients had stable disease and 7 progressed.[65]

The immune checkpoint inhibitor, nivolumab, a blocking antibody to programmed death-1 pathway, has been used in a small number of patients with T-cell lymphoma in a phase I study of relapsed/refractory hematologic malignancies. Five patients with PTCL (subtype[s] not specified) were included and 2 of them responded.[66] Future studies with a greater number of patients are needed to demonstrate any meaningful clinical benefit. With only modest results with single novel agents in PTCLs, including PTCL-NOS, there is interest in combining agents to enhance efficacy with multiple double and triplet studies currently underway. Given disease heterogeneity and evolving molecular subsets, it will be critical to incorporate biomarkers to assess the efficacy of this myriad of choices in relapsed disease and select promising agents to explore in the upfront setting.

FUTURE DIRECTIONS

Insights into the molecular basis of PTCL-NOS will hopefully aid future risk stratification, predict treatment response, and provide the basis for novel therapeutics. Given the modest efficacy of most agents, improving outcome will likely rely on drug combinations with complementary mechanisms of action. The key to moving toward better outcomes in PTCL-NOS will be the integration of correlative analysis into clinical trials to better understand the subgroup that benefits from a therapy.

REFERENCES

1. Swerdlow SH, Campo E, Harris NL, et al. WHO classification of tumours of hae-matopoietic and lymphoid tissue. 4th edition. Geneva (Switzerland): IARC; 2008.
2. Harris N, Jaffe ES, Stein H, et al. A revised European-American classification of lymphoid neoplasms: a proposal from the International Lymphoma Study Group. Blood 1994;84(5):1361–92.
3. Jaffe ES, Harris NL, Stein H, et al. World Health Organization classification: tu-mours of hematopoetic and lymphoid tissues. In: Jaffe ES, Harris NL, Stein H, et al, editors. Lyon (France): IARC Press; 2001.
4. Piccaluga PP, Agostinelli C, Califano A, et al. Gene expression analysis of periph-eral T cell lymphoma, unspecified, reveals distinct profiles and new potential ther-apeutic targets. J Clin Invest 2007;117(3):823–34.
5. Piccaluga PP, Agostinelli C, Tripodo C, et al. Peripheral T-cell lymphoma classifi-cation: the matter of cellular derivation. Expert Rev Hematol 2011;4(4):415–25.
6. Swerdlow SH, Campo E, Pileri SA, et al. The 2016 revision of the World Health Or-ganization classification of lymphoid neoplasms. Blood 2016;127(20):2375–90.
7. Hayashi E, Takata K, Sato Y, et al. Distinct morphologic, phenotypic, and clinical-course characteristics of indolent peripheral T-cell lymphoma. Hum Pathol 2013; 44(9):1927–36.
8. Yoshida N, Nishikori M, Izumi T, et al. Primary peripheral T-cell lymphoma, not otherwise specified of the thyroid with autoimmune thyroiditis. Br J Haematol 2013;161(2):214–23.
9. Iqbal J, Wright G, Wang C, et al. Gene expression signatures delineate biological and prognostic subgroups in peripheral T-cell lymphoma. Blood 2014;123(19):2915–23.
10. Savage KJ, Harris NL, Vose JM, et al. ALK-anaplastic large-cell lymphoma is clin-ically and immunophenotypically different from both ALK+ ALCL and peripheral T-cell lymphoma, not otherwise specified: report from the International Peripheral T-Cell Lymphoma Project. Blood 2008;111(12):5496–504.
11. de Leval L, Rickman DS, Thielen C, et al. The gene expression profile of nodal peripheral T-cell lymphoma demonstrates a molecular link between angioimmu-noblastic T-cell lymphoma (AITL) and follicular helper T (TFH) cells. Blood 2007;109(11):4952–63.
12. Martinez-Delgado B, Cuadros M, Honrado E, et al. Differential expression of NF-kappaB pathway genes among peripheral T-cell lymphomas. Leukemia 2005; 19(12):2254–63.
13. Martinez-Delgado B, Meléndez B, Cuadros M, et al. Expression profiling of T-cell lymphomas differentiates peripheral and lymphoblastic lymphomas and defines survival related genes. Clin Cancer Res 2004;10(15):4971–82.
14. Ballester B, Ramuz O, Gisselbrecht C, et al. Gene expression profiling identifies molecular subgroups among nodal peripheral T-cell lymphomas. Ann Oncol 2005;16(Supp 5):124a.
15. Cuadros M, Dave SS, Jaffe ES, et al. Identification of a proliferation signature related to survival in nodal peripheral T-cell lymphomas. J Clin Oncol 2007;25(22):3321–9.
16. Piccaluga PP, Fuligni F, De Leo A, et al. Molecular profiling improves classification and prognostication of nodal peripheral T-cell lymphomas: results of a phase III diagnostic accuracy study. J Clin Oncol 2013;31(24):3019–25.
17. de Leval L, Gaulard P. Cellular origin of T-cell lymphomas. Blood 2014;123(19): 2909–10.
18. Ishida T, Inagaki H, Utsunomiya A, et al. CXC chemokine receptor 3 and CC che-mokine receptor 4 expression in T-cell and NK-cell lymphomas with special

reference to clinicopathological significance for peripheral T-cell lymphoma, un-specified. Clin Cancer Res 2004;10(16):5494–500.

19. Tsuchiya T, Ohshima K, Karube K, et al. Th1, Th2, and activated T-cell marker and clinical prognosis in peripheral T-cell lymphoma, unspecified: comparison with AILD, ALCL, lymphoblastic lymphoma, and ATLL. Blood 2004;103(1):236–41.

20. Wang T, Feldman AL, Wada DA, et al. GATA-3 expression identifies a high-risk subset of PTCL, NOS with distinct molecular and clinical features. Blood 2014; 123(19):3007–15.

21. Palomero T, Couronné L, Khiabanian H, et al. Recurrent mutations in epigenetic regulators, RHOA and FYN kinase in peripheral T cell lymphomas. Nat Genet 2014;46(2):166–70.

22. Schatz JH, Horwitz SM, Teruya-Feldstein J, et al. Targeted mutational profiling of peripheral T-cell lymphoma not otherwise specified highlights new mechanisms in a heterogeneous pathogenesis. Leukemia 2015;29(1):237–41.

23. Vose J, Armitage J, Weisenburger D, et al. International Peripheral T-Cell and Nat-ural Killer/T-Cell Lymphoma Study: pathology findings and clinical outcomes. J Clin Oncol 2008;26(25):4124–30.

24. Abramson JS, Feldman T, Kroll-Desrosiers AR, et al. Peripheral T-cell lymphomas in a large US multicenter cohort: prognostication in the modern era including impact of frontline therapy. Ann Oncol 2014;25(11):2211–7.

25. Ellin F, Landström J, Jerkeman M, et al. Real world data on prognostic factors and treatment in peripheral T-cell lymphomas: a study from the Swedish lymphoma registry. Blood 2014;124(10):1570–7.

26. Schmitz N, Trümper L, Ziepert M, et al. Treatment and prognosis of mature T-cell and NK-cell lymphoma: an analysis of patients with T-cell lymphoma treated in studies of the German High-Grade Non-Hodgkin Lymphoma Study Group. Blood 2010;116(18):3418–25.

27. A predictive model for aggressive non-Hodgkin's lymphoma. The International Non-Hodgkin's Lymphoma Prognostic Factors Project. N Engl J Med 1993; 329(14):987–94.

28. Gallamini A, Stelitano C, Calvi R, et al. Peripheral T-cell lymphoma unspecified (PTCL-U): a new prognostic model from a retrospective multicentric clinical study. Blood 2004;103(7):2474–9.

29. Went P, Agostinelli C, Gallamini A, et al. Marker expression in peripheral T-cell lymphoma: a proposed clinical-pathologic prognostic score. J Clin Oncol 2006; 24(16):2472–9.

30. Gisselbrecht C, Gaulard P, Lepage E, et al. Prognostic significance of T-cell phenotype in aggressive non-Hodgkin's lymphomas. Groupe d'Etudes des Lym-phomes de l'Adulte (GELA). Blood 1998;92(1):76–82.

31. Savage KJ, Chhanabhai M, Gascoyne RD, et al. Characterization of peripheral T-cell lymphomas in a single North American institution by the WHO classification. Ann Oncol 2004;15(10):1467–75.

32. Asano N, Suzuki R, Kagami Y, et al. Clinicopathologic and prognostic signifi-cance of cytotoxic molecule expression in nodal peripheral T-cell lymphoma, un-specified. Am J Surg Pathol 2005;29(10):1284–93.

33. Dupuis J, Emile JF, Mounier N, et al. Prognostic significance of Epstein-Barr virus in nodal peripheral T-cell lymphoma, unspecified: a Groupe d'Etude des Lym-phomes de l'Adulte (GELA) study. Blood 2006;108(13):4163–9.

34. Weisenburger DD, Wilson WH, Vose JM. Peripheral T-cell Lymphoma, not other-wise specified: a clinicopathologic study of 340 cases from the International Pe-ripheral T-cell Lymphoma Project. Ann Oncol 2008;19(Supplement 4):113a.

35. Fisher RI, Gaynor ER, Dahlberg S, et al. Comparison of a standard regimen (CHOP) with three intensive chemotherapy regimens for advanced non-Hodgkin's lymphoma. N Engl J Med 1993;328(14):1002–6.
36. Briski R, Feldman AL, Bailey NG, et al. The role of front-line anthracycline-containing chemotherapy regimens in peripheral T-cell lymphomas. Blood Cancer J 2014;4:e214.
37. Simon A, Peoch M, Casassus P, et al. Upfront VIP-reinforced-ABVD (VIP-rABVD) is not superior to CHOP/21 in newly diagnosed peripheral T cell lymphoma. Results of the randomized phase III trial GOELAMS-LTP95. Br J Haematol 2010; 151(2):159–66.
38. Weisenburger DD, Savage KJ, Harris NL, et al. Peripheral T-cell lymphoma, not otherwise specified: a report of 340 cases from the International Peripheral T-cell Lymphoma Project. Blood 2011;117(12):3402–8.
39. Briski R, Feldman AL, Bailey NG, et al. Survival in patients with limited-stage peripheral T-cell lymphomas. Leuk Lymphoma 2015;56(6):1665–70.
40. Mahadevan D, List AF. Targeting the multidrug resistance-1 transporter in AML: molecular regulation and therapeutic strategies. Blood 2004;104(7):1940–51.
41. Mahadevan D, Unger JM, Spier CM, et al. Phase 2 trial of combined cisplatin, etoposide, gemcitabine, and methylprednisolone (PEGS) in peripheral T-cell non-Hodgkin lymphoma: Southwest Oncology Group Study S0350. Cancer 2013;119(2):371–9.
42. Kluin-Nelemans HC, van Marwijk Kooy M, Lugtenburg PJ, et al. Intensified alemtuzumab-CHOP therapy for peripheral T-cell lymphoma. Ann Oncol 2011; 22(7):1595–600.
43. Binder C, Ziepert M, Pfreundschuh M, et al. CHO(E)P-14 followed by alemtuzumab consolidation in untreated peripheral T cell lymphomas: final analysis of a prospective phase II trial. Ann Hematol 2013;92(11):1521–8.
44. Kim JG, Sohn SK, Chae YS, et al. Alemtuzumab plus CHOP as front-line chemotherapy for patients with peripheral T-cell lymphomas: a phase II study. Cancer Chemother Pharmacol 2007;60(1):129–34.
45. Gallamini A, Zaja F, Patti C, et al. Alemtuzumab (Campath-1H) and CHOP chemotherapy as first-line treatment of peripheral T-cell lymphoma: results of a GITIL (Gruppo Italiano Terapie Innovative nei Linfomi) prospective multicenter trial. Blood 2007;110(7):2316–23.
46. Trumper L, Wulf G, Ziepert M, et al. Alemtuzumab added to CHOP for treatment of peripheral T-cell lymphoma (pTNHL) of the elderly: final results of 116 patients treated in the international ACT-2 phase III trial. J Clin Oncol 2016;34(Suppl) [abstract: 7500].
47. Kim SJ, Shin DY, Kim JS, et al. A phase II study of everolimus (RAD001), an mTOR inhibitor plus CHOP for newly diagnosed peripheral T-cell lymphomas. Ann Oncol 2016;27(4):712–8.
48. Escalon MP, Liu NS, Yang Y, et al. Prognostic factors and treatment of patients with T-cell non-Hodgkin lymphoma. Cancer 2005;103(10):2091–8.
49. d'Amore F, Relander T, Lauritzsen GF, et al. Upfront autologuos stem-cell transplantation in peripheral T-cell lymphoma: NLG-T-01. J Clin Oncol 2012;30(25):3093–9.
50. Reimer P, Rüdiger T, Geissinger E, et al. Autologous stem-cell transplantation as first-line therapy in peripheral T-cell lymphomas: results of a prospective multicenter study. J Clin Oncol 2009;27(1):106–13.
51. Song KW, Mollee P, Keating A, et al. Autologous stem cell transplant for relapsed and refractory peripheral T-cell lymphoma: variable outcome according to pathological subtype. Br J Haematol 2003;120(6):978–85.

52. Smith SM, Burns LJ, van Besien K, et al. Hematopoietic cell transplantation for systemic mature T-cell non-Hodgkin lymphoma. J Clin Oncol 2013;31(25):3100–9.
53. Wei J, Xu J, Cao Y, et al. Allogeneic stem-cell transplantation for peripheral T-cell lymphoma: a systemic review and meta-analysis. Acta Haematol 2015;133(2):136–44.
54. Mak V, Hamm J, Chhanabhai M, et al. Survival of patients with peripheral T-cell lymphoma after first relapse or progression: spectrum of disease and rare long-term survivors. J Clin Oncol 2013;31(16):1970–6.
55. O'Connor OA, Pro B, Pinter-Brown L, et al. Pralatrexate in patients with relapsed or refractory peripheral T-cell lymphoma: results from the pivotal PROPEL study. J Clin Oncol 2011;29(9):1182–9.
56. Coiffier B, Pro B, Prince HM, et al. Results from a pivotal, open-label, phase II study of romidepsin in relapsed or refractory peripheral T-cell lymphoma after prior systemic therapy. J Clin Oncol 2012;30(6):631–6.
57. Coiffier B, Pro B, Prince HM, et al. Romidepsin for the treatment of relapsed/refractory peripheral T-cell lymphoma: pivotal study update demonstrates durable responses. J Hematol Oncol 2014;7:11.
58. O'Connor OA, Horwitz S, Masszi T, et al. Belinostat in patients with relapsed or refractory peripheral t-cell lymphoma: results of the pivotal phase II BELIEF (CLN-19) Study. J Clin Oncol 2015;33(23):2492–9.
59. Pro B, Advani R, Brice P, et al. Brentuximab vedotin (SGN-35) in patients with relapsed or refractory systemic anaplastic large-cell lymphoma: results of a phase II study. J Clin Oncol 2012;30(18):2190–6.
60. Horwitz SM, Advani RH, Bartlett NL, et al. Objective responses in relapsed T-cell lymphomas with single-agent brentuximab vedotin. Blood 2014;123(20):3095–100.
61. Horwitz SM, Peluso M, Faia K, et al. Duvelisib (IPI-145), a phosphoinositide-3-kinase-δ,γ inhibitor, shows activity in patients with relapsed/refractory T-cell lymphoma [abstract]. Blood 2014;124(21):803a.
62. Friedberg J, Mahadevan D, Jung JAh, et al. Phase 2 Trial of Alisertib (MLN8237), an investigational, potent inhibitor of aurora A kinase (AAK), in patients (pts) with aggressive B- and T-cell non-Hodgkin lymphoma (NHL). ASH Annu Meet Abstr 2011;118(21):95.
63. Barr PM, Li H, Spier C, et al. Phase II intergroup trial of alisertib in relapsed and refractory peripheral T-cell lymphoma and transformed mycosis fungoides: SWOG 1108. J Clin Oncol 2015;33(21):2399–404.
64. O'Connor OA, Ozcan M, Jacobsen ED, et al. First multicenter, randomized phase 3 study in patients (Pts) with relapsed/refractory (R/R) peripheral T-cell lymphoma (PTCL): Alisertib (MLN8237) versus investigator's choice (Lumiere trial; <a href="-pending:yes" l:ref-type="CLINTRIALGOV" l:ref="NCT01482962">NCT01482962</a>)</div>. Blood 2015;126(23):341.
65. Ogura M, Ishida T, Hatake K, et al. Multicenter phase II study of mogamulizumab (KW-0761), a defucosylated anti-cc chemokine receptor 4 antibody, in patients with relapsed peripheral T-cell lymphoma and cutaneous T-cell lymphoma. J Clin Oncol 2014;32(11):1157–63.
66. Lesokhin AM, Ansell SM, Armand P, et al. Nivolumab in Patients with relapsed or refractory hematologic malignancy: preliminary results of a phase Ib study. J Clin Oncol 2016;34(23):2698–704.

Management of Anaplastic Large Cell Lymphoma

Dai Chihara, MD, PhD[a,b], Michelle A. Fanale, MD[a],*

KEYWORDS

- Anaplastic large-cell lymphoma • Treatment • Brentuximab vedotin
- Stem cell transplant

KEY POINTS

- Anaplastic large cell lymphoma (ALCL) is the second most common peripheral T-cell lymphoma, and the incidence is higher in blacks than non-Hispanic whites.
- ALK (anaplastic lymphoma kinase)-positive and ALK-negative ALCL are distinct subtypes that have different characteristics and clinical outcomes; ALK-positive ALCL is more common in younger patients and has a better overall survival.
- Breast implant–associated ALCL is a rare lymphoma that has very good survival outcome, and recent study indicates that total capsulectomy is essential for treatment of this disease.
- Brentuximab vedotin (BV) is a standard therapy for relapsed or refractory ALCL.
- Overall response rate is about 80% to 90%; however, once a patient's disease progresses on BV, survival outcome is very poor with median overall survival of less than 2 months.

INTRODUCTION

Anaplastic large cell lymphoma (ALCL) is a distinct subtype of peripheral T-cell lymphoma (PTCL). ALCL accounts for 3% to 5% of all non-Hodgkin lymphoma and 10% to 20% of childhood lymphomas and consists of about 10% to 15% of PTCLs.[1] The age-adjusted incidence in the United States. for ALCL is 0.2 to 0.25 per 100,000 person-years.[2,3] Recently, a large study using population-based registry data suggested racial differences in the incidence of ALCL.[4] Asian/Pacific Islanders have significantly lower incidence compared with non-Hispanic whites (incidence rate ratio: 0.59, 95% confidence interval [CI]: 0.49–0.70), while blacks have significantly higher incidence of ALCL compared with non-Hispanic whites (incidence rate ratio: 1.17, 95% CI: 1.03–1.32). In the most recent World Health Organization classification,

The authors have nothing to disclose.
[a] Department of Lymphoma/Myeloma, The University of Texas MD Anderson Cancer Center, 1515 Holcombe Boulevard Unit 429, Houston, TX 77030, USA; [b] Department of Internal Medicine, The University of New Mexico, MSC10 5550, 1 University of New Mexico, Albuquerque, NM 87131, USA
* Corresponding author.
E-mail address: mfanale@mdanderson.org

3 types of noncutaneous ALCL are recognized.[5] One type associated with transloca-tions involving the ALK gene leading to ALK overexpression (ALK + ALCL) is well established. The other category is morphologically and phenotypically similar to ALK + ALCL but lacks ALK abnormalities of overexpression, and ALK-negative ALCL (ALK − ALCL), which was previously considered a provisional category, is now defined as definite entity based on gene expression profile (GEP) studies that showed that ALK − ALCL has similar features to that of ALK + ALCL and is distinct from other CD30-positive PTCLs.[6,7] Breast implant–associated ALCL (BIA-ALCL) was first described in 1997 and is now recognized as a distinct new entity, which usu-ally is associated with excellent outcomes.[8] Finally, primary cutaneous ALCL is a distinct subtype with a typically more indolent course and should be distinguished from systemic ALCL.

PATIENT AND DISEASE CHARACTERISTICS
ALK-Positive Anaplastic Large Cell Lymphoma

Patients with ALK + ALCL are commonly young, with a median age in the 30s; this is also one of the most common lymphoma diagnoses in children.[9,10] Patients with ALK + ALCL usually present with lymph node enlargement and have frequent extra-nodal involvement of skin, bone, soft tissue, lung, and liver. About 60% of cases pre-sent with advanced stage (stage III/IV) at presentation and often have B symptoms at diagnosis, particularly fever.

ALK + ALCL exhibits a wide histologic spectrum. Several morphologic patterns have been recognized: common type (60%), lymphohistiocytic (10%), small cell (5%–10%), Hodgkin-like (3%), and others as well as mixed or composite patterns (15%). The common type pattern is characterized by large lymphoma cells infiltrating sinuses and/or showing cohesive features (**Fig. 1**). In all variants, the lymphoma cells

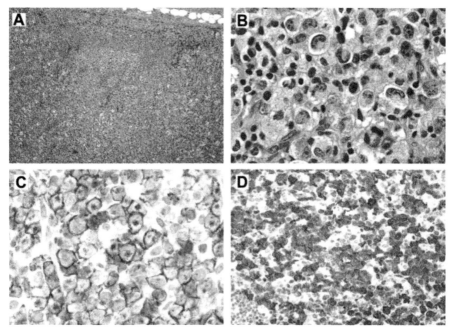

Fig. 1. (A) Sheets of lymphoma cells. (B) Atypical lymphocytes, so-called hallmark cells. (C) Immunohistochemical staining for CD30. (D) Immunohistochemical staining for ALK.

have eccentric, horseshoe- or kidney-shaped nuclei, often with an eosinophilic region near the nucleus (so-called hallmark cells). The cytoplasm is abundant and usually basophilic.

ALK + ALCL is a lymphoma of T-/null-cell lineage that is characterized by strong and diffuse CD30 and ALK expression. Most of cases are CD2+, CD4+, CD43+, and CD3−, CD8−, and BCL2−. CD15 and PAX5 are negative (unlike classical Hodgkin lymphoma). Typical genetic abnormality in ALK + ALCL is t(2;5)(p23;q35), which leads to nucleophosmin (NPM1)-ALK fusion protein and is present in 80% of the cases.[11] Different gene partners to ALK have been described, and the pattern of ALK expression by immunohistochemical staining, in part, can predict molecular abnormalities. ALK expression tends to be localized in both the cytoplasm and the nucleus in cases with NPM1-ALK fusion, whereas different partners with ALK show a cytoplasmic restricted or rarely a membranous pattern of expression.[12]

ALK + ALCL is associated with generally good prognosis, with the best outcome among systemic PTCLs.[1] Results from the International Peripheral T-Cell Lymphoma Study demonstrated a 5-year failure-free survival (FFS) and overall survival (OS) of 60% and 70%, respectively.[10] However, at relapse, the FFS for further therapies after relapse is not significantly different from ALK − ALCL.[13]

ALK-Negative Anaplastic Large Cell Lymphoma

Patients with ALK − ALCL are older, with a median age in the 50s. Similar to ALK + ALCL, patients present with advanced stage disease with lymph node enlargement, frequent extranodal involvement, and B symptoms. The morphologic spectrum of ALK − ALCL is similar to ALK + ALCL, except that the neoplastic cells may be more pleomorphic. The neoplastic cells have a T-/null-cell immunophenotype and strongly and uniformly express CD30, but are negative for ALK expression.

Studies have shown that ALK − ALCL is molecularly and genetically heterogeneous. Rearrangement of DUSP22, marked by t(6;7), was found in 30% of cases and is associated with excellent prognosis with 90% long-term survival, whereas TP63 rearrangement, marked by inv(3), was seen in 8% of cases and is associated with poor prognosis with only 17% long-term survival.[14,15] ERBB4 and COL29A1 are expressed in 24% of ALK − ALCL, mutually exclusive with TP63 rearrangement, and are associated with Hodgkin-like morphology.[16] However, several GEP studies have shown that ALK − ALCL has common signature with ALK + ALCL.[6,17–20] Crescenzo and colleagues[21] have shown kinase fusions and the presence of recurrent JAK1 and STAT3 somatic mutations that lead to constitutive activation of JAK/STAT3 pathway in ALK − ALCL. The JAK/STAT pathway is also a downstream signaling pathway of the ALK fusion proteins of ALK + ALCL. This study suggests the importance of the JAK/STAT3 pathway in the pathogenesis of ALCL and supports a rationale for the morphologic and phenotypic similarities between ALK + ALCL and ALK − ALCL.

The survival outcome of ALK − ALCL is worse than ALK + ALCL but better than PTCL-not other specified (PTCL-NOS). The International Peripheral T-Cell lymphoma Study has shown a 5-year FFS and OS of 49% and 36%, respectively.[10] The Group d'Etude des Lymphomes de l'Adulte (GELA) reported that age (<40 or ≥40) and beta 2-microglobulin were key prognostic indicators for ALK − ALCL.[9] The 8-year OS rates of patients in group 1 (age <40 years and beta 2-microglobulin <3 mg/L) and group 4 (age ≥40 years and beta 2-microglobulin ≥3 mg/L) were 84% and 22%, respectively.

Breast Implant–Associated Anaplastic Large Cell Lymphoma

BIA-ALCL usually presents as an accumulation of seroma fluid between the implant and the surrounding fibrous capsule. Greater than 90% of cases are limited stage

(stage I/II) at the time of diagnosis.[8] Both saline- and silicone-filled implants can be associated with BIA-ALCL, and the risk factors for developing this disease remain unclear. In a multicenter study of 60 patients, the median time from breast implant to ALCL was 9 years (range: 1–32 years).[8] The median OS in all patients was 12 years, and patients who presented with a mass lesion instead of only effusion had a shorter progression-free survival (PFS), although the median OS was still 12 years. A recent study showed significantly better OS and event-free survival (EFS) in patients who received total capsulectomy compared with patients who received partial capsulectomy, systemic chemotherapy, or radiation therapy.[22] Only 11.4% of patients who received total surgical excision without chemotherapy or radiation experienced events, whereas 54.5% of patients who received chemotherapy alone experienced events indicating the importance of surgical removal of breast implant in this disease. There are no data that suggest a survival benefit from removal of contralateral breast implant in nonbilateral limited stage BIA-ALCL; thus, the removal of contralateral breast implant remains controversial.

TREATMENT
Front-Line Treatment

There is no one standard treatment for both ALK + ALCL and ALK − ALCL due to a lack of randomized trials; however, CHOP (cyclophosphamide, doxorubicin, vincristine, and prednisone) has been the most commonly used chemotherapy, although the benefit of anthracycline in the treatment of PTCLs has been questioned.[1] The overall response rate (ORR) with CHOP is 70% to 80%, with complete response (CR) rates of around 50% in ALK − ALCL, and a higher response rate of around 90% in ALK + ALCL.[10,23] The long-term PFS rate for ALK − ALCL after CHOP is only about 30%, whereas ALK + ALCL has a relatively favorable outcome with 5-year PFS exceeding 60%.[1,10,23] Based on this survival outcome, ALK + ALCL is generally treated differently than other nodal PTCLs including ALK − ALCL.

Given the poor outcome with conventional chemotherapy, a more intensive approach has been investigated particularly in non-ALK + ALCL PTCLs. The MD Anderson Cancer Center (MDACC) conducted a phase II study of hyper-CVIDD/MA (cyclophosphamide, vincristine, pegylated liposomal doxorubicin, dexamethasone alternating with high-dose methotrexate and cytarabine) for the first-line therapy for non-ALK + ALCL PTCLs, to evaluate if intensive chemotherapy improves the outcome.[24] Although hyper-CVIDD/MA showed a high CR rate of 83% in patients with ALK − ALCL, median PFS was only 7.5 months with a 3-year PFS of 43%, which is not significantly different from historical data for CHOP therapy. The GELA group performed a retrospective review of patients with ALCL treated in 3 prospective trials. Almost all patients received anthracycline-based combination chemotherapy. Intensive chemotherapy (doxorubicin, cyclophosphamide, vindesine, bleomycin, and prednisone) was not associated with improved outcomes as compared with the CHOP regimen.[9]

Other studies showed a potential benefit from adding etoposide to CHOP.[25,26] The German High-Grade Non-Hodgkin Lymphoma Study Group evaluated the outcome of 320 patients with T-cell lymphoma enrolled in clinical trials. This study included 78 patients with ALK + ALCL and 113 patients with ALK − ALCL.[26] The addition of etoposide to CHOP (CHOEP, etoposide 100 mg/m^2 intravenously on days 1–3 in addition to standard CHOP) improved response rates and was associated with longer EFS in younger patients (18–60 years) with normal lactate dehydrogenase (LDH). In young patients with ALK + ALCL and a normal LDH, the 3-year EFS with CHOEP and with CHOP was 91% and 57%, respectively. In patients with non-ALK + ALCL PTCLs including ALK − ALCL, the 3-year EFS with CHOEP and CHOP was 61% and 48%, respectively. Ellin and colleagues[25] evaluated 755 patients with PTCLs (68 ALK + ALCL, 115 ALK − ALCL) in the Swedish Lymphoma Registry and confirmed that the addition of etoposide to CHOP was associated with superior PFS in patients age 60 or younger, even though no subtype-specific results were provided. Based on these studies, CHOEP is now increasingly used in the first-line treatment of ALCL.

About 30% to 40% of patients with ALK + ALCL and ALK − ALCL are diagnosed with early (stage I/II) stage disease. Currently, there are very limited data available to guide the management of these patients, and most patients are commonly treated similarly to those who have aggressive B-cell lymphoma minus the CD20-directed therapy rituximab. MDACC conducted a retrospective analysis of patients with early stage PTCLs and showed relatively favorable outcomes with 5-year PFS and OS of 74% and 79%, respectively.[27] The role of radiation therapy and the optimal number of chemotherapy cycles remain controversial and still need to be addressed.

Consolidative Stem Cell Transplant in First Remission

Given the favorable outcomes with chemotherapy, stem cell transplant as part of first-line treatment is not often considered in patients with ALK + ALCL. In fact, most clinical trials of stem cell transplant in first remission have excluded ALK + ALCL. For other non-ALK + ALCL PTCLs, several studies have evaluated the role of autologous stem cell transplant (auto-SCT) in first-line treatment either in single arm nonrandomized studies or in randomized studies including a minority of patients with PTCL.[28] A German study evaluated CHOP followed by auto-SCT in patients with newly diagnosed PTCLs (excluding ALK + ALCL).[23] Among 83 patients treated, the ORR after high-dose chemotherapy was 66% with a CR rate of 56%. The 3-year OS and PFS were 48% and 36%, respectively. For patients who actually underwent transplant (66% of patients), the 3-year OS was 71%.[23] By comparison, the Nordic group evaluated 6 cycles of CHOEP (etoposide was omitted for patients >60 years) followed by auto-SCT in patients with PTCLs (excluding ALK + ALCL).[29] Among 160 patients treated, the ORR after CHOEP was 82% with CR rate of 51%. By the subtype stratified analysis, 5-year OS of ALK − ALCL was 70%. These outcomes also seem better than historical patients treated by conventional chemotherapy like CHOP.[30] Based on these studies, auto-SCT in first remission in non-ALK + ALCL PTCLs is considered a reasonable option in clinical practice. There are also data suggesting the potential benefit of allogeneic stem cell transplant (allo-SCT) in first remission for patients with PTCLs.[31] Among 29 patients (4 ALK − ALCLs) who were able to undergo upfront allo-SCT, the 2-year OS was 72.5%, 1-year nonrelapse mortality (NRM) was 8.2%, and there seems to be a plateau in OS after 2 years although with short follow-up. However, allo-SCT is associated with significant toxicities, and this approach is still considered highly investigational and thus should only be performed on well-designed clinical trials (See Tejaswini M. Dhawale and Andrei R. Shustov's article, "Autologous and Allogeneic Hematopoietic Cell Transplantation in Peripheral T/NK-cell Lymphomas: A Histology-Specific Review," in this issue).

Treatment for Relapsed/Refractory Disease

Generally, the survival outcome of patients with PTCLs who experienced relapse or progression following first-line treatment is very poor. The British Columbia Cancer Agency analyzed 153 patients with relapsed/refractory PTCLs (11 ALK + ALCL, 27 ALK − ALCL) and showed that the median PFS and OS after the first recurrence or disease progression were only 3.1 and 5.5 months, respectively, without stem cell transplant.[32] Of note, patients who received chemotherapy after progression of relapse did not have significantly improved survival with a median OS and PFS of only 6.5 and 3.7 months, respectively. However, the study included patients who were diagnosed between 1976 and 2010, and none of the new agents described in later discussion were used during that time period. Notably, there was no difference in PFS and OS after first recurrence or disease progression by PTCL subtypes.

MDACC has assessed the survival outcome of patients with ALCL diagnosed between 1999 and 2014 who experienced disease progression or relapse after first-line and subsequent therapy.[13] A total of 176 patients (74 ALK + ALCL, 102 ALK − ALCL) diagnosed between 1999 and 2014 were retrospectively analyzed. The median age of the patients was 50 (range: 18–89). With a median follow-up of 64 months, 111 patients (38 ALK + ALCL, 73 ALK − ALCL) experienced progression/relapse after first-line therapy. The median PFS following second-line therapy in patients with ALK + ALCL and ALK − ALCL was 5.2 and 3.0 months, respectively (**Fig. 2**).

The median OS following second-line therapy in patients with ALK + ALCL and ALK − ALCL was 47.3 and 10.8 months, respectively. Interestingly, there was no significant difference in PFS following second-line treatment between ALK + ALCL and ALK − ALCL. This result potentially suggests relatively preserved chemosensitivity of recurrent ALK + ALCL, but interpretation needs to be cautious because of the small number of patients. Patients who experienced recurrent or refractory disease had a poor outcome, with less than 20% long-term disease control rate; however, there seems to be an improvement by newer treatment strategies for relapsed/refractory disease.

Brentuximab Vedotin

Brentuximab vedotin (BV) is an antibody-drug conjugate that consists of the CD30-specific monoclonal antibody conjugated with monomethyl auristatin E (MMAE) by a linker peptide. Binding of the antibody-drug conjugate to CD30 on the cell surface causes internalization of the drug by endocytosis, and the drug subsequently travels to the lysosome where proteases cleave the linker and release MMAE to cytosol.[33] Released MMAE binds to tubulin and disrupts microtubule polymerization, resulting in cell-cycle arrest and apoptotic death. BV is administered intravenously over 30 minutes at 1.8 mg/kg of body weight once every 3 weeks.

In a pivotal phase II study of patients with relapsed or refractory systemic ALCL, the ORR and CR rate were 86% and 57%, respectively.[34] BV was given up to 16 cycles, and the median number of cycles was 7 (range: 1–16). The median time to objective

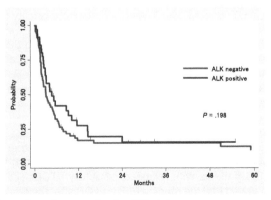

Fig. 2. PFS after first relapse/progression by ALK status.

response was 5.9 weeks, and the median time to CR was 11.9 weeks. The median PFS duration was 13.3 months, which was significantly longer than the PFS of the most recent prior therapy (hazard ratio [HR]: 0.48, P = .001). There was no difference in efficacy between ALK + ALCL and ALK − ALCL. Toxicity was generally manageable. Adverse events of grade 3 or higher were observed in 60% of patients, with the most common being neutropenia (21%), thrombocytopenia (14%), peripheral sensory neuropathy (12%), and anemia (7%). Long-term follow-up data from this study showed that the median duration of response for patients who achieved CR extended to 26.3 months, and 4-year OS was 64%.[35,36] On the basis of results from this trial, the US Food and Drug Administration (FDA) and subsequently the European Medicines Agency approved BV for the treatment of patients with ALCL in whom at least one prior multidrug chemotherapy regimen had failed.

In patients with ALCL who had previously responded to BV and experienced a recurrence after discontinuation of such therapy, retreatment with BV is very frequently effective.[37] In one reported study, objective response was observed in 7 of 8 patients (88%) with CR in 5 patients (63%). Median response duration was 12.3 months (range: 6.6–28.0+ months). Although the incidence of peripheral motor neuropathy was higher than that in the untreated population (28% vs 5%), toxicities were generally manageable with similar profiles.

BV also has been evaluated as a bridging agent to allogeneic transplantation in 24 patients with CD30-positive lymphomas refractory to at least 2 lines of chemotherapy or to auto-SCT.[38] In this study, among the 5 enrolled patients with ALCL, 3 achieved CR after 4 doses of BV, 2 of whom subsequently underwent an allogeneic stem cell transplantation. Although the number analyzed was small, this study suggests that BV can overcome some resistance to prior conventional treatment and provide an additional therapeutic option for patients for whom palliative therapy had previously been the only option.

In a retrospective MDACC study,[13] patients who received BV at some point during treatment after first-line therapy had significantly longer OS than those who did not (median OS after first progression or relapse: 49.9 vs 9.6 months, HR: 0.43 [95% CI: 0.23–0.80]). However, once disease progresses on BV, the median OS after BV failure was 1.4 months (95% CI: 0.5–9.5 months), indicating a high unmet need for new treatment strategies for patients with BV-refractory ALCL.

Other New Agents

Pralatrexate, an inhibitor of dihydrofolate reductase, is more than 10-fold more cytotoxic than methotrexate. A pivotal phase II study (PROPEL trial) enrolled 115 patients (17 ALK − ALCL) with relapsed/refractory PTCLs.[39] The ORR in patients with ALK − ALCL was 35% (95% CI: 14%–62%). The median PFS was 3.5 months in all patients, and 10.1 months in responding patients. Side effects such as severe mucositis (grade 3–4 in 22%) frequently resulted in dose delays or interruptions in pralatrexate.

Histone deacetylase inhibitors (HDAC inhibitors) are considered epigenetic modulating agents that induce accumulation of acetylated nucleosomal histones and induce differentiation and/or apoptosis in transformed cells. Two FDA-approved HDAC inhibitors for relapsed PTCLs are romidepsin and belinostat. A phase II study (N = 130) of romidepsin in relapsed/refractory PTCLs (21 ALK − ALCL) showed ORR of 24% with a CR rate of 19%.[40] The median PFS was 4 months overall. It should be noted, however, that responses were frequently durable with a median duration of response of 28 months.[41] A commonly associated adverse event was grade 3 to 4 thrombocytopenia, which is even more prevalent when combined with chemotherapy.[42] Belinostat was approved in 2014 by the FDA for the treatment of recurrent or refractory PTCLs based on the results of a phase II study (BELIEF trial).[43] This study enrolled patients with PTCLs after a failure of one or more prior systemic therapies. Among 129 patients enrolled (13 ALK − ALCL), the ORR was 15% (95% CI: 2%–45%) in patients with ALK − ALCL. The median response duration was 8.3 months. Grade 3/4 toxicity included thrombocytopenia (13%), neutropenia (13%), and anemia (10%).

The results and outcome of recent trials described above are summarized in **Table 1**.

Conventional Salvage Chemotherapy

Commonly used traditional salvage chemotherapy regimens for relapsed/refractory PTCLs are platinum containing, such as ICE (ifosfamide, carboplatin, and etoposide), DHAP (dexamethasone, cisplatin, and cytarabine), GDP (gemcitabine, dexamethasone and cisplatin), or GemOx (gemcitabine and oxaliplatin). The ORR with ICE ranges from 20% to 70% with a median PFS of 6 months.[44] The ORR was 40% with GDP[45] and 38% with GemOx with a median PFS of 10 months.[46] It should be again noted that the outcome of patients with relapsed/refractory PTCLs is historically dismal, and considering the high efficacy of BV, these chemotherapy regimens should be considered after BV. However, once patients have disease progression with BV, the median OS after BV failure is dismal at 1.4 months despite additional therapy, including the chemotherapy regimens described above.

Stem Cell Transplant After Progression or Relapse

The benefit of auto-SCT for PTCL at relapse as reported is rather disappointing, with a 5-year PFS less than 20%.[47] However, the 5-year OS after auto-SCT for relapsed/refractory ALCL was 57% in both ALK + ALCK and ALK − ALCL from an MDACC study,

Table 1
Summary of clinical trial data for recently approved drugs for anaplastic large cell lymphoma

	All PTCLs	ALK + ALCL	ALK − ALCL	ALCL	Refs.
Brentuximab Vedotin					
ORR	—	81%	88%	86%	Pro et al,[34] 2012;
CR rate	—	69%	52%	57%	Pro et al,[35] 2015
Median PFS	—	25.5 mo	20.0 mo	20.0 mo	
Median OS	—	—	—	4-y: 64%	
Pralatrexate					
ORR	29%	—	—	35%	O'Connor et al,[39] 2011
CR rate	11%	—	—	—	
Median PFS	3.5 mo	—	—	—	
Median OS	14.5 mo	—	—	—	
Romidepsin					
ORR	25%	—	24%	—	Coiffier et al,[40] 2012;
CR rate	15%	—	19%	—	Coiffier et al,[41] 2014
Median PFS	4.0 mo	—	—	—	
Median OS	11.3 mo	—	—	—	
Belinostat					
ORR	26%	0%	15%	—	O'Connor et al,[43] 2015
CR rate	11%	—	—	—	
Median PFS	1.6 mo	—	—	—	
Median OS	7.9 mo	—	—	—	

suggesting that ALCL patients who have chemosensitive disease can have benefit from auto-SCT.[13] Therefore, patients with ALCL who experience excellent disease response to salvage therapy can be considered for auto-SCT consolidation,[48] particularly if there is no option for allo-SCT, such as when no donor is available or for elderly patients.

There is also evidence that donor lymphocyte infusion can achieve long-term remission, and this is likely due to this graft-versus-lymphoma effect. Thus allo-SCT may provide effective disease control in relapsed/refractory PTCLs.[49–51] The French group has reported the outcome of 77 patients (27 ALCL) who received allo-SCT. The 5-year NRM was 33%, and 5-year OS and EFS were 55% and 48%, respectively, in patients with ALCL.[51] Patients with disease that achieved CR/PR showed significantly higher 5-year OS compared with patients who had stable disease or progressive disease (69% vs 29%); however, it is very interesting that even about 30% of chemorefractory patients can potentially achieve long-term remission. In a Japanese study, 354 patients (PTCL-NOS: N = 200, angioimmunoblastic T-cell lymphoma: N = 77, ALCL: N = 77) who received allo-SCT were analyzed.[52] The 3-year NRM rates and the 3-year OS rates in younger patients (16–49 years of age) who received myeloablative regimen were 22% and 42%, respectively, whereas patients who received reduced-intensity conditioning regimen were 14% and 56%, respectively.[52] These studies suggest the efficacy of allo-SCT. However, the results of a retrospective analysis using Center for International Blood and Marrow Transplant Research registry data comparing auto-SCT and allo-SCT (112 ALCL) showed that survival outcome following auto-SCT is better than following allo-SCT in both 3-year PFS (55% vs 35%) and 3-year OS (68% vs 41%) in patients with ALCL.[53] This low PFS and OS were likely influenced by the NRM at 3 years of 34% in patients who received allo-SCT. Given these results, even though allo-SCT is associated with long-term remissions and has a potential for cure, benefits versus risks of this treatment should be carefully discussed with each patient being considered for an allo-SCT (See Tejaswini M. Dhawale and Andrei R. Shustov's article, "Autologous and Allogeneic Hematopoietic Cell Transplantation in Peripheral T/NK-cell Lymphomas: A Histology-Specific Review," in this issue, for more details).

FUTURE DIRECTIONS

Despite the drastic, very positive change in the treatment strategy for ALCL by BV, the survival outcome is still not satisfactory particularly for patients with ALK − ALCL. Future management of ALCL in the first-line treatment is evolving and will likely involve a combination of cytotoxic chemotherapy plus newer targeted agents, most likely BV with its known very high efficacy in ALCL. A phase I study of CHOP or CHP (CHOP without vincristine) plus BV (sequential or in combination) showed very promising results with manageable toxicities.[54] Of note, in 19 patients with ALCL who received BV plus CHP as combination therapy, the ORR was 100% with CR rate of 84%. Following a median follow-up period of 21.4 months, 9 of 19 ALCL patients did experience progression of disease or death, suggesting a role for a consolidative treatment strategy. Given these very promising results, a phase III study comparing BV plus CHP versus CHOP for first-line treatment in patients with CD30-positive PTCLs (ECHELON-2) is ongoing (NCT01777152).

For ALK + ALCL, the ALK inhibitor crizotinib showed significant activity in pediatric patients with ALK + ALCL.[55] Nine patients with ALK + ALCL were enrolled in a phase I study as a part of a larger trial of crizotinib in ALK-positive malignancies, and 8 of 9 responded (ORR: 88%), with 7 CRs (CR rate: 78%). In adults, crizotinib was given as a compassionate use to chemoresistant patients with ALK + ALCL, and the CR rate was 100%.[56] Crizotinib was mostly well tolerated without significant grade 3 to 4 toxicities. Trials for adults in the first-line and relapsed/refractory settings are ongoing (NCT02487316, NCT01524926).

For the relapsed/refractory patients, the current goal of treatment is to improve salvage treatment to achieve CR and consolidate with either auto-SCT or allo-SCT in fit patients for long-term remission. Many clinical trials are ongoing, mostly using combinations of targeted agents and cytotoxic chemotherapy. BV was combined with bendamustine in patients with relapsed/refractory Hodgkin lymphoma and ALCL (NCT01657331), although only one patient with ALCL was enrolled to this study at the time of this article.[57] A phase I study of romidepsin in combination with ICE is also ongoing, and preliminary results showed an ORR of 78% with a CR rate of 64% (NCT01590732).[58] However, only 2 patients with ALCL were enrolled in this trial.

Immune therapy such as chimeric antigen receptor (CAR) T-cell therapy and checkpoint inhibitors are now under evaluation in PTCLs after impressive successes in other lymphomas.[59,60] Clinical trials evaluating BV in combination with nivolumab (NCT02581631) and CAR T-cell therapy (NCT02274584) in patients with CD30-positive non- Hodgkin lymphomas are ongoing.

In the future, it is hoped as well that the emerging understanding of the molecular pathogenesis of ALCL not only will further refine the ability to classify subtypes of ALCL and more fully predict prognosis but also open up further therapeutic options by directly being able to target molecular abnormalities. Although the recent approval of 4 new therapies for the management of relapsed ALCL has been a huge therapeutic advance, there still remains a continued need to help improve outcomes for this patient population.

SUMMARY

ALCL is a distinct subtype of PTCL that recently had a drastic change in treatment strategy as a result of the efficacy of BV in relapsed/refractory disease. Survival outcomes of patients with relapsed/refractory ALK+ and ALK − ALCL have improved after BV became available. However, patients who fail BV have dismal outcomes, and new treatment strategies to consolidate or maintain the response after BV and to develop safe and effective therapeutic options are needed. It is still strongly recommended that patients receive treatment on clinical trials so that progress can be made in the management of this very rare lymphoma. Risk stratification, targeted therapies based on recent findings in molecular biology, and novel agents may offer further improvement in survival outcomes of patients with ALCL.

REFERENCES

1. Vose J, Armitage J, Weisenburger D, International T-Cell Lymphoma Project. International peripheral T-cell and natural killer/T-cell lymphoma study: pathology findings and clinical outcomes. J Clin Oncol 2008;26(25):4124–30.
2. Chihara D, Ito H, Matsuda T, et al. Differences in incidence and trends of haematological malignancies in Japan and the United States. Br J Haematol 2014; 164(4):536–45.
3. Morton LM, Wang SS, Devesa SS, et al. Lymphoma incidence patterns by WHO subtype in the United States, 1992-2001. Blood 2006;107(1):265–76.
4. Adams SV, Newcomb PA, Shustov AR. Racial patterns of peripheral T-cell lymphoma incidence and survival in the United States. J Clin Oncol 2016;34(9): 963–71.
5. Swerdlow SH, Campo E, Pileri SA, et al. The 2016 revision of the World Health Organization classification of lymphoid neoplasms. Blood 2016;127(20):2375–90.

6. Piccaluga PP, Fuligni F, De Leo A, et al. Molecular profiling improves classification and prognostication of nodal peripheral T-cell lymphomas: results of a phase III diagnostic accuracy study. J Clin Oncol 2013;31(24):3019–25.

7. Agnelli L, Mereu E, Pellegrino E, et al. Identification of a 3-gene model as a powerful diagnostic tool for the recognition of ALK-negative anaplastic large-cell lymphoma. Blood 2012;120(6):1274–81.

8. Miranda RN, Aladily TN, Prince HM, et al. Breast implant-associated anaplastic large-cell lymphoma: long-term follow-up of 60 patients. J Clin Oncol 2014; 32(2):114–20.

9. Sibon D, Fournier M, Briere J, et al. Long-term outcome of adults with systemic anaplastic large-cell lymphoma treated within the Groupe d'Etude des Lymphomes de l'Adulte trials. J Clin Oncol 2012;30(32):3939–46.

10. Savage KJ, Harris NL, Vose JM, et al. ALK- anaplastic large-cell lymphoma is clinically and immunophenotypically different from both ALK+ ALCL and peripheral T-cell lymphoma, not otherwise specified: report from the international peripheral T-Cell lymphoma project. Blood 2008;111(12):5496–504.

11. Duyster J, Bai RY, Morris SW. Translocations involving anaplastic lymphoma kinase (ALK). Oncogene 2001;20(40):5623–37.

12. Falini B, Pulford K, Pucciarini A, et al. Lymphomas expressing ALK fusion protein(s) other than NPM-ALK. Blood 1999;94(10):3509–15.

13. Chihara D, Fanale M, Noorani M, et al. The survival outcome of the patients with relapsed/refractory anaplastic large-cell lymphoma. Blood 2015;126(23) [abstract: 2738].

14. King RL, Dao LN, McPhail ED, et al. Morphologic features of ALK-negative anaplastic large cell lymphomas with DUSP22 rearrangements. Am J Surg Pathol 2016;40(1):36–43.

15. Parrilla Castellar ER, Jaffe ES, Said JW, et al. ALK-negative anaplastic large cell lymphoma is a genetically heterogeneous disease with widely disparate clinical outcomes. Blood 2014;124(9):1473–80.

16. Scarfo I, Pellegrino E, Mereu E, et al. Identification of a new subclass of ALK-negative ALCL expressing aberrant levels of ERBB4 transcripts. Blood 2016; 127(2):221–32.

17. Iqbal J, Wright G, Wang C, et al. Gene expression signatures delineate biological and prognostic subgroups in peripheral T-cell lymphoma. Blood 2014;123(19): 2915–23.

18. Piva R, Agnelli L, Pellegrino E, et al. Gene expression profiling uncovers molecular classifiers for the recognition of anaplastic large-cell lymphoma within peripheral T-cell neoplasms. J Clin Oncol 2010;28(9):1583–90.

19. Iqbal J, Weisenburger DD, Greiner TC, et al. Molecular signatures to improve diagnosis in peripheral T-cell lymphoma and prognostication in angioimmunoblastic T-cell lymphoma. Blood 2010;115(5):1026–36.

20. Lamant L, de Reynies A, Duplantier MM, et al. Gene-expression profiling of systemic anaplastic large-cell lymphoma reveals differences based on ALK status and two distinct morphologic ALK+ subtypes. Blood 2007;109(5):2156–64.

21. Crescenzo R, Abate F, Lasorsa E, et al. Convergent mutations and kinase fusions lead to oncogenic STAT3 activation in anaplastic large cell lymphoma. Cancer cell 2015;27(4):516–32.

22. Clemens MW, Medeiros LJ, Butler CE, et al. Complete surgical excision is essential for the management of patients with breast implant-associated anaplastic large-cell lymphoma. J Clin Oncol 2016;34(2):160–8.

23. Reimer P, Rudiger T, Geissinger E, et al. Autologous stem-cell transplantation as first-line therapy in peripheral T-cell lymphomas: results of a prospective multi-center study. J Clin Oncol 2009;27(1):106–13.

24. Chihara D, Pro B, Loghavi S, et al. Phase II study of HCVIDD/MA in patients with newly diagnosed peripheral T-cell lymphoma. Br J Haematol 2015;171(4): 509–16.

25. Ellin F, Landstrom J, Jerkeman M, et al. Real-world data on prognostic factors and treatment in peripheral T-cell lymphomas: a study from the Swedish Lymphoma Registry. Blood 2014;124(10):1570–7.

26. Schmitz N, Trumper L, Ziepert M, et al. Treatment and prognosis of mature T-cell and NK-cell lymphoma: an analysis of patients with T-cell lymphoma treated in studies of the German High-Grade Non-Hodgkin Lymphoma Study Group. Blood 2010;116(18):3418–25.

27. Lee HK, Wilder RB, Jones D, et al. Outcomes using doxorubicin-based chemo-therapy with or without radiotherapy for early-stage peripheral T-cell lymphomas. Leuk Lymphoma 2002;43(9):1769–75.

28. Stiff PJ, Unger JM, Cook JR, et al. Autologous transplantation as consolidation for aggressive non-Hodgkin's lymphoma. N Engl J Med 2013;369(18):1681–90.

29. d'Amore F, Relander T, Lauritzsen GF, et al. Up-front autologous stem-cell trans-plantation in peripheral T-cell lymphoma: NLG-T-01. J Clin Oncol 2012;30(25): 3093–9.

30. Abouyabis AN, Shenoy PJ, Sinha R, et al. A systematic review and meta-analysis of front-line anthracycline-based chemotherapy regimens for peripheral T-cell lymphoma. ISRN Hematol 2011;2011:623924.

31. Loirat M, Chevallier P, Leux C, et al. Upfront allogeneic stem-cell transplantation for patients with nonlocalized untreated peripheral T-cell lymphoma: an intention-to-treat analysis from a single center. Ann Oncol 2015;26(2):386–92.

32. Mak V, Hamm J, Chhanabhai M, et al. Survival of patients with peripheral T-cell lymphoma after first relapse or progression: spectrum of disease and rare long-term survivors. J Clin Oncol 2013;31(16):1970–6.

33. Sutherland MS, Sanderson RJ, Gordon KA, et al. Lysosomal trafficking and cysteine protease metabolism confer target-specific cytotoxicity by peptide-linked anti-CD30-auristatin conjugates. J Biol Chem 2006;281(15):10540–7.

34. Pro B, Advani R, Brice P, et al. Brentuximab vedotin (SGN-35) in patients with relapsed or refractory systemic anaplastic large-cell lymphoma: results of a phase II study. J Clin Oncol 2012;30(18):2190–6.

35. Pro B, Advani RH, Brice P, et al. Four-year survival data from an ongoing pivotal phase 2 study of brentuximab vedotin in patients with relapsed or refractory sys-temic anaplastic large cell lymphoma. Blood 2014;124(21) [abstract: 3095].

36. Pro B, Advani RH, Brice P, et al. Three-year survival results from an ongoing phase 2 study of brentuximab vedotin in patients with relapsed or refractory sys-temic anaplastic large cell lymphoma. Blood 2013;122 [abstract: 1809].

37. Bartlett NL, Chen R, Fanale MA, et al. Retreatment with brentuximab vedotin in patients with CD30-positive hematologic malignancies. J Hematol Oncol 2014; 7:24.

38. Gibb A, Jones C, Bloor A, et al. Brentuximab vedotin in refractory CD30+ lym-phomas: a bridge to allogeneic transplantation in approximately one quarter of patients treated on a Named Patient Programme at a single UK center. Haema-tologica 2013;98(4):611–4.

39. O'Connor OA, Pro B, Pinter-Brown L, et al. Pralatrexate in patients with relapsed or refractory peripheral T-cell lymphoma: results from the pivotal PROPEL study. J Clin Oncol 2011;29(9):1182–9.

40. Coiffier B, Pro B, Prince HM, et al. Results from a pivotal, open-label, phase II study of romidepsin in relapsed or refractory peripheral T-cell lymphoma after prior systemic therapy. J Clin Oncol 2012;30(6):631–6.

41. Coiffier B, Pro B, Prince HM, et al. Romidepsin for the treatment of relapsed/refractory peripheral T-cell lymphoma: pivotal study update demonstrates durable responses. J Hematol Oncol 2014;7(1):11.

42. Chihara D, Oki Y, Fayad L, et al. Phase I Study of Romidepsin in Combination with ICE (Ifosfamide, Carboplatin and Etoposide) in patients with relapsed or refractory peripheral T-cell lymphoma. Blood 2014;124(21):1748.

43. O'Connor OA, Horwitz S, Masszi T, et al. Belinostat in patients with relapsed or refractory peripheral t-cell lymphoma: results of the pivotal Phase II BELIEF (CLN-19) study. J Clin Oncol 2015;33(23):2492–9.

44. Zelenetz AD, Hamlin P, Kewalramani T, et al. Ifosfamide, carboplatin, etoposide (ICE)-based second-line chemotherapy for the management of relapsed and refractory aggressive non-Hodgkin's lymphoma. Ann Oncol 2003;14(Suppl 1): i5–10.

45. Emmanouilides C, Colovos C, Pinter-Brown L, et al. Pilot study of fixed-infusion rate gemcitabine with cisplatin and dexamethasone in patients with relapsed or refractory lymphoma. Clin Lymphoma 2004;5(1):45–9.

46. Yao YY, Tang Y, Zhu Q, et al. Gemcitabine, oxaliplatin and dexamethasone as salvage treatment for elderly patients with refractory and relapsed peripheral T-cell lymphoma. Leuk Lymphoma 2013;54(6):1194–200.

47. Smith SD, Bolwell BJ, Rybicki LA, et al. Autologous hematopoietic stem cell transplantation in peripheral T-cell lymphoma using a uniform high-dose regimen. Bone Marrow Transplant 2007;40(3):239–43.

48. Kim MK, Kim S, Lee SS, et al. High-dose chemotherapy and autologous stem cell transplantation for peripheral T-cell lymphoma: complete response at transplant predicts survival. Ann Hematol 2007;86(6):435–42.

49. Kim SW, Yoon SS, Suzuki R, et al. Comparison of outcomes between autologous and allogeneic hematopoietic stem cell transplantation for peripheral T-cell lymphomas with central review of pathology. Leukemia 2013;27(6):1394–7.

50. Jacobsen ED, Kim HT, Ho VT, et al. A large single-center experience with allogeneic stem-cell transplantation for peripheral T-cell non-Hodgkin lymphoma and advanced mycosis fungoides/Sezary syndrome. Ann Oncol 2011;22(7):1608–13.

51. Le Gouill S, Milpied N, Buzyn A, et al. Graft-versus-lymphoma effect for aggressive T-cell lymphomas in adults: a study by the Societe Francaise de Greffe de Moelle et de Therapie Cellulaire. J Clin Oncol 2008;26(14):2264–71.

52. Aoki K, Suzuki R, Chihara D, et al. Reduced-intensity conditioning of allogeneic transplantation for nodal peripheral T-cell lymphomas. ASH Annual Meeting Abstracts 2014:124 [abstract: 2585].

53. Smith SM, Burns LJ, van Besien K, et al. Hematopoietic cell transplantation for systemic mature T-cell non-Hodgkin lymphoma. J Clin Oncol 2013;31(25): 3100–9.

54. Fanale MA, Horwitz SM, Forero-Torres A, et al. Brentuximab vedotin in the frontline treatment of patients with CD30+ peripheral T-cell lymphomas: results of a phase I study. J Clin Oncol 2014;32(28):3137–43.

55. Mosse YP, Lim MS, Voss SD, et al. Safety and activity of crizotinib for paediatric patients with refractory solid tumours or anaplastic large-cell lymphoma: a

Children's Oncology Group phase 1 consortium study. Lancet Oncol 2013;14(6): 472–80.

56. Gambacorti Passerini C, Farina F, Stasia A, et al. Crizotinib in advanced, chemo-resistant anaplastic lymphoma kinase-positive lymphoma patients. J Natl Cancer Inst 2014;106(2):djt378.

57. Sawas A, Connors JM, Kuruvilla J, et al. The combination of Brentuximab Vedotin (Bv) and Bendamustine (B) demonstrates marked activity in heavily treated pa-tients with relapsed or refractory Hodgkin lymphoma (HL) and anaplastic large T-Cell lymphoma (ALCL): results of an international multi center phase I/II EXPE-RIENCE. Blood 2015;126(23) [abstract: 586].

58. Chihara D, Oki Y, Fayad L, et al. High response rate of romidepsin in combination with ICE (Ifosfamide, Carboplatin and Etoposide) in patients with relapsed or re-fractory peripheral T-cell lymphoma: updates of phase I trial. Blood 2015;126(23) [abstract: 3987].

59. Kochenderfer JN, Dudley ME, Kassim SH, et al. Chemotherapy-refractory diffuse large B-cell lymphoma and indolent B-cell malignancies can be effectively treated with autologous T cells expressing an anti-CD19 chimeric antigen recep-tor. J Clin Oncol 2015;33(6):540–9.

60. Ansell SM, Lesokhin AM, Borrello I, et al. PD-1 blockade with nivolumab in relapsed or refractory Hodgkin's lymphoma. N Engl J Med 2015;372(4):311–9.

Angioimmunoblastic T-Cell Lymphoma

 CrossMark

Alessandro Broccoli, MD, Pier Luigi Zinzani, MD, PhD*

KEYWORDS

- Angioimmunoblastic T-cell lymphoma • Autologous stem cell transplantation
- Brentuximab vedotin • CHOP • *DNMT3A* • Follicular T-helper • *IDH2*
- Lenalidomide

KEY POINTS

- Angioimmunoblastic T-cell lymphoma is a follicular T-helper–derived neoplasm, sharing many of its features with a proportion of peripheral T-cell lymphomas, not otherwise specified.
- New mutations have been recently described (*TET2, DNMT3A, IDH2, RHOA*), and fresh biological insights into the molecular pathogenesis of the disease are now available.
- Anthracycline-containing regimens represent the most widely adopted first-line option, to be followed by a consolidative autologous transplantation whenever possible.
- Newly approved agents and off-label compounds (romidepsin, belinostat, brentuximab vedotin, lenalidomide) seem active in pretreated patients but response durations are short.
- Innovative induction strategies (CHOP + biologic agent) should be designed to enhance response quality, facilitate autoSCT and prolong survival.

INTRODUCTION AND EPIDEMIOLOGY

An angioimmunoblastic lymphadenopathy with dysproteinemia was first described by the group of Henry Rappaport in the 1970s.[1] At that time, it was not recognized as a malignant condition because some patients seemed to gain long-term benefit from steroid treatment. Some investigators reported, however, that this condition was prone to progression to an overt lymphoma,[2,3] and underscored the difficulty of pathologists in establishing a clear-cut distinction between a "benign" and a "malignant" lesion based on morphology alone. Angioimmunoblastic T-cell lymphoma (AITL) is an acknowledged entity since the 1994 Revised European American Lymphoma (REAL) Classification.[4] Given that a number of recurrent mutations and a peculiar gene

Disclosure Statement: The authors have nothing to disclose.
Institute of Hematology "L. e A. Seràgnoli", University of Bologna, Via Massarenti, 9, Bologna 40138, Italy
* Corresponding author.
E-mail address: pierluigi.zinzani@unibo.it

Hematol Oncol Clin N Am 31 (2017) 223–238
http://dx.doi.org/10.1016/j.hoc.2016.12.001
0889-8588/17/© 2016 Elsevier Inc. All rights reserved.

signature characterize a significant proportion of AITL cases (see next paragraph for details), as well as some cases of peripheral T-cell lymphoma (PTCL), not otherwise specified (NOS), which manifest a follicular T-helper (T_{FH}) phenotype, the 2016 revision of the World Health Organization classification unifies under a common heading AITL, follicular T-cell lymphoma, and nodal PTCL with T_{FH} phenotype.[5]

AITL is a rare disease, which accounts for only 1% to 2% of non-Hodgkin lymphomas and 15% to 20% of PTCL.[6,7] Incidence is low, with 0.05 new cases diagnosed per 100,000 patients in the United States per year. Disease incidence is higher in Europe (29% of all cases of PTCL), followed by Asia (18%) and North America (16%): the reasons for this heterogeneity in different parts of the world are unexplained. AITL is generally regarded as the second most common PTCL entity, although it was the prevalent subtype in 2 recently published French datasets, in which it represented 36.1% of all PTCL cases.[8] This may be explained by a geographic heterogeneity of incidence across Europe, but more likely reflects a refined classification of PTCL-NOS cases by the use of novel molecular tools in more recent studies.

The purpose of this article is to provide a brief overview of the new biological insights of AITL, to discuss patients' management, and to review the currently adopted treatment strategies for newly diagnosed, relapsed, and refractory disease.

MORPHOLOGY AND MOLECULAR FEATURES

The architecture of the affected lymph node is completely effaced by a T-cell infiltrate of polymorphous small to medium-sized lymphocytes, usually with clear cytoplasm, which extends beyond the node capsule although characteristically sparing the subcapsular sinus, which appears open and dilated.[9] Regressed follicles may be appreciated, especially in earlier stages of the disease, indicating that the disease arises in association with germinal centers with the extension to extrafollicular regions as it progresses.[10] T-cell–associated antigens are demonstrated by immunohistochemistry, although neoplastic cells may show an aberrant phenotype in many instances. CD3, CD4, CD10, PD1, and sometimes BCL6 are the most frequently encountered antigens, whereas CD5 and CD7 are frequently absent. Using immunohistochemistry, it also has been demonstrated that tumor elements almost invariably express CXCL13,[11] a chemokine characteristic of T_{FH} cells, normally present in germinal centers with a helper function to follicular B-lymphocytes.

Neoplastic cells are admixed with reactive small lymphocytes, eosinophils, plasma cells, and an abundant amount of follicular dendritic cells, which represent the accompanying non-neoplastic populations. Scattered large CD20^{+} immunoblastic cells, usually staining positively for Epstein-Barr virus (EBV)-encoded RNA (EBNA), are found in most cases (**Fig. 1**). The prominent proliferation of high endothelial venules with a tendency to arborization is a characteristic feature of AITL and reflects the overexpression of the vascular endothelial growth factor (*VEGF*) *A* gene both in lymphoma and endothelial cells.[12]

From the molecular point of view, AITL displays a peculiar signature characterized by a strong microenvironment imprint, made up of the overexpression of genes related to B cells, plasma cells, follicular dendritic cells, extracellular matrix molecules (laminin, collagen, fibronectin), enzymes, and factors involved in extracellular matrix synthesis and remodeling (transforming growth factor-β, fibroblast growth factor, matrix metalloproteinases), cell adhesion molecules (cadherins, integrins), vasculogenesis (*VEGF-A*), and coagulation.[10,12] This particular gene signature distinguishes AITL from PTCL-NOS.

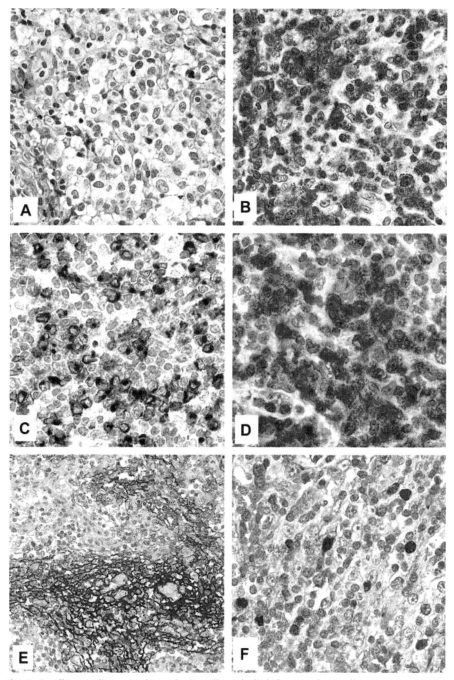

Fig. 1. Small to medium-sized neoplastic cells with slightly irregular nuclear contours, coarse chromatin, small nucleoli, and a rather large rim of clear cytoplasm (Giemsa stain, ×400, *A*). AITL lymphomatous elements expressing T$_{FH}$ markers PD1 (×400, *B*), CXCL13 (×400, *C*), CD10 (×400, *D*). Antibodies against CD21 showing aberrant follicular dendritic cell mesh works (×200, *E*). Activated B-lymphocytes carrying EBV infection demonstrated by EBER (Epstein-Barr virus-Encoded small RNAs) in situ hybridization (×400, *F*). (*Courtesy of* Prof. Claudio Agostinelli, University of Bologna.)

Several genes overexpressed in AITL (such as *CD200*, *PDCD1*, *CD40L*, *NFATC1*, *LIF*) have been reported as overexpressed in T_{FH} compared with other T-cell subsets, thus supporting the AITL derivation from T_{FH} cells.[10] The detection of at least 3 T_{FH}-associated molecules by immunohistochemistry (CD10, BCL6, PD1, CXCL13, CCR5, SAP, ICOS), which is a surrogate for gene expression profiling, is considered sufficient to suggest the derivation of a given T-cell neoplasm from T_{FH}. This is generally true for AITL, but also from a proportion of PTCL-NOS.[5,13–15]

The AITL mutational landscape is complex, and again the same genes appear mutated also in some cases of PTCL-NOS, although prevalence is different.[16] *TET2*, *IDH2*, *DNMT3A*, and *RHOA* are among the most relevant mutated genes,[17–20] whose alteration may play a significant role in T-cell lymphomagenesis. Mutations of the ten-eleven translocation 2 (*TET2*) gene are the most prevalent among AITL (one-half to three-quarters of the cases) and generally correlate with advanced-stage disease, high International Prognostic Index (IPI) score, thrombocytopenia, elevated lactate dehydrogenase (LDH), and shortened survival.[17,21] Interestingly, nearly 40% of PTCL-NOS share the same mutations, specifically those with T_{FH} marker expression or morphologic similarity to AITL. *TET2* and DNA methyltransferase 3A (*DNMT3A*) mutations seem to occur at an early stage of hematopoietic differentiation, and may represent early events of lymphomagenesis.[18] Isocitrate dehydrogenase 2 (*IDH2*) mutations at R172 are also characteristic of AITL (which is different from acute myeloid leukemias, in which mutations are at R140 and *IDH1* is also affected), and tend to co-occur with *TET2* mutations.[19,21] Moreover, $IDH2^{R172}$ mutations define a unique subgroup of AITL with distinct gene expression, and *IDH2/TET2* double-mutant cases display a significantly more polarized T_{FH} phenotype, with an upregulation of T_{FH}-associated genes (*IL21*, *ICOS*), and downregulation of genes correlating with a T-helper 1 (Th1), Th2, and Th17 phenotype.[22] In addition, $IDH2^{R172}$ mutations are associated with hypermethylation of genes involved in T-cell receptor (TCR) signaling and T-cell differentiation, suggesting a possible pathogenetic correlation.[22] Somatic *RHOA* mutations encoding a Gly17Val substitution also have been described in nearly 70% of AITL, constantly co-occurring with *TET2* and very often with *DNMT3A* mutations.[23] RHOA is activated downstream of TCR engagement in mature T-lymphocytes, and when mutated it shows an impaired GTP-ase function that also inhibits its wild-type form.[20] The coexistence of these mutations occurring at different times of a multistep model of lymphomagenesis, the cooperation of the aberrant encoded proteins, along with other mutations affecting genes related to TCR signaling that deregulate TCR activation may cooperate in the pathogenesis of AITL and other T_{FH}-derived PTCL.[24]

CLINICAL FEATURES, DIAGNOSIS AND PATIENT EVALUATION

AITL is a disease of older adults, with a median age at onset of 65 years, with a slight male predominance. It generally presents with advanced Ann Arbor stage III to IV, with generalized lymphadenopathy in approximately 75% of cases accompanied by hepatosplenomegaly in one-third of cases and with the involvement of at least 2 extranodal sites in up to one-fifth of patients.[7,25] Skin lesions are the most common extranodal manifestations, ranging from macular rash to papular and plaque/nodular lesions, with an incremental increase in the density of the dermal infiltrate and with the detection of lymphocyte cytologic atypia over time.[26]

Lymphoma-related symptoms can be found in nearly 70% of patients at disease onset, thus indicating the clinical aggressiveness of the disease. Peripheral edema, pleural or peritoneal effusion, joint pain, or cold agglutinin disease can be associated phenomena. At least 65% of patients are anemic at diagnosis: Coombs-positive auto-immune hemolytic anemia is diagnosed in 10% to 40% of cases, and a bone marrow infiltration may be appreciated in approximately 60% of anemic patients. Peculiar laboratory abnormalities include hypergammaglobulinemia (more than 12 g/dL) in 30% to 50% of cases, sometimes accompanied by the presence of monoclonal serum immunoglobulin, elevated serum LDH, and the detection of autoimmune markers, such as rheumatoid factor, circulating immunocomplexes, and anti–smooth muscle antibodies.[7,25,27]

The diagnosis is established on the biopsy of the involved tissue (lymph node or skin lesion in selected cases); review of slides or paraffin block by a pathologist with expertise in the diagnosis of T-cell lymphomas is always encouraged. Molecular studies are optional because none of the known molecular alterations dictates treatment decisions at present. The complete staging workup is outlined in **Box 1**.

[18]F-fluorodeoxyglucose (FDG) PET scan is not mandatory in this context, although it has proven to be helpful in detecting FDG-avid nodal or extranodal lesions that can be missed by a computed tomography (CT) scan evaluation. PET is able to change the disease stage in nearly 5% of patients at diagnosis as compared with CT, but this change does not translate into any treatment alteration because systemic chemotherapy in nodal PTCL is generally used regardless of tumor extent. It should be noted, however, that PET positivity found at the end of induction treatment and in patients who have received autologous stem cell transplantation (autoSCT) is a strong predictor of reduced survival.[28–30]

PROGNOSIS

Among the 243 patients with AITL evaluated by Federico and colleagues,[7] who represented 18.5% of the entire cohort of 1314 patients collected within the International

---

Box 1
Patient evaluation overview

- Histologically confirmed diagnosis of angioimmunoblastic T-cell lymphoma made by an expert hematopathologist (excisional biopsy of a suspect nodal mass in a compatible clinical context).

- Full patient's history, particularly focusing on the presence of lymphoma-related symptoms.

- Complete physical examination (seek for superficial lymph nodes, hepatic or splenic enlargement, abdominal or pleural effusion, skin lesions; inspect the oral cavity; listen to heart sounds and murmurs).

- Laboratory: full blood counts, ferritin, C-reactive protein, erythrocyte sedimentation rate, creatinine, uric acid, lactate dehydrogenase, transaminases, blood proteins with electrophoresis, and serum immunofixation; serology for hepatitis B and C viruses and human immunodeficiency virus. Reticulocytes and bilirubin (total and fractionated) are useful markers in case of suspect hemolytic anemia.

- Autoimmune markers: direct Coombs test, nonorganospecific antibodies, rheumatoid factor, circulating immunocomplexes.

- Computed tomography scan of neck, thorax, abdomen, and pelvis (with contrast) and fluorodeoxyglucose PET scan (the latter is optional, but appears useful to establish the depth of response on treatment completion).

- Bone marrow biopsy.

- Transthoracic echocardiogram, to evaluate the fitness of the patient in receiving anthracyclines.

Peripheral T-cell and Natural Killer/T-cell Lymphoma Study,[6] 14% presented with an IPI score of 0 to 1, 59% with a score of 2 to 3, and 28% with a score of 4 to 5. Patients were largely treated frontline with anthracycline-containing combination chemotherapy, mainly cyclophosphamide, doxorubicin, vincristine, and prednisone (CHOP) and CHOP-like regimens, obtaining a 5-year overall and failure-free survival of 33% and 18%, which did not differ from what was observed in a case series of 157 French patients.[27] The 5-year overall survival (OS) for those with an IPI score of 0 to 1 was 56%, whereas it was 25% for patients with a score of 4 to 5. However, only age older than 60 years, performance status greater than 2, and the presence of extranodal involvement (>1 site) were predictive of OS, thus indicating that IPI score was not particularly informative in patients with AITL. An alternative prognostic model based on age (>60 years), performance status (>2), extranodal site involvement ($\geq$2 sites), presence of B-symptoms, and platelet count (<150,000/mm^3) was proposed (prognostic index for AITL, PIAI [Prognostic Index for Angio-Immunoblastic]) and was more predictive of OS in patients with lower (score 0–1) and higher (score 3–5) risk (P = .0065).[7] Anemia (hemoglobin <12 g/dL), mediastinal lymphadenopathy,[27,31] white blood cell count (>10,000/mmc), and immunoglobulin A concentration (>400 mg/dL)[31] also have shown a significant impact on prognosis.

FIRST-LINE TREATMENT APPROACH

Once the diagnosis has been clearly established and a complete disease staging thoroughly accomplished, the first aspect to be considered is to determine whether the patient is a suitable candidate for an autoSCT approach (**Box 2**). As is true of

---

Box 2
First-line treatment approach

- Enrollment in a clinical trial is encouraged at any time.
- Determine whether the patient is a suitable candidate for autologous stem cell transplantation (autoSCT) (age, comorbidities, performance status).

For transplant candidates:

- An anthracycline-containing regimen (cyclophosphamide, doxorubicin, vincristine, and prednisone [CHOP], CHOP-like) is the most suitable induction treatment. Consider to add etoposide (CHOEP) if age <60 years.
- Perform peripheral blood stem cell mobilization, either primed with chemotherapy or with granulocyte-colony stimulating factor stimulation ($\pm$plerixafor).
- Evaluate response before conditioning (as treatment response before transplantation is a major outcome predictor).
- Repeat response evaluation at least 2 months after autoSCT.

For nontransplant candidates:

- An anthracycline-containing regimen remains the recommended approach, provided the patient shows an adequate cardiac function. Liposomal doxorubicin formulations may be an alternative for patients with mild cardiac impairment.
- Response should be evaluated at the end of the induction regimen.
- Responding patients require posttreatment careful monitoring.

For patients unfit for chemotherapy:

- Single-agent prednisone may provide disease control as well as single-agent cyclosporine.

other subtypes of nodal PTCL, patients with AITL appear to benefit from frontline consolidation with autoSCT when at least a partial response (PR) to induction is achieved[32–34] (See the article by Tejaswini M. Dhawale and Andrei R. Shustov's article, "Autologous and Allogeneic Hematopoietic Cell Transplantation in Peripheral T/NK-cell Lymphomas: A Histology-Specific Review," in this issue, for further detail). As a second point, it is important to select and apply the most appropriate induction regimen to ensure adequate control of the disease and to maximize the probability of a good-quality response.

Three retrospective autoSCT experiences specifically involving patients with AITL have been published.[35–37] Schetelig and colleagues[35] treated 29 patients in the 1990s: 48% received autoSCT as part of first-line treatment, and although without reaching statistical significance and with the possible limitations related to a retrospective analysis, patients transplanted in first remission showed a more favorable trend in terms of OS than those transplanted as second (or later) line (60% vs 44% at 5 years). Rodríguez and colleagues[36] reported in 2007 on 19 patients with AITL (median age 46 years, range 16–65) who received autoSCT after a previous anthracycline-containing regimen: 79% of them were transplanted first-line, either in complete response (CR) or PR. All patients transplanted in CR maintained a CR after transplantation; among those in PR at the time of autoSCT, 80% could upgrade their final status to a CR. OS at 3 years was 60%, with a 3-year progression-free survival (PFS) of 55%. Last, the experience of Kyriakou and colleagues[37] puts in evidence that patients transplanted in first CR can perform significantly better than those transplanted during salvage treatment, even if with chemosensitive disease, with PFS rates of 70% and 42% at 2 years, respectively. These data are in line with the results of prospective studies enrolling diverse subtypes of PTCL and contemplating autoSCT as first-line consolidation,[32,34] and in particular with the survival outcomes reported for the AITL subset by d'Amore and colleagues[34] (5-year OS and PFS of 52% and 49%, respectively).

Given that age at disease onset is generally advanced, most patients are unsuitable for autoSCT, as demonstrated in the article by Federico and colleagues[7] by the relatively low percentage of cases (8%) in which transplantation was considered as part of the initial treatment. Moreover, it clearly emerges from published clinical trials that a significant proportion of patients fail to obtain a proper clinical response or progress during induction or immediately before transplantation,[32–34] thus having precluded an effective consolidation.

Which chemotherapy combination provides the best induction strategy is still a matter of debate. Anthracycline-containing regimens, however, are regarded as the most effective and widely adopted approach in patients with nodal PTCL, including AITL.[38] On the one hand, it should be noted that according to the International Peripheral T-cell and Natural Killer/T-cell Lymphoma Study the CR rate observed in patients receiving an anthracycline-based induction was 61%,[7] however without any significant survival advantage for those receiving anthracyclines if compared with patients treated with anthracycline-free schedules.[6] On the other hand, different data sets provide the evidence that anthracycline-containing regimens are associated with improved OS and PFS in patients with PTCL, particularly with the AITL and PTCL-NOS subtypes, and that the benefit is reinforced by first-line consolidation with autoSCT.[39] It is noteworthy that according to the German experience, the addition of etoposide to the standard CHOP regimen (CHOEP), given either every 14 or 21 days, improved response and event-free survival (EFS) rates in young patients with normal LDH levels (3-year EFS was 70.5% after CHOEP and 51.0% after CHOP, $P = .004$), although 3-year OS did not significantly differ (81.3% for CHOEP vs 75.2% for CHOP, P = .285). In patients with AITL, in particular, OS and EFS rates at 5 years were 67.5% and 50.0%, respectively.[40] No enhanced benefit, however, could be appreciated in patients older than 60 years (median age for patients with AITL in this study was 64, range 22–77), for whom neither dose intensification nor the addition of etoposide could improve OS or EFS. When CHOP was compared with an upfront reinforced induction schedule including etoposide, ifosfamide, and cisplatin, alternating with doxorubicin, bleomycin, vinblastine, and dacarbazine (VIP-rABVD)[41] in a randomized phase 3 trial involving 88 patients with untreated PTCL lymphoma, including 17% patients with AITL, no significant difference emerged between the 2 arms in terms of EFS at 2 years. CHOP was therefore confirmed as the reference regimen for all patients with nodal PTCL, serving as the backbone for possible newer drug combinations.

Patients considered unfit for autoSCT should also receive an anthracycline-containing induction, provided they have adequate cardiac function, unless a clinical trial is available. Those who are considered unfit for chemotherapy may be treated with single-agent cyclosporine or prednisone. Cyclosporine, in particular, has yielded an overall response rate (ORR) of 67% (with 25% CR) in a series of 12 patients who were previously untreated or had just received steroids or chemotherapy, when given for 6 to 8 weeks at the dosage of 3 to 5 mg/kg and then tapered by 50 mg every 1 to 3 weeks.[42]

MANAGEMENT OF RELAPSED AND REFRACTORY DISEASE

Patients with relapsed or refractory PTCL are always a challenge for treating physicians, and the best therapeutic approach represents an unmet medical need. Median survival rates are only a few months, being comparable for both relapsed and refractory patients and without relevant differences among PTCL subtypes. In a survey from the British Columbia Cancer Agency on 153 patients with relapsed or refractory PTCL, 21 patients with AITL showed a median second PFS and OS of 3.8 and 6.5 months, respectively.[43] Notably, patients who could receive salvage chemotherapy did only marginally better than those who received steroids or supportive care.

This clearly indicates that drugs displaying novel mechanisms of actions and lacking significant cross-resistance with previously administered chemotherapy agents are urgently needed. Three next-generation compounds (pralatrexate, romidepsin, and belinostat) have been approved by the Food and Drug Administration for the treatment of relapsed and refractory PTCL, including AITL. However, approvals were based on response rates alone, as none of these drugs has demonstrated an increase in OS.[44–46] Response rates obtained in patients with AITL to any of these agents within each pivotal trial are summarized in **Table 1**.

Patients with AITL enrolled in the romidepsin and belinostat trials achieved a clinical response in a substantial proportion of cases, ranging from 30% with romidepsin to 46% with belinostat.[45,46] Both drugs are histone deacetylase (HDAC) inhibitors, both given intravenously: the former specifically inhibits class 1 HDAC, whereas the latter has a broader spectrum of action, being active on class 1, 2, and 4 HDAC. Of note, among the 27 patients with AITL enrolled in the pivotal romidepsin trial, 5 of the 9 responders (56%) achieved a remission lasting more than 12 months. Moreover, at least 50% of patients who were refractory to their last prior therapy could obtain a response, which was a CR in 40% of cases.[47] More disappointing results were obtained with the dihydrofolate reductase and thymidylate synthase

Table 1
Selected experiences with approved single agents and off-label compounds in peripheral
T-cell lymphoma patients, including AITL (shaded column)

Treatment	AITL		PTCL-NOS		ALCL		Reference
	ORR, %	CR, %	ORR, %	CR, %	ORR, %	CR, %	
Pralatrexate[a]	8	—	32	—	35	—	O'Connor et al,[44] 2011
Romidepsin[a]	30	19	29	14	24	19	Coiffier et al,[45] 2012
Belinostat[a]	46	—	23	—	15	—	O'Connor et al,[46] 2015
Brentuximab vedotin[b]	54	38	33	14	86	57	Pro et al,[48] 2012; Horwitz et al,[49] 2014
Lenalidomide	31	15	20	—	—	—	Morschhauser et al,[50] 2013
	33	11	43	14	10	0	Toumishey et al,[51] 2015
Alisertib	33	0	31	8	50	0[c]	Barr et al,[52] 2015
Mogamulizumab	50	25	19	6	100	100[d]	Ogura et al,[53] 2014

Abbreviations: AITL, angioimmunoblastic T-cell lymphoma; ALCL, anaplastic large cell lymphoma; CR, rate of complete responses (if available); ORR, overall response rate; PTCL-NOS, peripheral T-cell lymphoma, not otherwise specified.

[a] Indicates that the drug has received Food and Drug Administration approval in patients with relapsed and refractory peripheral T-cell lymphoma.

[b] Indicates that the drug has received Food and Drug Administration approval in patients with CD30+ relapsed or refractory anaplastic large cell lymphoma.

[c] Response is established on 2 patients who are ALK-negative.

[d] Response is established on 1 patient who is ALK-negative.

inhibitor pralatrexate: only 8% of patients with AITL responded, in spite of an ORR of at least 32% for other PTCL subtypes.[44]

Relevant results also have been obtained with brentuximab vedotin, an anti-CD30 drug-conjugated monoclonal antibody currently approved for relapsed and refractory anaplastic large-cell lymphoma.[48] In a study from Horwitz and colleagues,[49] single-agent brentuximab vedotin in PTCL-NOS and AITL produced an ORR of 33% and 54%, respectively, with CR in 14% and 38% of cases. Clinical benefit also was seen in cases with undetectable CD30 expression on central review, raising the possibility that responses may be to some extent independent of the presence of CD30 on tumor cells.

Among off-label compounds, lenalidomide has shown promising results in patients with AITL due to its antiproliferative, immunomodulator, and antiangiogenetic effects. Response rates varied between 22% and 30%, with CR rates ranging from 8% to 30% in heavily pretreated patients with nodal forms of PTCL: more specifically, at least 1 of 3 patients with AITL responded,[50,51] with CR reported in 11% to 15% of cases. Response durations were, however, short (3.6–5.0 months) and not substantially different from those documented with pralatrexate, romidepsin, and belinostat.

Alisertib and mogamulizumab are 2 innovative compounds with clinical activity in relapsed and refractory PTCL. Among individuals treated with alisertib, an Aurora A kinase inhibitor that determines mitotic spindle defects during mitosis, 3 of 9 heavily pretreated patients with AITL obtained a PR, although without any CR, and disease stability was documented in 2 cases, yielding a disease control rate of 56%.[52] Also mogamulizumab, an anti-CC chemokine receptor 4 (CCR4) monoclonal antibody, was able to induce a clinical response in 6 of 12 pretreated patients with AITL, being able to induce 3 CR and 3 PR, with an overall disease control rate of 75%.[53] Again, observed median OS rates were short and not exceeding 14 months, with median PFS ranging from 2 to 3 months for mogamulizumab and alisertib, respectively. Preliminary results of an ongoing phase 3 randomized trial comparing alisertib with investigator's choice (gemcitabine, pralatrexate, romidepsin) in patients with relapsed or refractory PTCL (NCT01482962) showed no superiority of alisertib to comparators.[54] Please see Enrica Marchi and colleagues' article, "Novel Agents in the Treatment of Relapsed or Refractory Peripheral T-Cell Lymphoma," in this issue for additional detail on new drugs in development.

Allogeneic bone marrow transplantation (alloSCT) is putatively the only strategy that may provide a cure for relapsed and refractory AITL.[25,55,56] This is substantiated by the fact that allogeneic hematopoietic stem cells are free of tumor contamination and that donor-derived immune cells are potentially capable of an antitumor effect, that is, graft-versus-lymphoma. Patients in remission at the time of transplantation can be cured of their disease, as demonstrated by OS curves that reach a plateau after approximately 18 months. This seems particularly true for patients with AITL, which displayed an OS probability of 80% at 5 years in a French experience published in 2008.[55] Kyriakou and colleagues[56] confirmed in a retrospective trial on 45 patients with AITL that alloSCT was able to induce durable responses, with OS and PFS curves reaching a plateau over time and yielding a 3-year OS and PFS rate of 64% and 53%, respectively. Differences were not appreciated in terms of conditioning regimen (myeloablative vs reduced intensity), but disease status at transplantation (sensitive vs refractory disease) and the presence of chronic graft-versus-host disease significantly impacted on relapse rate, thus confirming a possibly relevant role of a graft-versus-lymphoma effect.

At present, alloSCT is feasible in just a few cases of relapsed AITL, principally because of age at presentation, but also as most patients rapidly progress or show clinical decay and chemoresistance, all factors that may preclude a timely and effective application of this approach. In this sense, new drugs should be considered an option for a selected proportion of patients to gain disease control before being timely addressed to alloSCT. Please see Tejaswini M. Dhawale and Andrei R. Shustov's article, "Autologous and Allogeneic Hematopoietic Cell Transplantation in Peripheral T/NK-cell Lymphomas: A Histology-Specific Review," in this issue for additional detail.

NEWER APPROACHES TO TREATMENT-NAÏVE PATIENTS

Newer first-line strategies, such as the incorporation of a new agent with some activity in AITL into an anthracycline-containing regimen (CHOP or CHOEP), should be designed to increase the rate of postinduction CR. The goal of this strategy would be to allow a higher proportion of patients to undergo autoSCT in first remission when appropriate, or more generally prolong survival in patients who are not candidates for autoSCT. Several new approaches have just been tested in patients with AITL, as CHOP has already been combined with rituximab,[57] bevacizumab,[58] belinostat,[59] and alemtuzumab.[60–62] However, these strategies for the most part have proven unsuccessful. Some ongoing phase 2 and 3 clinical trials with lenalidomide, romidepsin, and brentuximab vedotin in patients with PTCL also allow AITL cases to be enrolled. The published preliminary results of these studies, along with the underlying rationale for their application in AITL, are provided in **Table 2**.

Table 2
Combination regimens including new agents for the first-line treatment of patients with PTCL, with a particular focus on AITL

Combination	Patients with AITL	Study status	Rationale for application in AITL	Available results in AITL	Reference or NCT
Rituximab + CHOP	100%	Completed	Variable amounts of CD20⁺ large B-blasts, often infected by EBV, are found in tumor tissue. The disruption of putative B-T interactions or the depletion of the EBV reservoir can enhance the clinical outcome.	Phase 2 study. 25 patients enrolled. ORR 80%; CR 44%; DOR 25 mo; 2-y PFS 42%; 2-y OS 62%. No clear benefit of the addition of rituximab to conventional chemotherapy.	Delfau-Larue et al,[57] 2012
Bevacizumab + CHOP	44%	Completed	*VEGF-A* gene is overexpressed in AITL cells and accompanying endothelial cells. Prominent high endothelial vasculature is a morphologic hallmark of AITL. Bevacizumab given at the dosage of 15 mg/kg on day 1 every 21 d.	39 patients enrolled, 17 with AITL. ORR 90%; CR 49% (53% in AITL); 1-y PFS 44% (57% in AITL); 1-y OS 88% in AITL. No significant improvement of combination therapy over CHOP alone. Significant toxicity: Neutropenia, thrombocytopenia, cardiac toxicity, infections.	Ganjoo et al,[58] 2014
Lenalidomide + CHOP	100%	Ongoing	Lenalidomide is active in pretreated AITL; it exerts antiangiogenic activity through the inhibition of VEGF and has immuno-modulatory functions.	Final data collection for primary outcome measures: March 2018.	NCT01553786
Romidepsin + CHOP	—	Ongoing	Romidepsin induces durable responses in relapsed or refractory patients with AITL when given as single agent. Romidepsin is given at 12 mg/m² on day 1 and 8 every 3 wk.	Phase 3, randomized study to compare efficacy of romidepsin + CHOP vs CHOP in untreated PTCL. Final data collection for primary outcome measures: July 2019.	NCT01796002

(continued on next page)

Table 2
(continued)

Combination	Patients with AITL	Study status	Rationale for application in AITL	Available results in AITL	Reference or NCT
Brentuximab + CHP	—	Ongoing	CD30 is variably expressed in AITL. Single agent brentuximab produces relevant objective response rates in relapsed and refractory patients, also in case of low CD30 expression.	Phase 3 randomized, placebo-controlled study to compare efficacy of brentuximab vedotin + CHP (without vincristine to avoid excessive neurotoxicity) vs CHOP in CD30-positive mature T-cell lymphoma (ECHELON-2 trial). Final data collection for primary outcome measures: December 2017.	NCT01777152
Belinostat + CHOP	39%	Completed	Belinostat shows relevant activity in relapsed and refractory AITL, in which mutations in genes affecting the DNA epigenetic changes are considered pathogenetically significant.	Phase 1 study. 23 patients enrolled, 9 with AITL. Belinostat MTD was 1000 mg/m², days 1–5 (cohort 5). ORR (18 evaluable patients) 89%; CR 72%.	Johnston et al,[59] 2015
Alemtuzumab + CHOP	30%	Completed	CD52 is highly expressed on the surface of malignant T-lymphocytes.	20 patients enrolled, 6 with AITL. ORR 90% (100% for AITL); 2-y EFS 30% (50% for AITL); 2-y OS 55% (83% for AITL). Alemtuzumab given at 90 mg/cycle for 8 cycles every 2 wk.	Kluin-Nelemans et al,[60] 2011
	—	Ongoing	Same as above.	Phase 3 randomized study to compare efficacy of alemtuzumab (A) + CHOP vs CHOP, followed by autoSCT (patients' age <60 y). Estimated study completion date: December 2016.	d'Amore et al,[61] 2012, NCT00646854
	41%	Completed	Same as above.	For all the 116 patients enrolled: CR 60% (A-CHOP) vs 43% (CHOP); 3-y PFS 26% (A-CHOP) vs 29% (CHOP); 3-y OS 38% (A-CHOP) vs 56% (CHOP). Differences in PFS and OS do not reach statistical significance. Survival not improved mostly due to treatment toxicity.	Trumper et al,[62] 2016

Abbreviations: A-CHOP, alemtuzumab + CHOP; AITL, angioimmunoblastic T-cell lymphoma; autoSCT, autologous transplantation; CHOP, cyclophosphamide, doxorubicin, vincristine, and prednisone; CR, complete response; DOR, duration of response; EBV, Epstein-Barr virus; EFS, event-free survival; MTD, maximum tolerated dose; ORR, overall response rate; OS, overall survival; PFS, progression-free survival; PTCL, peripheral T-cell lymphoma; VEGF, vascular endothelial growth factor.

Data from https://clinicaltrials.gov. Accessed November 13, 2016.

SUMMARY

AITL is a T_{FH}-derived neoplasm, sharing many features with a proportion of PTCL-NOS. It displays a peculiar morphologic appearance and is biologically complex. Several new mutations have been recently described, which are now elucidating the possible underlying pathogenetic mechanisms and may hopefully suggest innovative treatment targets. Given the aggressiveness of the disease and the poor outcomes with anthracycline-containing induction regimens, autoSCT in first remission should be offered whenever possible. Relapsed patients and refractory cases should be enrolled in clinical trials, as newer approaches and novel drugs are urgently required in this context. Newly approved agents seem active in pretreated patients, although response durations are short. Innovative induction strategies, made up of a standard CHOP (or CHOEP) regimen combined with a biologic agent should be designed to enhance the rate of CRs, to increase the number of patients that can benefit from autoSCT and to prolong survival.

REFERENCES

1. Frizzera G, Moran EM, Rappaport H. Angioimmunoblastic lymphadenopathy with dysproteinaemia. Lancet 1974;1:1070–3.
2. Lukes RJ, Tindle BH. Immunoblastic lymphadenopathy. A hyperimmune entity resembling Hodgkin's disease. N Engl J Med 1975;292:1–8.
3. Nathwani BN, Rappaport H, Moran EM, et al. Malignant lymphoma arising in angioimmunoblastic lymphadenopathy. Cancer 1978;41:578–606.
4. Harris NL, Jaffe ES, Stein H, et al. A revised European-American classification of lymphoid neoplasms: a proposal from the International Lymphoma Study Group. Blood 1994;84:1361–92.
5. Swerdlow SH, Campo E, Pileri SA, et al. The 2016 revision of the World Health Organization classification of lymphoid neoplasms. Blood 2016;127:2375–90.
6. Vose J, Armitage J, Weisenburger D. International T-Cell Lymphoma Project. International peripheral T-cell and natural killer/T-cell lymphoma study: pathology findings and clinical outcomes. J Clin Oncol 2008;26:4124–30.
7. Federico M, Rudiger T, Bellei M, et al. Clinicopathologic characteristics of angioimmunoblastic T-cell lymphoma: analysis of the International Peripheral T-cell lymphoma project. J Clin Oncol 2012;31:240–6.
8. de Leval M, Parrens M, Le Bras F, et al. Angioimmunoblastic T-cell lymphoma is the most common T-cell lymphoma in two distinct French information data sets. Haematologica 2015;100:e361–4.
9. Dogan A, Gaulard P, Jaffe ES, et al. Angioimmunoblastic T-cell lymphoma. In: Swerdlow SH, Campo E, Harris NL, et al, editors. World Health Organization classification of tumors of haematopoietic and lymphoid tissues. 4th edition. Lyon (France): IARC Press; 2008. p. 309–11.
10. de Leval M, Rickman DS, Thielen C, et al. The gene expression profile of nodal peripheral T-cell lymphoma demonstrates a molecular link between angioimmunoblastic T-cell lymphoma (AITL) and follicular helper T (T_{FH}) cells. Blood 2007;109:4952–63.
11. Dupuis J, Boye K, Martin N, et al. Expression of CXCL13 by neoplastic cells in angioimmunoblastic T-cell lymphoma (AITL). Am J Surg Pathol 2006;30:490–4.
12. Piccaluga PP, Agostinelli C, Califano A, et al. Gene expression analysis of angioimmunoblastic lymphoma indicates derivation from T follicular helper cells and vascular endothelial growth factor deregulation. Cancer Res 2007;67:10703–10.
13. Laurent C, Fazilleau N, Brousset P. A novel subset of T-helper cells : follicular T-helper cells and their markers. Haematologica 2010;95:356–8.

14. Agostinelli C, Hartmann S, Klapper W, et al. Peripheral T cell lymphomas with follicular T helper phenotype: a new basket or a distinct entity? Revising Karl Lennert's personal archive. Histopathology 2011;59:679–91.

15. Pileri SA. Follicular helper T cell-related lymphomas. Blood 2015;8:1733–4.

16. Iqbal J, Wilcox R, Naushad H, et al. Genomic signatures in T-cell lymphoma: how can these improve precision in diagnosis and inform prognosis? Blood Rev 2016; 30:89–100.

17. Lemonnier F, Couronné L, Parrens M, et al. Recurrent TET2 mutations in peripheral T-cell lymphomas correlate with TFH-like features and adverse clinical parameters. Blood 2012;120:1466–9.

18. Couronné L, Bastard C, Bernard OA. TET2 and DNMT3A mutations in human T-cell lymphoma. N Engl J Med 2012;366:95–6.

19. Cairns RA, Iqbal J, Lemonnier F, et al. IDH2 mutations are frequent in angioimmunoblastic T-cell lymphoma. Blood 2012;119:1901–3.

20. Palomero T, Couronné L, Khiabanian H, et al. Recurrent mutations in epigenetic regulators, RHOA and FYN kinase in peripheral T cell lymphomas. Nat Genet 2014;46:166–70.

21. Odejide O, weigert O, Lane AA, et al. A targeted mutational landscape of angioimmunoblastic T-cell lymphoma. Blood 2014;123:1293–6.

22. Wang C, McKeithan TW, Gong Q, et al. IDH2^{R172} mutations define a unique subgroup of patients with angioimmunoblastic T-cell lymphoma. Blood 2015;126: 1741–52.

23. Sakata-Yanagimoto M, Enami T, Yoshida K, et al. Somatic RHOA mutation in angioimmunoblastic T cell lymphoma. Nat Genet 2014;46:171–5.

24. Vallois D, Dobay MPD, Morin RD, et al. Activating mutations in genes related to TCR signalling in angioimmunoblastic and other follicular helper T-cell-derived lymphomas. Blood 2016;128:1490–502.

25. Zinzani PL, Broccoli A. T-cell lymphoproliferative disorders. In: Hoffbrand V, Higgs DR, Keeling DM, et al, editors. Postgraduate hematology. 7th edition. Hoboken (NJ): Wiley Blackwell; 2016. p. 524–36.

26. Botros N, Cerroni L, Shawwa A, et al. Cutaneous manifestations of angioimmunoblastic T-cell lymphoma: clinical and pathological characteristics. Am J Dermatopathol 2015;37:274–83.

27. Mourad N, Mounier N, Brière J, et al. Clinical, biologic, and pathologic features in 157 patients with angioimmunoblastic T-cell lymphoma treated within the Groupe d'Etude des Lymphomes de l'Adulte (GELA) trials. Blood 2008;111:4463–70.

28. Casulo C, Schöder H, Feeney J, et al. ^{18}F-fluorodeoxyglucose positron emission tomography in the staging and prognosis of T cell lymphoma. Leuk Lymphoma 2013;54:2163–7.

29. El-Galaly TC, Pedersen MB, Hutchings M, et al. Utility of interim and end-of-treatment PET/CT in peripheral T-cell lymphomas: a review of 124 patients. Am J Hematol 2015;90:975–80.

30. Tomita N, Hattori Y, Fujisawa S, et al. Post-therapy ^{18}F-fluorodeoxyglucose positron emission tomography for predicting outcome in patients with peripheral T cell lymphoma. Ann Hematol 2015;94:4316.

31. Tokunaga T, Shimada K, Yamamoto K, et al. Retrospective analysis of prognostic factors for angioimmunoblastic T-cell lymphoma: a multicentre cooperative study in Japan. Blood 2012;119:2837–43.

32. Reimer P, Rüdiger T, Geissinger E, et al. Autologous stem-cell transplantation as first-line therapy in peripheral T-cell lymphomas: results of a prospective multicentre study. J Clin Oncol 2009;27:106–13.

33. Wilhelm M, Smetak M, Reimer P, et al. First-line therapy of peripheral T-cell lymphoma: extension and long-term follow-up of a study investigating the role of autologous stem cell transplantation. Blood Cancer J 2016;6:e452.
34. d'Amore F, Relander T, Lauritzsen GF, et al. Up-front autologous stem-cell transplantation in peripheral T-cell lymphoma: NLG-T-01. J Clin Oncol 2012;30:3093–9.
35. Schetelig J, Fetscher S, Reichle A, et al. Long-term disease-free survival in patients with angioimmunoblastic T-cell lymphoma after high-dose chemotherapy and autologous stem cell transplantation. Haematologica 2003;88:1272–8.
36. Rodríguez J, Conde E, Gutiérrez A, et al. Prolonged survival of patients with angioimmunoblastic T-cell lymphoma after high-dose chemotherapy and autologous stem cell transplantation. The GELTAMO experience. Eur J Haematol 2007;78:290–6.
37. Kyriakou C, Canals C, Goldstone A, et al. High-dose therapy and autologous stem-cell transplantation in angioimmunoblastic lymphoma: complete remission at transplantation is the major determinant of outcome-lymphoma working party of the European Group for Blood and Marrow Transplantation. J Clin Oncol 2008;26:218–24.
38. Abramson JS, Feldman T, Kroll-Desrosiers AR, et al. Peripheral T-cell lymphomas in a large US multicentre cohort: prognostication in the modern era including impact of frontline therapy. Ann Oncol 2014;25:2211–7.
39. Briski R, Feldman AL, Bailey NG, et al. The role of front-line anthracycline-containing chemotherapy regimens in peripheral T-cell lymphomas. Blood Cancer J 2014;4:e214.
40. Schmitz N, Trümper L, Ziepert M, et al. Treatment and prognosis of mature T-cell and NK-cell lymphoma: an analysis of patients with T-cell lymphoma treated in studies of the German High-Grade Non-Hodgkin Lymphoma Study Group. Blood 2010;116:3418–25.
41. Simon A, Peoch M, Casassus P, et al. Upfront VIP-reinforced-ABVD (VIP-rABVD) is not superior to CHOP/21 in newly diagnosed peripheral T cell lymphoma. Results of the randomized phase III trial GOELAMS-LTP95. Br J Haematol 2010;151:159–66.
42. Advani RH, Horwitz S, Zelenetz A, et al. Angioimmunoblastic T cell lymphoma: treatment experience with cyclosporine. Leuk Lymphoma 2007;48:521–5.
43. Mak V, Hamm J, Chhanabhai M, et al. Survival of patients with peripheral T-cell lymphoma after first relapse or progression: spectrum of disease and rare long-term survivors. J Clin Oncol 2013;31:1970–6.
44. O'Connor OA, Pro B, Pinter-Brown L, et al. Pralatrexate in patients with relapsed or refractory peripheral T-cell lymphoma: results from the pivotal PROPEL study. J Clin Oncol 2011;29:1182–9.
45. Coiffier B, Pro B, Prince HM, et al. Results from a pivotal, open-label, phase II study of romidepsin in relapsed or refractory peripheral T-cell lymphoma after prior systemic therapy. J Clin Oncol 2012;30:631–6.
46. O'Connor OA, Horwitz S, Masszi T, et al. Belinostat in patients with relapsed or refractory peripheral T-cell lymphoma: results of the pivotal phase II BELIEF (CLN-19) study. J Clin Oncol 2015;33:2492–9.
47. Pro B, Horwitz SM, Prince HM, et al. Romidepsin induces durable responses in patients with relapsed or refractory angioimmunoblastic T-cell lymphoma. Hematol Oncol 2016. [Epub ahead of print].
48. Pro B, Advani R, Brice P, et al. Brentuximab vedotin (SGN-35) in patients with relapsed or refractory systemic anaplastic large-cell lymphoma: results of a phase II study. J Clin Oncol 2012;30:2190–6.

49. Horwitz S, Advani RH, Bartlett NL, et al. Objective responses in relapsed T-cell lymphomas with single-agent brentuximab vedotin. Blood 2014;123:3095–100.

50. Morschhauser F, Fitoussi O, Haioun C, et al. A phase 2, multicentre, single-arm, open-label study to evaluate the safety and efficacy of single-agent lenalidomide (Revlimid®) in subjects with relapsed or refractory peripheral T-cell non-Hodgkin lymphoma: the EXPECT trial. Eur J Cancer 2013;49:2869–76.

51. Toumishey E, Prasad A, Dueck G, et al. Final report of a phase 2 clinical trial of lenalidomide monotherapy for patients with T-cell lymphoma. Cancer 2015;121: 716–23.

52. Barr PM, Li H, Spier C, et al. Phase II intergroup trial of alisertib in relapsed and refractory peripheral T-cell lymphoma and transformed mycosis fungoides: SWOG 1108. J Clin Oncol 2015;33:2399–404.

53. Ogura M, Ishida T, Hatake K, et al. Multicenter phase II study of mogamulizumab (KW-0761), a defucosylated anti-CC chemokine receptor 4 antibody, in patients with relapsed peripheral T-cell lymphoma and cutaneous T-cell lymphoma. J Clin Oncol 2014;32:1157–63.

54. O'Connor OA, Özcan M, Jacobsen ED, et al. First multicentre, randomized phase 3 study in patients (pts) with relapsed/refractory (R/R) peripheral T-cell lymphoma (PTCL): alisertib (MLN8237) versus investigator's choice (Lumiere trial; NCT01482962). In: 57th ASH annual meeting abstracts. Orlando, December 5–8, 2015. [abstract: 341].

55. Le Gouill S, Milpied N, Buzyn A, et al. Graft-versus-lymphoma effect for aggressive T-cell lymphoma in adults: a study by the Société Française de Greffe de Moëlle et de Thérapie Cellulaire. J Clin Oncol 2008;26:2264–71.

56. Kyriakou C, Canals C, Finke J, et al. Allogeneic stem cell transplantation is able to induce long-term remissions in angioimmunoblastic T-cell lymphoma: a retrospective study from the Lymphoma Working Party of the European Group for Blood and Marrow Transplantation. J Clin Oncol 2009;27:3951–8.

57. Delfau-Larue MH, de Leval L, Joly B, et al. Targeting intratumoral B cells with rituximab in addition to CHOP in angioimmunoblastic T-cell lymphoma. A clinicobiological study of the GELA. Haematologica 2012;97:1594–602.

58. Ganjoo K, Hong F, Horning SJ, et al. Bevacizumab and cyclosphosphamide, doxorubicin, vincristine and prednisone in combination for patientswith peripheral T-cell or natural killer cell neoplasms: an Eastern Cooperative Oncology Group study (E2404). Leuk Lymphoma 2014;55:768–72.

59. Johnston PB, Cashen AF, Nikolinakos PG, et al. Safe and effective treatment of patients with peripheral T-cell lymphoma (PTCL) with the novel HDAC inhibitor, belinostat, in combination with CHOP: results of the Bel-CHOP phase 1 trial. In: 57th ASH annual meeting abstracts. Orlando, December 5–8, 2015. [abstract: 253].

60. Kluin-Nelemans HC, van Marwijk Kooy M, Lugtenburg PJ, et al. Intensified alemtuzumab-CHOP therapy for peripheral T-cell lymphoma. Ann Oncol 2011; 22:1595–600.

61. d'Amore F, Leppä S, Gomes da Silva M, et al. First interim efficacy and safety analysis of an international phase III randomized trial in newly diagnosed systemic peripheral T-cell lymphoma treated with chemotherapy with or without alemtuzumab and consolidated with high dose therapy. In: 54th ASH annual meeting abstracts. Atlanta, December 8–11, 2012. [abstract: 57].

62. Trumper LH, Wulf G, Ziepert M, et al. Alemtuzumab added to CHOP for treatment of peripheral T-cell lymphoma (pTNHL) of the elderly: final results of 116 patients treated in the international ACT-2 phase 3 trial. In: 2016 ASCO annual meeting. Chicago, June 3–7, 2016. [abstract: 7500].

Clinical Features and Current Optimal Management of Natural Killer/T-Cell Lymphoma

 CrossMark

Shinichi Makita, MD, PhD*, Kensei Tobinai, MD, PhD

KEYWORDS

- Lymphoma • Extranodal NK/T-cell lymphoma • ENKL • CCRT • DeVIC • SMILE
- EBV

KEY POINTS

- Extranodal NK/T-cell lymphoma, nasal type (ENKL) is a predominantly extranodal lymphoma and is associated with Epstein-Barr virus.
- ENKL is a rare subtype of lymphoma (<1% of all NHL) with poor treatment outcome.
- Concurrent chemoradiotherapy containing MDR-nonrelated agents is recommended as an initial therapy in patients with newly diagnosed localized nasal ENKL.
- L-Asparaginase-containing regimen (eg, SMILE, AspaMetDex) is recommended as an induction therapy in patients with advanced or relapsed/refractory disease.

INTRODUCTION

Natural killer (NK)/T-cell lymphoma is formally named as extranodal NK/T-cell lymphoma, nasal type (ENKL) in the World Health Organization (WHO) classification 2008.[1] ENKL is a predominantly extranodal lymphoma associated with Epstein-Barr virus (EBV). It is a rare subtype of non-Hodgkin lymphoma (NHL), and its incidence is less than 1% of all NHL in Western countries,[2,3] whereas it is 3% to 9% in Asian countries.[4–6] Therefore, several prospective clinical trials of ENKL have been conducted mainly in Asian countries. The successful results of these clinical trials have completely changed the management of ENKL.

This article describes the general features of ENKL, and then discusses current optimal management of ENKL based on the obtained results from recent clinical trials.

Disclosure Statement: The authors have nothing to disclose.
Department of Hematology, National Cancer Center Hospital, 5-1-1 Tsukiji, Chuo-ku, Tokyo 104-0045, Japan
* Corresponding author.
E-mail address: smakita@ncc.go.jp

Hematol Oncol Clin N Am 31 (2017) 239–253
http://dx.doi.org/10.1016/j.hoc.2016.11.007
0889-8588/17/© 2016 Elsevier Inc. All rights reserved.

hemonc.theclinics.com

CLINICAL CHARACTERISTICS

Median age at diagnosis of ENKL ranges from 46 to 52 years.[7–10] As its name suggests, the most frequently involved site at presentation is the nasal cavity. Nasal obstruction, nasal discharge, and epistaxis caused by nasal mass lesions are common initial symptoms.[1]

Although 75% of patients have localized disease at initial presentation, the disease disseminates rapidly to various sites, such as the skin, gastrointestinal tract, testis, and lymph nodes during its clinical course.

Approximately 40% of patients have B symptoms, which is a higher incidence than other aggressive lymphomas.[9,10] Also of note, ENKL is one of the common causes of hemophagocytic syndrome, which is associated with poor outcome and a high mortality rate.[11]

PATHOLOGIC FINDINGS

A diffuse growth pattern of atypical lymphocytes, which are medium-sized cells or a mixture of medium and large cells, is observed. Necrosis and an angiocentric growth pattern or an angiodestructive growth pattern is frequently present. In some cases, florid pseudoepitheliomatous hyperplasia is observed. Because the hyperplasia closely resembles squamous cell carcinoma, squamous cell carcinoma is one of the differential diagnoses, although it is a nonhematopoietic tumor.

Immunohistochemically, the lymphoma cells are positive for cytoplasmic CD3, CD56, and cytotoxic molecules, such as granzyme B, TIA1, and perforin. When CD56, a representative NK-cell marker, is negative, both a positive EBV status and the expression of cytotoxic molecules are required for diagnosis of ENKL.

To make a definite diagnosis of ENKL, clear evidence of positive EBV status is important. EBV-encoded small RNA1 in situ hybridization (EBER1 ISH) is the most reliable and widely used method to confirm the infected EBV in tumor cells. Lymphoma cells are diffusely and strongly positive for EBER1 ISH. If EBV is negative in tumor cells, a diagnosis of ENKL should be reconsidered (**Fig. 1**).

PROGNOSTIC FACTORS
Natural Killer/T-cell Lymphoma Prognostic Index

Because the clinical significance of the International Prognostic Index is low in patients with ENKL, a Korean group proposed an original prognostic scoring system, the NK/T-cell Lymphoma Prognostic Index (NK-PI), in 2006.[7] The NK-PI was developed based on data from a retrospective study of 262 patients with ENKL treated with CHOP (cyclophosphamide, doxorubicin, vincristine, and prednisone)-like regimens and/or radiotherapy (RT). Four independent factors associated with overall survival (OS) were identified: (1) presence of B symptoms, (2) advanced stage, (3) elevated serum lactate dehydrogenase level, and (4) lymph node involvement. However, the NK-PI might not be relevant for patients receiving non-anthracycline-containing chemotherapy.

Prognostic Index for Natural Killer–Cell Lymphoma

To establish a novel prognostic model based on the therapeutic results of patients treated with non-anthracycline-containing chemotherapy, Kim and colleagues[12] conducted an international retrospective study. Based on the multivariate analyses of 527 patients with newly diagnosed ENKL, the Prognostic Index for NK-cell lymphoma was established. The investigators identified four independent prognostic factors: (1) age greater than 60 years, (2) stage III/IV, (3) distant lymph node involvement, and

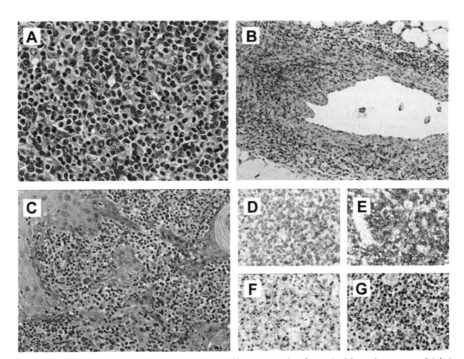

Fig. 1. Histologic features of ENKL. (*A*) The diffuse growth of atypical lymphocytes, which is a mixture of medium and large cells, is observed (hematoxylin and eosin [H&E], original magnification ×400). (*B*) Angiocentric growth patterns are frequently observed (H&E, original magnification ×100). (*C*) In some cases, florid pseudoepitheliomatous hyperplasia is observed (H&E, original magnification ×200). Immunohistochemically, the lymphoma cells are positive for cytoplasmic CD3 (*D*, original magnification ×400), CD56 (*E*, original magnification ×400), and granzyme B (*F*, original magnification ×400). EBV-encoded small RNA1 in situ hybridization demonstrates positive nuclei in lymphoma cells (*G*, original magnification ×400). (*Courtesy of* Dr Akiko M. Maeshima, Department of Pathology, National Cancer Center Hospital, Tokyo, Japan.)

(4) nonnasal-type disease. According to the number of corresponding risk factors, patients are categorized into low-risk (no risk factor), intermediate-risk (one risk factor), or high-risk (two or more risk factors) groups. The 3-year OS rate of each risk group was 81%, 62%, and 25%, respectively.

Quantitative Polymerase Chain Reaction of Epstein-Barr Virus DNA

Because ENKL is associated with EBV infection, EBV-DNA can be detected in the peripheral blood by polymerase chain reaction (PCR) and has been shown to be useful for quantification of tumor burden. Some studies have reported the prognostic implication of the circulating EBV-DNA level in ENKL.[13,14]

The NK-cell Tumor Study Group analyzed 33 patients with ENKL prospectively, and showed pretreatment high plasma EBV-DNA level (>1000 copies/mL) is associated with significantly lower OS.[14] The international study conducted by Kim and colleagues[12] also showed that a detectable viral DNA titer is an independent prognostic factor, but the impact of quantitative PCR was not assessed because the method was not validated in the study. Further accumulation of data is needed.

Soluble Interleukin-2 Receptor

The serum level of soluble interleukin-2 receptor (sIL-2R) is known to reflect the tumor volume or activity in aggressive NHL.[15] Yamaguchi and colleagues retrospectively analyzed the outcomes of 146 patients with localized nasal ENKL who were treated with concurrent RT and dexamethasone, etoposide, ifosfamide, and carboplatin (DeVIC). In this study, a pretreatment sIL-2R greater than the upper limit of normal was an independent risk factor for worse OS and progression-free survival (PFS).[16]

sIL-2R might be a useful prognostic factor in our practice because measurement of serum sIL-2R is easier and cheaper than other techniques, such as quantitative PCR of EBV-DNA.

STAGING

The clinical stage of ENKL is determined mainly according to the Ann Arbor classification or the Lugano classification.[17] However, the staging of nasal ENKL is often problematic. For example, the primary-nasal mass lesion with involvement extending to paranasal sinus, nasopharynx, and orbit is defined as stage IV according to the Ann Arbor classification, whereas such a contiguous involvement is conventionally considered to be stage IE in ENKL.

Typically stage IIE nasal ENKL is considered to be the primary site with cervical lymph node involvement. Stage IIE disease with axillary lymph nodes or mediastinal lesions is treated as advanced disease.

The staging procedures of ENKL are similar to those of other NHLs. Thus, a whole-body contrast-enhanced computed tomography scan is essential. To evaluate local invasion around the nasal cavity, MRI is thought to be more useful than a computed tomography scan alone. ENKL is an ^{18}F-fluorodeoxyglucose-avid tumor, as with other aggressive NHLs.[18] Therefore, ^{18}F-fluorodeoxyglucose PET is a useful device to evaluate the tumor distribution (**Box 1**).

Bone marrow biopsy or aspiration should also be performed. To evaluate the bone marrow involvement precisely, EBER1 ISH of bone marrow clot sections or biopsy is recommended.[19,20]

TREATMENT OF LOCALIZED EXTRANODAL NATURAL KILLER/T-CELL LYMPHOMA, NASAL TYPE
Background

The results of retrospective studies in patients with localized ENKL are summarized in **Table 1**.[21–31] The outcomes of CHOP or CHOP-like chemotherapy alone were poor; the complete remission (CR) rates were 25% to 50% and the 5-year OS rates were

---

Box 1
Required tests for the staging and initial evaluation of ENKL

- Whole-body computed tomography
- MRI including primary nasal disease
- ^{18}F-Fluorodeoxyglucose PET scan
- Bone marrow aspiration or biopsy (EBER1 ISH is recommended)
- Quantitative PCR of plasma or blood EBV-DNA level (if possible)

Table 1					
Reports of retrospective studies on localized ENKL					
Authors, Year	**Stage**	**No. of Patients**	**Treatment**	**CR Rate (%)**	**5-year OS Rate (%)**
Kim et al,[21] 2000	I-II	92	RT	66	40
Li et al,[22] 2004	I-II	11	RT	55	50
Huang et al,[23] 2008	I-II	9	RT	100	56
Yang et al,[24] 2015	I-II	253	RT	82	70
	I[a]	90	RT	NA	89
Li et al,[22] 2004	I-II	18	Cx	50	15
You et al,[25] 2004	I-II	22	Cx	NA	23
Huang et al,[23] 2008	I-II	8	Cx	25	0
Yang et al,[24] 2015	I-II	131	Cx	25	34
Kwong et al,[26] 1997	I	18	Cx → RT	—	28
Ribrag et al,[27] 2001	I-II	12	Cx → RT	—	<50
Yamaguchi et al,[28] 2001	I-II	7	Cx → RT	—	14
Cheung et al,[29] 2002	I-II	61	Cx → RT	—	40
You et al,[25] 2004	I-II	18	Cx → RT	—	38
Huang et al,[23] 2008	I-II	43	Cx → RT	—	48
Yang et al,[24] 2015	I[b]-II	509	Cx → RT	—	58
Nakamura et al,[30] 1997	I-II	11	RT → Cx	—	45
Avilés et al,[31] 2000	I-II	57	RT → Cx	—	87[c]
Ribrag et al,[27] 2001	I-II	8	RT → Cx	—	100
Huang et al,[23] 2008	I-II	31	RT → Cx	—	68
Yang et al,[24] 2015	I[b]-II	155	RT → Cx	—	72

Abbreviations: CR, complete remission; Cx, CHOP or CHOP-like chemotherapy; Cx → RT, frontline Cx followed by RT; LDH, lactate dehydrogenase; PS, performance status; RT → Cx, frontline RT followed by Cx or concurrent use of RT and Cx.
  [a] Clinical stage I without any risk factors: age greater than 60, PS 2 to 4, or elevated LDH.
  [b] Clinical stage I with 1 or more risk factors.
  [c] 8-year OS.

0% to 34%.[22–25] ENKL cells express P-glycoprotein derived from the multidrug resistance 1 (MDR1) gene.[32–34] This is thought to be one reason why CHOP or CHOP-like regimens are inadequate against ENKL, because P-glycoprotein acts as an efflux pump of various drugs including doxorubicin and vincristine.

However, RT is one of the most reliable treatment methods of localized ENKL; the CR rates of RT alone were 66% to 100% and the 5-year OS rates were 40% to 70%.[21–24] However, the high rates of relapse remain a problem.

Therefore, a combined modality treatment has been validated. Although anthracycline-containing chemotherapy followed by irradiation has been established as the standard of care for localized aggressive B-cell NHLs, the same therapeutic strategy was ineffective against localized ENKL: 5-year OS rates were 14% to 58%.[23–29] These poor outcomes are caused by an insufficient response to frontline chemotherapy. Frontline RT followed by chemotherapy or concurrent chemoradiotherapy (CCRT) is more effective compared with frontline chemotherapy alone: 5-year OS rates were 45% to 100%.[23,24,27,30,31] The efficacy of various chemotherapy regimens is discussed in the following sections.

Prospective Trials of Localized Extranodal Natural Killer/T-Cell Lymphoma, Nasal Type

JCOG0211 study

To explore a more effective treatment of localized nasal ENKL, the Lymphoma Study Group of the Japan Clinical Oncology Group (JCOG-LSG) conducted a phase I/II study of novel CCRT for newly diagnosed localized nasal ENKL (JCOG0211 study).[35,36]

In this study, patients with stage IE disease or contiguous stage IIE disease with cervical lymph node involvement were eligible. The protocol treatment consisted of concurrently used RT (50–50.4 Gy) and three cycles of DeVIC (**Fig. 2**). DeVIC was originally designed as salvage chemotherapy for aggressive NHLs.[37] Because the regimen is comprised of MDR-nonrelated agents (ifosfamide and carboplatin) and etoposide, which is known to be effective against EBV-associated diseases,[38] DeVIC was expected to be effective against ENKL.

In phase I, the safety of two dose-levels (full dose and two-third dose) of DeVIC was evaluated with the concurrent use of irradiation. Three patients that received two-third doses of DeVIC (2/3DeVIC) did not develop dose-limiting toxicities, whereas four of six patients that received full dose developed dose-limiting toxicities, such as prolonged myelosuppression and grade 3 infection. Therefore, 2/3DeVIC was selected as the recommended dose for use in phase II. In total, 27 patients were treated with RT-2/3DeVIC and the efficacy was assessed in 26 patients: CR rate was 77% and the ORR (overall response rate) was 81%. One patient was not evaluable for response because the target lesion was taken by biopsy. Survival was evaluable in all 27 patients: 5-year OS rate was 70% and the PFS rate was 63% with a median follow-up duration of 67 months. Seventy percent of the patients that achieved CRs had long-term durable remission without any consolidative therapy, such as autologous stem cell transplantation (SCT). No treatment-related death (TRD) was observed. Among these 27 patients, the most common grade 3 nonhematologic toxicity was mucositis related to irradiation (30%), but it was transient and manageable in most patients.

Furthermore, Yamaguchi and colleagues[16] reported the retrospective treatment outcomes of 149 patients with localized nasal ENKL who were treated with RT-DeVIC in a clinical practice setting. With a median follow-up of 4.9 years, the 5-year OS and PFS

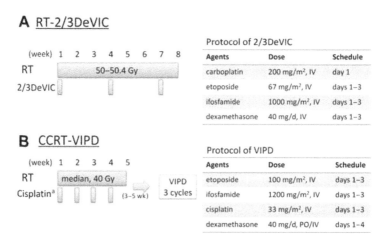

Fig. 2. Treatment protocols of RT-2/3DeVIC (*A*) and CCRT-VIPD (*B*). [a] Weekly infusion of cisplatin (30 mg/m^2, Days 1, 8, 15, and 22). IV, intravenous infusion; PO, oral administration; VIPD, etoposide, ifosfamide, cisplatin, and dexamethasone.

rates of the 149 patients were 71% and 60%, respectively. These results validate the efficacy of RT-DeVIC in a large number of patients with long-term follow-up.

Clinical trials conducted by Korean group

In addition to the JCOG0211 study, several prospective trials to assess CCRT have been conducted in East Asia (summarized in **Table 2**).[39–43] A Korean group (Consortium for Improving Survival of Lymphoma) reported the promising results of a phase II study that assessed the efficacy of weekly cisplatin concurrently used with RT (median dose, 40 Gy) followed by three cycles of VIPD (etoposide, ifosfamide, cisplatin, and dexamethasone) for localized nasal ENKL (see **Fig. 2**).[39] In the 30 evaluable patients, CR rate was 80% and the estimated 3-year OS and PFS rates were 86% and 85%, respectively. As for grade 3/4 toxicities, one patient experienced grade 3 nausea during the CCRT phase, and 12 of 29 patients experienced grade 4 neutropenia in the VIPD phase. Two TRDs caused by infection were observed during the VIPD phase.

Consortium for Improving Survival of Lymphoma subsequently conducted a phase II study of CCRT with weekly cisplatin followed by two cycles of VIDL (etoposide, ifosfamide, dexamethasone, and L-asparaginase).[40] VIDL is similar to the VIPD therapy, but uses L-asparaginase instead of cisplatin. L-Asparaginase is known to be a key agent for ENKL and several reports have indicated its efficacy against advanced or relapsed/refractory ENKL as a single agent or in combination with other agents.[44,45] In the 30 evaluable patients, CCRT-VIDL demonstrated a CR rate of 90%. The estimated 5-year OS and PFS rates were 60% and 73%, respectively, with a median follow-up duration of 44 months.

Clinical trials conducted by Chinese study groups

Recently, Chinese groups also have reported the results of several phase II studies to evaluate their original regimens, such as LVP (L-asparaginase, vincristine, and prednisolone) or GELOX (gemcitabine, etoposide, L-asparaginase, and oxaliplatin) with "sandwiched" RT.[42,43] However, the long-term efficacy of these strategies remains unclear.

Recommended Management for Localized Extranodal Natural Killer/T-Cell Lymphoma, Nasal Type

Based on the results obtained from prospective clinical trials, CCRT containing MDR-nonrelated agents is thought to be the most suitable standard of care for patients with localized nasal ENKL. Although the most suitable chemotherapeutic regimen in the CCRT is unclear, the Japanese Society of Hematology recommends RT-2/3DeVIC in its clinical practice guideline, not only because it is based on the results of a Japanese clinical trial, but also because (1) mature long-term follow-up data are available, (2) time to completion of the treatment is shorter than for other regimens (eg, 9 weeks in RT-2/3DeVIC vs 16–18 weeks in CCRT-VIPD), and (3) short-term and long-term toxicities are manageable.

TREATMENT OF NEWLY DIAGNOSED ADVANCED OR NONNASAL EXTRANODAL NATURAL KILLER/T-CELL LYMPHOMA AND RELAPSED/REFRACTORY EXTRANODAL NATURAL KILLER/T-CELL LYMPHOMA, NASAL TYPE

Background

Patients with newly diagnosed advanced or nonnasal ENKL have shown poor outcomes in the past; the 1-year OS rate of patients treated with anthracycline-containing regimens was less than 20%.[10] This is also the case in relapsed/refractory patients.

Table 2
Selected prospective clinical trials on ENKL

Disease	Study Group	Treatment	Study Design	No of Patients	CR Rate (%)	OS (%)	PFS (%)	Median Follow-Up Duration (mo)
Localized nasal disease	JCOG-LSG	RT + 2/3DeVIC	Phase I/II	27	77	70 (5-y)	63 (5-y)	67
	CISL	CCRT-VIPD	Phase II	30	80	86 (3-y)	85 (3-y)	24
	CISL	CCRT-VIDL	Phase II	30	87	60 (5-y)	73 (5-y)	44
	Ma et al.	CEOP → RT vs	Randomized phase II	38	21	73 (2-y)	66 (2-y)	30
		CEOP + S → RT		37	27	62 (2-y)	62 (2-y)	
	Jiang et al.	LVP → RT → LVP		26	81	89 (2-y)	81 (2-y)	27
	Wang et al.	GELOX → RT → GELOX	Phase II	27	74	86 (2-y)	86 (2-y)	27
Advanced disease or R/R	Yamaguchi et al.	SMILE	Phase II	38	45	55 (1-y) 47 (5-y)	53 (1-y) 39 (5-y)	24 74
R/R	GELA/GOELAMS	AspaMetDex	Phase II	18	61	40 (2-y)	40 (2-y)	24

Abbreviations: AspaMetDex, L-astaraginase, methotrexate, and dexamethasone; CEOP, cyclophosphamide, epirubicin, vincristine, and prednisolone; CISL, Consortium for Improving Survival of Lymphoma; GELA, Groupe d'Etude des Lymphomes de l'Adulte; GELOX, gemcitabine, oxaliplatin, and L-asparaginase; GOELAMS, Groupe Ouest-Est d'études des Leucémies Aigües et autres Maladies du Sang; LVP, L-asparaginase, vincristine, and prednisolone; R/R relapsed or refractory; S, semustine; SMILE, dexamethasone, methotrexate, ifosfamide, L-asparaginase, and etoposide; VIDL, etoposide, ifosfamide, dexamethasone, and L-asparaginase; VIPD, etoposide, ifosfamide, cisplatin, and dexamethasone.

Several retrospective studies have reported the efficacy of L-asparaginase-containing regimens,[44,45] whereas the number of prospective clinical trials of L-asparaginase-containing regimens has been limited (see **Table 2**).

SMILE Therapy

To overcome the poor outcomes in advanced and relapsed/refractory ENKL, NK-cell Tumor Study Group of Japan and colleagues in East Asia designed a novel regimen, named SMILE (dexamethasone, methotrexate, ifosfamide, L-asparaginase, and etoposide) in 2004 (**Table 3**). Subsequent to a dose-finding phase I study,[46] a phase II study of SMILE therapy in patients with newly diagnosed stage IV or relapsed/refractory ENKL was conducted.[47] Thirty-eight eligible patients were treated with two cycles of SMILE, accompanied by the physician's choice of additional SMILE and/or autologous/allogeneic SCT.

Because the initial two patients died of grade 5 infections, the protocol was revised to include more careful assessment of infection and to incorporate a lymphocyte count of 500/μL or more into the eligibility criteria. There were no subsequent TRDs. The most common toxicity was grade 4 neutropenia, which was observed in 92% of treated patients despite prophylactic granulocyte colony–stimulating factor use. The most common grade 3 or 4 nonhematologic toxicity was infection (61%).

The ORR in the 38 eligible patients was 79% and the CR rate was 45%. According to the long-term follow-up data presented at the 13th International Conference on Malignant Lymphoma, the 5-year OS and PFS rates were 47% and 39%, respectively, with a median follow-up duration of 74 months.[48] These results indicate the high efficacy of SMILE in this unfavorable population, and this regimen is now widely used in clinical practice. However, careful monitoring for myelosuppression and infection is essential when using this regimen. Prophylactic antibiotics, such as fluoroquinolones, are acceptable, but physical examination and frequent laboratory testing might be more important for the early diagnosis and treatment of infection.

AspaMetDex Therapy

A French group (Groupe d'Etude des Lymphomes de l'Adulte/Groupe Ouest-Est d'études des Leucémies Aigües et Autres Maladies du Sang) also reported the promising results of their multicenter phase II study examining another L-asparaginase-containing regimen that used L-asparaginase, methotrexate, and dexamethasone

Table 3
Treatment protocols of SMILE therapy and AspaMetDex therapy

Regimen		Protocol			Reference
SMILE	Dexamethasone	40 mg/d	IV or orally	Days 2–4	Yamaguchi et al,[46] 2008; Yamaguchi et al,[47] 2011; Suzuki et al,[48] 2015
	Methotrexate	2000 mg/m^2	IV	Day 1	
	Ifosfamide	1500 mg/m^2	IV	Days 2–4	
	L-Asparaginase	6000 U/m^2	IV	Days 8, 10, 12, 14, 16, 18, and 20	
	Etoposide	100 mg/m^2	IV	Days 2–4	
AspaMetDex	L-Asparaginase	6000 U/m^2	IM	Days 2, 4, 6, and 8	Jaccard et al,[49] 2011
	Methotrexate	3000 mg/m^2	IV	Day 1	
	Dexamethasone	40 mg/d	orally	Days 1–4	

Abbreviations: IM, intramuscular injection; IV, intravenous infusion.

(AspaMetDex) in relapsed/refractory patients (see **Table 3**).[49] Nineteen patients received three cycles of AspaMetDex in this study. Of note, these relapsed/refractory patients received CHOP or CHOP-like regimens as a frontline therapy. Among the 18 evaluable patients, 14 patients (78%) responded to the therapy including 11 CRs (61%). The median survival time was 12.2 months and the median PFS was 12.2 months with a median follow-up duration of 26.2 months. The main toxicities were hepatic dysfunction, anaphylactic reaction to L-asparaginase, and hematologic toxicities. Although this study only included a small number of patients and the follow-up duration was relatively short, AspaMetDex is recommended for treatment of patients who are unfit for SMILE therapy.

Role of Hematopoietic Stem Cell Transplantation

Several retrospective studies have shown that several patients with advanced or relapsed/refractory ENKL that underwent consolidative SCT achieved durable remissions.[50–53] Therefore, consolidative SCT is thought to be a potentially curable treatment modality in this population. However, the optimal source of stem cells (allogeneic or autologous) remains controversial. According to the analysis of the Japanese Society for Hematopoietic Cell Transplantation registry data, 60 patients with ENKL who received autologous-SCT showed superior OS compared with 74 patients who received allogeneic SCT. However, the OS adjusted for disease status and PS at SCT, and clinical stage at the presentation, showed no significant difference between autologous and allogeneic SCT.[54] Further accumulation of data is expected.

Recommended Management of Advanced or Nonnasal Extranodal Natural Killer/T-Cell Lymphoma and Relapsed/Refractory Extranodal Natural Killer/T-Cell Lymphoma, Nasal Type

SMILE therapy is recommended as an induction therapy in this population. In patients who are unfit for SMILE (elderly patients, lymphocyte count $<500/\mu L$, impaired organ function), other L-asparaginase-containing regimens (eg, AspaMetDex) or MDR-nonrelated regimens (eg, DeVIC) are alternative options. If a patient achieved CR after induction therapy, consolidative SCT is recommended, because it might be a curative treatment modality.

In transplant-ineligible patients, four to six cycles of chemotherapy might be appropriate, but the optimal number of cycles depends on the patient condition and response. If localized PET-positive residual disease is present after the chemotherapy, RT might be a treatment option.

NEW AGENT DEVELOPMENT

There have been few clinical trials of novel agents in ENKL. However, some novel agents for peripheral T-cell lymphomas (PTCLs) are expected to be effective. Because ENKL is positive for CD30 in 60% to 70% of cases,[55,56] brentuximab vedotin, an anti-CD30 antibody-drug conjugate, could be a promising agent for treatment of ENKL.[57,58]

Because ENKL is associated with EBV infection, cell therapy targeting EBV-related antigens, such as latent membrane protein (LMP), represents a possible novel treatment. Bollard and colleagues[59] reported the efficacy of autologous LMP-specific cytotoxic T lymphocytes (CTL). Fifty patients with EBV-positive lymphoma including 11 patients with ENKL (six with active disease and five with remission) received LMP-specific CTL infusion. Among six patients with active ENKL, four patients achieved

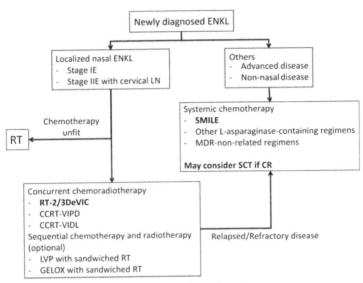

Fig. 3. Treatment algorithm of ENKL. LN, lymph node lesion.

CR and three of them showed durable response. Five patients with remission after chemotherapy received consolidative LMP-specific CTL infusion and all of them continued CR without any severe toxicities. The Korean group also reported the efficacy of LMP-specific CTL infusion as a postremission therapy in 10 patients with ENKL.[60] Anti-LMP chimeric antigen receptor engineered T-cell therapy also is under development.[61] Cell therapy targeting EBV-related antigen might be an alternative consolidative therapy to SCT in the future.

Although ENKL is an entity of mature T-NK-cell neoplasms, potentially effective novel agents for PTCLs sometimes show different toxicity profiles in patients with ENKL. For example, Kim and colleagues[62] reported severe EBV reactivation in ENKL patients treated with romidepsin, a histone deacetylase inhibitor that was already approved by the US Food and Drug Administration for relapsed/refractory PTCLs. Considering its unique pathophysiology, clinical management of ENKL should be considered separately from that of other PTCLs.

SUMMARY

Several recent well-designed clinical trials have reported improved outcomes for ENKL in the last decade. The recommended current management of ENKL is summarized in **Fig. 3**. Continued efforts should be made to further improve chemotherapy, to find the optimal method of irradiation, to define the role of SCT, and to find effective novel agents. As ENKL is a rare subtype of lymphoma, it is not easy to conduct well-designed prospective trials. International collaboration will be needed to achieve further improvements in the treatment of ENKL.

ACKNOWLEDGMENTS

The authors thank Dr Akiko M. Maeshima (Department of Pathology, National Cancer Center Hospital, Tokyo, Japan) for providing the photomicrographs in **Fig. 1**.

REFERENCES

1. Swerdlow SH, Campo E, Harrris NL, et al, editors. World Health Organization classification of tumours and haematopoietic and lymphoid tissues. Lyon (France): IARC; 2008.
2. Anderson JR, Armitage JO, Weisenburger DD. Epidemiology of the non-Hodgkin's lymphomas: distributions of the major subtypes differ by geographic locations. Non-Hodgkin's Lymphoma Classification Project. Ann Oncol 1998;9:717–20.
3. A clinical evaluation of the International Lymphoma Study Group classification of non-Hodgkin's lymphoma. The Non-Hodgkin's Lymphoma Classification Project. Blood 1997;89:3909–18.
4. The world health organization classification of malignant lymphomas in japan: incidence of recently recognized entities. Lymphoma Study Group of Japanese Pathologists. Pathol Int 2000;50:696–702.
5. Oshimi K. Progress in understanding and managing natural killer-cell malignancies. Br J Haematol 2007;139:532–44.
6. Perry AM, Diebold J, Nathwani BN, et al. Non-Hodgkin lymphoma in the Far East: review of 730 cases from the international non-Hodgkin lymphoma classification project. Ann Hematol 2016;95:245–51.
7. Lee J, Suh C, Park YH, et al. Extranodal natural killer T-cell lymphoma, nasal-type: a prognostic model from a retrospective multicenter study. J Clin Oncol 2006;24: 612–8.
8. Kim TM, Lee SY, Jeon YK, et al. Clinical heterogeneity of extranodal NK/T-cell lymphoma, nasal type: a national survey of the Korean Cancer Study Group. Ann Oncol 2008;19:1477–84.
9. Au WY, Weisenburger DD, Intragumtornchai T, et al. Clinical differences between nasal and extranasal natural killer/T-cell lymphoma: a study of 136 cases from the International Peripheral T-Cell Lymphoma Project. Blood 2009;113:3931–7.
10. Suzuki R, Suzumiya J, Yamaguchi M, et al. Prognostic factors for mature natural killer (NK) cell neoplasms: aggressive NK cell leukemia and extranodal NK cell lymphoma, nasal type. Ann Oncol 2010;21:1032–40.
11. Han AR, Lee HR, Park BB, et al. Lymphoma-associated hemophagocytic syndrome: clinical features and treatment outcome. Ann Hematol 2007;86:493–8.
12. Kim SJ, Yoon DH, Jaccard A, et al. A prognostic index for natural killer cell lymphoma after non-anthracycline-based treatment: a multicentre, retrospective analysis. Lancet Oncol 2016;17:389–400.
13. Chan KC, Zhang J, Chan AT, et al. Molecular characterization of circulating EBV DNA in the plasma of nasopharyngeal carcinoma and lymphoma patients. Cancer Res 2003;63:2028–32.
14. Suzuki R, Yamaguchi M, Izutsu K, et al. Prospective measurement of Epstein-Barr virus-DNA in plasma and peripheral blood mononuclear cells of extranodal NK/T-cell lymphoma, nasal type. Blood 2011;118:6018–22.
15. Rubin LA, Nelson DL. The soluble interleukin-2 receptor: biology, function, and clinical application. Ann Intern Med 1990;113:619–27.
16. Yamaguchi M, Suzuki R, Oguchi M, et al. Treatments and outcomes of patients with extranodal natural killer/T-cell lymphoma diagnosed between 2000 and 2013: A cooperative study in Japan. J Clin Oncol 2016. [Epub ahead of print].
17. Cheson BD, Fisher RI, Barrington SF, et al. Recommendations for initial evaluation, staging, and response assessment of Hodgkin and non-Hodgkin lymphoma: the Lugano classification. J Clin Oncol 2014;32:3059–68.

18. Kako S, Izutsu K, Ota Y, et al. FDG-PET in T-cell and NK-cell neoplasms. Ann Oncol 2007;18:1685–90.
19. Lee J, Suh C, Huh J, et al. Effect of positive bone marrow EBV in situ hybridization in staging and survival of localized extranodal natural killer/T-cell lymphoma, nasal-type. Clin Cancer Res 2007;13:3250–4.
20. Kwong YL, Anderson BO, Advani R, et al. Management of T-cell and natural-killer-cell neoplasms in Asia: consensus statement from the Asian Oncology Summit 2009. Lancet Oncol 2009;10:1093–101.
21. Kim GE, Cho JH, Yang WI, et al. Angiocentric lymphoma of the head and neck: patterns of systemic failure after radiation treatment. J Clin Oncol 2000;18:54–63.
22. Li CC, Tien HF, Tang JL, et al. Treatment outcome and pattern of failure in 77 patients with sinonasal natural killer/T-cell or T-cell lymphoma. Cancer 2004;100:366–75.
23. Huang MJ, Jiang Y, Liu WP, et al. Early or up-front radiotherapy improved survival of localized extranodal NK/T-cell lymphoma, nasal-type in the upper aerodigestive tract. Int J Radiat Oncol Biol Phys 2008;70:166–74.
24. Yang Y, Zhu Y, Cao JZ, et al. Risk-adapted therapy for early-stage extranodal nasal-type NK/T-cell lymphoma: analysis from a multicenter study. Blood 2015; 126:1424–32.
25. You JY, Chi KH, Yang MH, et al. Radiation therapy versus chemotherapy as initial treatment for localized nasal natural killer (NK)/T-cell lymphoma: a single institute survey in Taiwan. Ann Oncol 2004;15:618–25.
26. Kwong YL, Chan AC, Liang R, et al. CD56+ NK lymphomas: clinicopathological features and prognosis. Br J Haematol 1997;97:821–9.
27. Ribrag V, Ell Hajj M, Janot F, et al. Early locoregional high-dose radiotherapy is associated with long-term disease control in localized primary angiocentric lymphoma of the nose and nasopharynx. Leukemia 2001;15:1123–6.
28. Yamaguchi M, Ogawa S, Nomoto Y, et al. Treatment outcome of nasal NK-cell lymphoma: a report of 12 consecutively-diagnosed cases and a review of the literature. J Clin Exp Hematop 2001;41:93–9.
29. Cheung MM, Chan JK, Lau WH, et al. Early stage nasal NK/T-cell lymphoma: clinical outcome, prognostic factors, and the effect of treatment modality. Int J Radiat Oncol Biol Phys 2002;54:182–90.
30. Nakamura K, Uehara S, Omagari J, et al. Primary non-Hodgkin lymphoma of the sinonasal cavities: correlation of CT evaluation with clinical outcome. Radiology 1997;204:431–5.
31. Avilés A, Díaz NR, Neri N, et al. Angiocentric nasal T/natural killer cell lymphoma: a single centre study of prognostic factors in 108 patients. Clin Lab Haematol 2000;22:215–20.
32. Drénou B, Lamy T, Amiot L, et al. CD3- CD56+ non-Hodgkin's lymphomas with an aggressive behavior related to multidrug resistance. Blood 1997;89:2966–74.
33. Egashira M, Kawamata N, Sugimoto K, et al. P-glycoprotein expression on normal and abnormally expanded natural killer cells and inhibition of P-glycoprotein function by cyclosporin A and its analogue, PSC833. Blood 1999;93:599–606.
34. Yamaguchi M, Kita K, Miwa H, et al. Frequent expression of P-glycoprotein/MDR1 by nasal T-cell lymphoma cells. Cancer 1995;76:2351–6.
35. Yamaguchi M, Tobinai K, Oguchi M, et al. Phase I/II study of concurrent chemoradiotherapy for localized nasal natural killer/T-cell lymphoma: Japan Clinical Oncology Group Study JCOG0211. J Clin Oncol 2009;27:5594–600.
36. Yamaguchi M, Tobinai K, Oguchi M, et al. Concurrent chemoradiotherapy for localized nasal natural killer/T-cell lymphoma: an updated analysis of the Japan clinical oncology group study JCOG0211. J Clin Oncol 2012;30:4044–6.

37. Okamoto M, Maruyama F, Tsuzuki M, et al. Salvage chemotherapy for relapsed/refractory aggressive non-Hodgkin's lymphoma with a combination of dexamethasone, etoposide, ifosfamide and carboplatin. Rinsho Ketsueki 1994;35:635–41.

38. Imashuku S, Kuriyama K, Teramura T, et al. Requirement for etoposide in the treatment of Epstein-Barr virus-associated hemophagocytic lymphohistiocytosis. J Clin Oncol 2001;19:2665–73.

39. Kim SJ, Kim K, Kim BS, et al. Phase II trial of concurrent radiation and weekly cisplatin followed by VIPD chemotherapy in newly diagnosed, stage IE to IIE, nasal, extranodal NK/T-Cell Lymphoma: Consortium for Improving Survival of Lymphoma study. J Clin Oncol 2009;27:6027–32.

40. Kim SJ, Yang DH, Kim JS, et al. Concurrent chemoradiotherapy followed by L-asparaginase-containing chemotherapy, VIDL, for localized nasal extranodal NK/T cell lymphoma: CISL08-01 phase II study. Ann Hematol 2014;93:1895–901.

41. Ma X, Guo Y, Pang Z, et al. A randomized phase II study of CEOP with or without semustine as induction chemotherapy in patients with stage IE/IIE extranodal NK/T-cell lymphoma, nasal type in the upper aerodigestive tract. Radiother Oncol 2009;93:492–7.

42. Jiang M, Zhang H, Jiang Y, et al. Phase 2 trial of "sandwich" L-asparaginase, vincristine, and prednisone chemotherapy with radiotherapy in newly diagnosed, stage IE to IIE, nasal type, extranodal natural killer/T-cell lymphoma. Cancer 2012;118:3294–301.

43. Wang L, Wang ZH, Chen XQ, et al. First-line combination of gemcitabine, oxaliplatin, and L-asparaginase (GELOX) followed by involved-field radiation therapy for patients with stage IE/IIE extranodal natural killer/T-cell lymphoma. Cancer 2013;119:348–55.

44. Yong W, Zheng W, Zhu J, et al. L-asparaginase in the treatment of refractory and relapsed extranodal NK/T-cell lymphoma, nasal type. Ann Hematol 2009;88:647–52.

45. Jaccard A, Petit B, Girault S, et al. L-asparaginase-based treatment of 15 western patients with extranodal NK/T-cell lymphoma and leukemia and a review of the literature. Ann Oncol 2009;20:110–6.

46. Yamaguchi M, Suzuki R, Kwong YL, et al. Phase I study of dexamethasone, methotrexate, ifosfamide, L-asparaginase, and etoposide (SMILE) chemotherapy for advanced-stage, relapsed or refractory extranodal natural killer (NK)/T-cell lymphoma and leukemia. Cancer Sci 2008;99:1016–20.

47. Yamaguchi M, Kwong YL, Kim WS, et al. Phase II study of SMILE chemotherapy for newly diagnosed stage IV, relapsed, or refractory extranodal natural killer (NK)/T-cell lymphoma, nasal type: the NK-Cell Tumor Study Group study. J Clin Oncol 2011;29:4410–6.

48. Suzuki R, Kwong YL, Maeda Y, et al. 5-year follow-up of the SMILE phase II study for newly-diagnosed stage IV, relapsed or refractory extranodal NK/T-cell lymphoma, nasal type. Hematol Oncol 2015;33:140 [Abstract 075].

49. Jaccard A, Gachard N, Marin B, et al. Efficacy of L-asparaginase with methotrexate and dexamethasone (AspaMetDex regimen) in patients with refractory or relapsing extranodal NK/T-cell lymphoma, a phase 2 study. Blood 2011;117:1834–9.

50. Murashige N, Kami M, Kishi Y, et al. Allogeneic haematopoietic stem cell transplantation as a promising treatment for natural killer-cell neoplasms. Br J Haematol 2005;130:561–7.

51. Suzuki R, Suzumiya J, Nakamura S, et al. Hematopoietic stem cell transplantation for natural killer-cell lineage neoplasms. Bone Marrow Transpl 2006;37:425–31.

52. Kim SJ, Park S, Kang ES, et al. Induction treatment with SMILE and consolidation with autologous stem cell transplantation for newly diagnosed stage IV extranodal natural killer/T-cell lymphoma patients. Ann Hematol 2015;94:71–8.
53. Yokoyama H, Yamamoto J, Tohmiya Y, et al. Allogeneic hematopoietic stem cell transplant following chemotherapy containing l-asparaginase as a promising treatment for patients with relapsed or refractory extranodal natural killer/T cell lymphoma, nasal type. Leuk Lymphoma 2010;51:1509–12.
54. Suzuki R, Kako S, Hyo R, et al. Comparison of autologous and allogeneic hematopoietic stem cell transplantation for extranodal NK/T-cell lymphoma, nasal type: analysis of the japan society for hematopoietic cell transplantation (JSHCT) Lymphoma Working Group. Blood 2011;118(21): [Abstract 503].
55. Pongpruttipan T, Sukpanichnant S, Assanasen T. Extranodal NK/T-cell lymphoma, nasal type, includes cases of natural killer cell and $\alpha\beta$, $\gamma\delta$, and $\alpha\beta/\gamma\delta$ T-cell origin: a comprehensive clinicopathologic and phenotypic study. Am J Surg Pathol 2012;36:481–99.
56. Kim WY, Nam SJ, Kim S, et al. Prognostic implications of CD30 expression in extranodal natural killer/T-cell lymphoma according to treatment modalities. Leuk Lymphoma 2015;56:1778–86.
57. Kim HK, Moon SM, Moon JH, et al. Complete remission in CD30-positive refractory extranodal NK/T-cell lymphoma with brentuximab vedotin. Blood Res 2015; 50:254–6.
58. Poon LM, Kwong YL. Complete remission of refractory disseminated NK/T cell lymphoma with brentuximab vedotin and bendamustine. Ann Hematol 2016; 95(5):847–9.
59. Bollard CM, Gottschalk S, Torrano V, et al. Sustained complete responses in patients with lymphoma receiving autologous cytotoxic T lymphocytes targeting Epstein-Barr virus latent membrane proteins. J Clin Oncol 2014;32:798–808.
60. Cho SG, Kim N, Sohn HJ, et al. Long-term outcome of extranodal NK/T cell lymphoma patients treated with postremission therapy using EBV LMP1 and LMP2a-specific CTLs. Mol Ther 2015;23:1401–9.
61. Tang X, Zhou Y, Li W, et al. T cells expressing a LMP1-specific chimeric antigen receptor mediate antitumor effects against LMP1-positive nasopharyngeal carcinoma cells in vitro and in vivo. J Biomed Res 2014;28:468–75.
62. Kim SJ, Kim JH, Ki CS, et al. Epstein-Barr virus reactivation in extranodal natural killer/T-cell lymphoma patients: a previously unrecognized serious adverse event in a pilot study with romidepsin. Ann Oncol 2016;27:508–13.

Adult T-cell Leukemia/Lymphoma

A Problem Abroad and at Home

Christopher Dittus, DO, MPH[a],*, J. Mark Sloan, MD[b]

KEYWORDS

- Lymphoma • Leukemia • HTLV-1 • Rare cancer • T-cell lymphoma
- Aggressive lymphoma • Hypercalcemia

KEY POINTS

- Adult T-cell leukemia/lymphoma (ATLL) is a rare and, often, aggressive lymphoma that is causally linked to chronic infection with human T-cell lymphotropic virus type 1.
- Four subtypes have been described: acute, lymphomatous, chronic, and smoldering. The acute and lymphomatous subtypes comprise the aggressive variants.
- Patients often require extensive supportive care designed to manage hypercalcemia, tumor lysis syndrome, and infectious complications.
- Prognosis is poor for the aggressive subtypes, and treatment strategies have traditionally focused on antiviral therapy with zidovudine and interferon-alfa, as well as combination chemotherapy.
- Novel therapeutic approaches include monoclonal antibody therapy with brentuximab vedotin, anti–CC chemokine receptor 4 therapy with mogamulizumab, and immunomodulatory therapy with lenalidomide.

INTRODUCTION

Adult T-cell leukemia/lymphoma (ATLL) is a severe, yet fascinating, disease that develops in a small proportion of individuals who are chronically infected with human T-cell lymphotropic virus type 1 (HTLV-1). ATLL is epidemiologically unique because of this association with HTLV-1, which is the first described human retrovirus.[1,2] Clinically, ATLL has protean manifestations, with each of 4 variants possessing a distinct

Disclosures: Dr C. Dittus has nothing to disclose. Dr J.M. Sloan has received grants from Molecular Templates, Stemline Pharmaceuticals.
[a] Division of Hematology and Oncology, University of North Carolina at Chapel Hill, 170 Manning Drive, Campus Box 7305, Chapel Hill, NC 27599-7305, USA; [b] Division of Hematology and Oncology, Boston University Medical Center, 820 Harrison Avenue, FGH Building, 1st Floor, Boston, MA 02118, USA
* Corresponding author.
E-mail address: cedittus@gmail.com

constellation of symptoms. The aggressive variants have an unrelenting progressive course, with primary refractory disease proving to be the norm.

This article reviews the epidemiology of ATLL, as well as the clinical manifestations, diagnostic considerations, traditional approach to therapy, and recent data on novel therapeutic agents.

EPIDEMIOLOGY

The geographic distribution of ATLL is rooted in the epidemiology of HTLV-1. HTLV-1 infection is common, with an estimated 15 million to 20 million people worldwide living with chronic infection.[3] These individuals predominantly live in endemic regions. The areas with an HTLV-1 seroprevalence of at least 1% to 5% include Japan, Iran, the Caribbean islands, Honduras, Brazil, Peru, Ecuador, and many west African nations (**Fig. 1**).[4] Specific communities have hyperendemic HTLV-1; notably the Shikoku and Kyushu islands of Japan, as well as the Okinawa Prefecture, have seroprevalences of up to 37%. These regions stand out even compared with other high-prevalence regions, such as Jamaica, which has a rate of 5%. In contrast, France has a very low seroprevalence, ranging from 0.004% to 0.007% in blood donors,[5] as does the United States with a seroprevalence of 0.018%.[6]

HTLV-1 persists in these endemic regions primarily because of vertical transmission of the virus from mother to child via breastfeeding, with a transmission rate of roughly 20%.[3] HTLV-1 can also be transmitted via blood transfusion, sexual contact, and parenterally via shared needles. Most patients who develop ATLL acquire HTLV-1 via breastfeeding, which is likely related to the early age of infection.[7] Individuals who develop HTLV-associated myelopathy/tropical spastic paresis are more likely to have acquired the virus as a blood-borne pathogen. In Nagasaki, an HTLV-1 screening program that included prenatal testing and counseling on breastfeeding

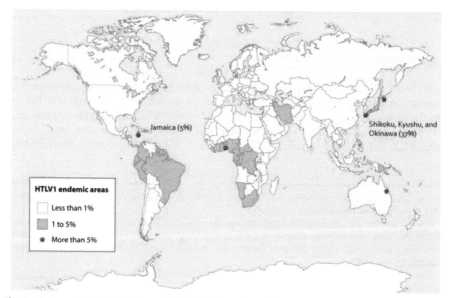

Fig. 1. Geographic distribution of HTLV-1. (*From* Goncalves DU, Proietti FA, Ribas JGR, et al. Epidemiology, treatment, and prevention of human T-cell leukemia virus 1-associated diseases. Clin Microbiol Rev 2010;23(3):579; with permission.)

avoidance for HTLV-1–positive mothers decreased transmission of the virus by 80%.[8] Blood transfusion was a major source of HTLV-1 transmission before universal screening measures.

In contrast with HTLV-1 infection, ATLL is a rare malignancy. The lifetime risk of a patient with HTLV-1 developing ATLL is 2% to 4%, and the average latency period from infection to ATLL onset is 60 years in Japan and 40 years in Jamaica.[7] Worldwide, there were 2100 cases of ATLL in 2008, and most of these cases were clustered in the HTLV-1–endemic regions described earlier.[9] ATLL is most prevalent in the Kyushu region of Japan, with an age-standardized incidence of 2 per 100,000 individuals in 2008.[10] ATLL accounted for 36.8% of all lymphoma cases from 2003 to 2008 in Kyushu. ATLL is very common in the Kyushu region, even compared with Japan as a whole (0.3 per 100,000 individuals), and particularly compared with the United States where ATLL is exceedingly rare (0.02 per 100,000 individuals). In addition, ATLL accounts for only 0.2% of all lymphoma cases in the United States.[10] However, the rate of ATLL seems to be increasing. From 2002 and 2011, there was an annual percentage change (APC) of 6.2%, which is a statistically significant increase. In Kyushu, where screening programs have helped decrease transmission of HTLV-1, the APC is 0%. The increasing trend in the United States is driven by increased emigration from endemic regions, with certain cities on the eastern seaboard reporting a higher incidence of ATLL than the rest of the country.

MECHANISM

HTLV-1 is a human retrovirus that has the capacity to directly transform CD4-positive T cells. Mechanistic research, coupled with extensive epidemiologic, clinical, and experimental (animal) research, has led the International Agency for Research on Cancer (IARC) to classify HTLV-1 as a group 1 carcinogen, meaning this exposure is carcinogenic to humans.[7]

Extensive basic research has identified that the viral transactivator protein, Tax, plays a key role in carcinogenesis. Tax activates the viral promoter, as well as the cyclic AMP and nuclear factor kappa-B pathways. In addition, antiapoptotic proteins are upregulated and p53 is suppressed. Most recently, researchers have shown that Tax can induce the epigenetic reprogramming of more than half the cellular genes via activation of enhancer of zeste homolog 2 (EZH2) and subsequent alteration of trimethylation at histone H3Lys27.[11,12] Ultimately, a T cell is transformed into a cancer cell, and there is expansion of the malignant clone.

Tax protein expression is often undetectable in circulating ATLL cells, whereas the HTLV-1 basic leucine zipper factor (HBZ) is consistently expressed.[13,14] In the study described earlier, the researchers were able to reproduce their findings via Tax transduction into normal T lymphocytes, whereas HBZ was not able to induce these epigenetic changes.[11] In addition, the epigenetic profile persisted into the late stages of disease. Therefore, it seems that Tax plays an ongoing role in driving ATLL, but it is unclear whether this is caused by an initial activating event or continuous Tax expression, which may be possible if the methods of detection are lacking in sensitivity. Ultimately, these findings may have clinical implications because agents targeting Tax and/or EZH2 have shown preliminary efficacy.[12]

CLINICAL PRESENTATION

The clinical presentation of ATLL is highly variable, but correlates with various subtypes of disease that were first described by Shimoyama[15] (**Table 1**). The 4 subtypes

Table 1
Shimoyama[15] classification

	Acute	Chronic[a]	Smoldering	Lymphoma
HTLV-1	Yes	Yes	Yes	Yes
Skin	Yes	Yes	Yes	Yes
Flower Cells	Yes	Yes	Yes	No
Lymphocytosis	Yes	Yes	No	No
Lymphadenopathy/Spleen	Yes	Mild	None	Yes
Hypercalcemia	Yes (70%)	No	No	Less
LDH Level	Increased	Normal/mild	Normal/mild	Increased

Abbreviation: LDH, lactate dehydrogenase.

[a] Chronic unfavorable (≥1 factor): LDH level > upper limit of normal (ULN); blood urea nitrogen level > ULN; albumin level < lower limit of normal.

Adapted from Shimoyama M. Diagnostic criteria and classification of clinical subtypes of adult T-cell leukaemia-lymphoma. Br J Haematol 1991;79:428–37; with permission.

of ATLL are (1) acute, (2) lymphomatous, (3) chronic, and (4) smoldering. The chronic subtype is further divided into unfavorable and favorable, based on the presence or absence of several factors. The unfavorable risk factors are a serum lactate dehydrogenase (LDH) level greater than the upper limit of normal (ULN), serum blood urea nitrogen level greater than the ULN, and serum albumin level lower than the lower limit of normal.[16] The smoldering, chronic, and acute types of ATLL can be viewed on a continuum of leukemic involvement, with the smoldering subtype representing the mildest form of the disease, and the acute type representing the most aggressive form of the disease. The lymphomatous subtype is also very aggressive, but lacks a leukemic component by definition. The smoldering subtype has atypical lymphocytes, termed flower cells (**Fig. 2**), but does not have a lymphocytosis (absolute lymphocyte count [ALC] <4000 mcL). In addition, these patients have no lymphadenopathy (LAD), splenomegaly, or significant increase in LDH level. The chronic subtype differs from the smoldering type in that there is an increased ALC greater than or equal to 4000, and patients may have mild LAD, splenomegaly, or increased LDH level. The acute type has an atypical lymphocytosis and often presents with diffuse LAD,

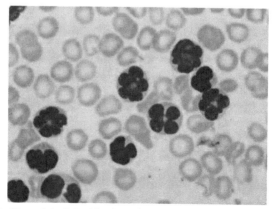

Fig. 2. Flower cells. (*From* Jain P, Prabhash K. Flower cells of leukemia. Blood 2010;115:1668; with permission.)

splenomegaly, significantly increased LDH level, and hypercalcemia. Lastly, the lymphomatous subtype often presents with rapidly growing LAD and splenomegaly without a leukemic component. The LDH level is typically markedly increased in the lymphomatous subtype, but hypercalcemia is less frequent. All subtypes of ATLL can have variable dermatologic manifestations (**Fig. 3**).

The acute and lymphomatous subtypes are often grouped together as aggressive ATLL. Progression is rapid in these patients, and they often present in organ failure or respiratory compromise from rapidly enlarging lymph node masses and visceral organ invasion. Even after therapy is initiated, aggressive ATLL often progresses, resulting in primary refractory disease. In addition, patients with aggressive ATLL are at risk for central nervous system (CNS) involvement, and any neurologic deficits at presentation warrant further evaluation. As in other aggressive lymphomas, tumor lysis syndrome (TLS) is a concern, both spontaneously and after initiation of therapy.

A distinctive finding in ATLL is a profoundly increased calcium level at presentation. Calcium levels more than 20 mg/mL are common in acute-type ATLL. Such high calcium levels are less common in the lymphomatous, chronic, and smoldering forms of the disease. Pathologic studies have revealed that patients with ATLL with hypercalcemia often have an increased number of osteoclasts, as well as increased bone resorption.[17] Parathyroid hormone–related protein has been suggested as a driver of bone resorption in ATLL,[18] although increased transcription of receptor activator of nuclear factor kB (RANK) ligand seems to correlate more precisely in patients with ATLL with hypercalcemia.[17] More recently, researchers have found that ATLL cells overexpress Wnt5a, which induces osteoclastogenesis,[19] and this could be responsible for both the osteolytic lesions and hypercalcemia found in many patients with ATLL.

All patients with ATLL are immunosuppressed and at risk for infections, which frequently complicates therapy. In his initial description of the ATLL subtypes, Shimoyama[15] quantified this risk. In the acute type, 27% of patients had an infection at diagnosis. The infection was most commonly bacterial (12%), followed by fungal (8%), parasitic (5%), and viral (3%). The nematode *Strongyloides stercoralis* is commonly identified in patients with ATLL, and causes severe, disseminated disease. Because of the risk of severe infection in patients with ATLL, prophylaxis against bacterial, fungal, and viral pathogens is appropriate and prompt diagnosis and management of infectious complications are paramount.

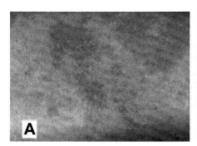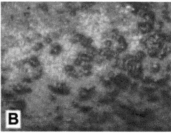

Fig. 3. Dermatologic manifestations of ATLL. Dermatologic findings include erythema (*A*) and papules (*B*). (*From* Ohshima K, Jaffe ES, Kikuchi M. Adult T-cell leukaemia/lymphoma. In: Swerdlow SH, Campo E, Harris NL, et al, editors. WHO classification of tumours of haematopoietic and lymphoid tissues. 4th edition. Lyon (France): International Agency for Research on Cancer (IARC); 2008; with permission.)

MAKING THE DIAGNOSIS

The diagnosis of ATLL begins with the historical evaluation. Although it is possible for someone who is not from an endemic country to become infected with HTLV-1, it is highly unlikely; almost all patients with ATLL were born in an endemic country. Therefore, in evaluating a patient with either a leukemic or lymphomatous presentation, ATLL must be considered for any patient emigrating from an endemic country. A profound hypercalcemia (>20 mg/mL), although not 100% specific, can point toward a diagnosis of ATLL. In addition, about 20% of patients with ATLL have an eosinophilia, which can be severe.[20] If there is a leukemic component, the diagnosis can be made if flower cells are visualized on the peripheral smear because these cells are pathognomonic for ATLL. Any case suspicious for ATLL must have HTLV-1 serologic testing. Although a positive test does not confirm ATLL, a negative test does rule-out ATLL. Flow cytometry sent on a peripheral blood sample is the confirmatory test of choice for any ATLL with a leukemic component. The characteristic flow cytometry pattern is positive for CD2, CD3, CD4, CD5, and CD25. Typically, CD7, CD8, and CD56 are negative, and CD30 is variable (positive in 20%–50%) (**Table 2**). Lymphomatous presentations depend on an excisional lymph node biopsy for diagnosis, which should have flow cytometry and immunohistochemical (IHC) testing. Additional IHC tests include anaplastic lymphoma kinase (ALK), paired box 5 (PAX5) and terminal deoxynucleotidyl transferase (TdT) which are all negative in ATLL. The Ki-67 proliferation index is very high in aggressive ATLL. Bone marrow aspiration and biopsy may be performed to obtain a diagnosis or to complete the staging.

FURTHER WORK-UP

In addition to the complete blood count with differential, complete metabolic panel, and peripheral blood smear, all patients with ATLL should have a LDH test performed, as well as a TLS panel, including uric acid, phosphate, calcium, potassium, and creatinine levels. Glucose-6-phosphate dehydrogenase (G6PD) testing should also be sent with the initial work-up in order to evaluate for the presence of a hereditary deficiency that would preclude the use of the recombinant urate oxidase enzyme rasburicase. A viral panel consisting of human immunodeficiency virus, hepatitis B virus, and hepatitis C virus serology should be sent for all patients with leukemia/lymphoma. In addition, all patients with aggressive ATLL should have human leukocyte antigen (HLA) typing of their siblings in preparation for allogeneic stem cell transplant. This process should start immediately on diagnosis of aggressive ATLL, because the process can take time and remissions do not last long in this disease.

Table 2 Adult T-cell leukemia/lymphoma immunophenotype			
	Flow Cytometry	**IHC Stains**	**Other Tests**
Positive	CD2 CD3 CD4 CD5 CD25 CD30 (+/−)	Ki-67 High	HTLV-1
Negative	CD7 CD8 CD56	ALK PAX5 TdT	

Abbreviation: IHC, immunohistochemical.

All patients should have imaging to evaluate the extent of lymphadenopathy, splenomegaly, organ infiltration, and skeletal involvement. Even patients with acute-type ATLL can have massive LAD that can impair organ function. Imaging with either computed tomography (CT) with intravenous contrast or PET is acceptable. Note that because of the rapid progression of this disease, treatment should not be delayed to obtain PET imaging unless it is readily available. In this situation, CT imaging is prudent. Aggressive ATLL often invades the CNS. Therefore, all patients newly diagnosed with either the acute or lymphomatous types of ATLL should have brain imaging (CT or MRI), as well as a lumbar puncture (LP) sent for cytology and flow cytometry. Intrathecal chemotherapy should be given at the time of the initial LP.

PROGNOSIS

The prognosis for ATLL depends on the subtype, with the smoldering and chronic variants having improved survival compared with the aggressive subtypes[15] (**Fig. 4**). In addition, the chronic variant has been divided into favorable and unfavorable types, with the unfavorable type correlating with a poorer survival. Importantly, a recent study reexamined the original Shimoyama[15] prognostic groups and found that the median survival times were 8.3, 10.6, 31.5, and 55 months for the acute, lymphomatous, chronic, and smoldering types, respectively.[21] Four-year overall survival (OS) rates were 11%, 16%, 36%, and 52%, respectively. These data show an improvement in the 4-year OS for the aggressive subtypes, but the smoldering type had worse than expected survival.

Efforts have been made to apply prognostic scores to ATLL. One study applied the commonly used International Prognostic Index (IPI) for lymphoma to patients with ATLL.[22] This score takes into account 5 factors (age >60 years, stage III/IV, Eastern Collaborative Oncology Group [ECOG] score ≥2, increased LDH level, >1 extranodal region), with prognosis worsening with the presence of a greater number of factors. Most patients evaluated in the ATLL study had the lymphomatous subtype (89%). More specific prognostic scores have been evaluated, including the simplified ATLL prognostic index (ATL-PI).[23] This study reviewed data from 807 patients with newly diagnosed acute and lymphomatous type ATLL. Five variables were identified that correlated with worse survival: stage III/IV (2 points), ECOG score 2 to 4 (1 point),

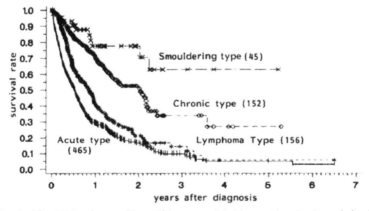

Fig. 4. Survival by ATLL subtype. (*From* Shimoyama M. Diagnostic criteria and classification of clinical subtypes of adult T-cell leukaemia-lymphoma. Br J Haematol 1991;79:428–37; with permission.)

age greater than 70 years (1 point), serum albumin level less than 3.5 g/dL (1 point), and soluble interleukin 2 receptor (sIL-2R) level greater than 20,000 U/mL (1 point). A low score (0–2 points) correlated with a median OS of 16.2 months, an intermediate score (3–4 points) correlated with a median OS of 7 months, and a high score (5–6 points) correlated with a median OS of 4.6 months.

In addition to prognostic scores, several studies have identified various other poor prognostic factors. Takasaki and colleagues[24] evaluated the impact that visceral and cytologic abnormalities have on survival. In this study of 168 patients with ATLL, bone marrow involvement, skin involvement, and monocytosis correlated with poorer survival in patients with aggressive ATLL. Bone marrow involvement coupled with additional visceral organ involvement worsened prognosis further. Eosinophilia has also been associated with a poor prognosis.[25]

CD30 positivity not only has therapeutic implications but also has prognostic importance in the acute and unfavorable chronic types. A study evaluating 68 patients with ATLL found that 22.1% of these patients were positive for CD30.[26] In the acute/unfavorable chronic group, the median survival of CD30-positive patients was 10.1 weeks, whereas CD30-negative patients had a median survival of 33.7 weeks. CD30 was not a significant prognostic marker in patients with lymphomatous ATLL.

MANAGEMENT

Treatment of ATLL is notoriously difficult. Patients with aggressive ATLL have disease that is often refractory to intensive regimens. If a remission can be induced, patients typically relapse quickly, often while still on their initial regimen (**Table 3**). It is therefore imperative to begin planning for allogeneic stem cell transplant (alloSCT) as soon as the diagnosis of aggressive ATLL is confirmed. The goal for all of these patients should be expedited alloSCT in first remission. In addition, patients with ATLL are immunosuppressed and have a course complicated by recurrent bacterial, viral, and fungal infections. Metabolic derangements, including hypercalcemia and TLS, also complicate management.

Antiretroviral Therapy

The smoldering and favorable chronic types of ATLL respond well to antiretroviral therapy. The primary antiretroviral agents studied in ATLL are zidovudine (AZT) and interferon-alfa (IFN). The best evidence for the combination of AZT/IFN comes from

Table 3 Treatment regimens for aggressive adult T-cell leukemia/lymphoma					
	N	Study	ORR (%)	CR (%)	OS (mo)
AZT/IFN	19	Phase II	76.5	53	11
CHOP-14	61	Rand phase II	66	21	11
LSG15	57	Rand phase II	72	40	13
Lenalidomide	26	Phase II	42	19	20.3
BV-CHP	2	Phase I	100	100	—
Mogamulizumab	27	Phase II	50	31	13.7
Mogamulizumab-LSG15	29	Rand phase II	86	52	NR

Abbreviations: AZT, zidovudine; BV, brentuximab vedotin; CHOP, cyclophosphamide, doxorubicin, vincristine, and prednisone; CHP, cyclophosphamide, doxorubicin, and prednisone; CR, complete response; IFN, interferon; NR, not reported; ORR, overall response rate.

a small phase II trial.[27] Nineteen patients with ATLL (15 acute and 4 lymphomatous) received AZT 1 g/d and IFN 9 million units/d for a minimum of 2 months. The response rate (RR) was 76.5%, with a complete response (CR) rate of 53%. This finding applied to both acute and lymphomatous subtypes. Responders went on to receive maintenance therapy with AZT 600 mg daily and IFN 4.5 million units daily for 1 year. Event-free survival was 7 months for the entire study population, and this increased to 10 months when only the patients receiving initial therapy were included (N = 13). Median OS was 11 months for the study population. Although this study only included aggressive forms of ATLL, the results have been extrapolated to the smoldering and favorable chronic types with excellent effect.

An important meta-analysis evaluated the use of AZT/IFN in 3 groups of patients with ATLL: smoldering/chronic, acute, and lymphomatous.[28] The study compared 207 patients who received either AZT/IFN or chemotherapy as initial therapy, as well as those who received chemotherapy followed by AZT/IFN. The median OS for those receiving AZT/IFN as initial therapy (N = 75) was 17 months, with a 5-year OS of 46%. Patients who received chemotherapy as initial therapy (N = 77) had a median OS of 10 months, with a 5-year OS of 20%. Patients who received chemotherapy followed by AZT/IFN (N = 55) had a median OS of 15 months, with a 5-year OS of 12%. When the data were evaluated by ATLL subtype, there was a particularly impressive improvement in OS for the smoldering/chronic group that received up-front AZT/IFN. These patients had a 5-year OS of 100% (N = 17), whereas those who received chemotherapy initially had a 5-year OS of 42% (N = 6). Patients with acute-type ATLL who received up-front AZT/IFN had a 5-year OS of 28% (N = 45). Patients who received initial chemotherapy had a 5-year OS of 10% (N = 53). Because the most aggressive cases of acute ATLL were more likely to receive chemotherapy at a higher rate than patients with ATLL with a more indolent presentation, this may impart a selection bias that works in favor of AZT/IFN. In addition, patients with lymphomatous-type ATLL who received AZT/IFN initially did poorly, with no patients living at 5 years (N = 13). Patients who received chemotherapy as initial treatment had an improved 5-year OS of 18% (N = 71). Based on these data, the use of AZT/IFN has become the standard of care for the smoldering and favorable chronic subtypes of ATLL. Initial use of AZT/IFN is reasonable for the acute-type ATLL, but this study did not support the use of AZT/IFN in the lymphomatous type.

In 2011, a retrospective study evaluated the effect of AZT/IFN in the aggressive types of ATLL.[29] AZT/IFN given anytime throughout the treatment course correlated with a survival advantage in both the acute and lymphomatous types of ATLL. Interestingly, the investigators also reported a survival advantage for patients with either acute or lymphomatous ATLL who received concurrent chemotherapy and low-dose AZT/IFN compared with those who received chemotherapy alone. The recommended low-dose regimen was IFN 3 million units daily and AZT 250 mg twice daily, but the dosing and intervals were variable. More prospective data are required to determine whether AZT/IFN given with concurrent chemotherapy is an appropriate treatment approach.

Other research has evaluated the use of arsenic trioxide and IFN with or without AZT. Arsenic trioxide has been shown to synergize with IFN to induce cell-cycle arrest and apoptosis in leukemia cells from patients with ATLL.[30] A small phase 2 trial evaluating arsenic trioxide with IFN in 7 patients with relapsed ATLL resulted in 1 CR and 3 partial responses (PRs).[31] When arsenic trioxide was combined with AZT/IFN in 10 patients with chronic ATLL, there was a 100% RR (7 CR, 2 CR with >5% circulating atypical lymphocytes, 1 PR).[32] This result for chronic-type ATLL is impressive, but these patients generally respond well to AZT/IFN and it is hard to discern the impact of arsenic trioxide without a randomized trial.

Chemotherapy

Although a trial of AZT/IFN may be pursued in otherwise stable patients with aggressive ATLL, eventually all of these patients require more aggressive treatment with combination chemotherapy. A review of the National Comprehensive Cancer Network (NCCN) guidelines will prove disappointing, because there are no category 1 recommendations for ATLL.[33] Instead, there is an alphabetical listing of 4 regimens: CHOP (cyclophosphamide, doxorubicin, vincristine, and prednisone), CHOEP (cyclophosphamide, doxorubicin, vincristine, etoposide, and prednisone), dose-adjusted EPOCH (etoposide, prednisone, vincristine, cyclophosphamide, and doxorubicin), and hyper-CVAD (cyclophosphamide, vincristine, doxorubicin, and dexamethasone) alternating with high-dose methotrexate and cytarabine. These recommendations are based on either an extrapolation from evidence in other types of lymphoma and/or case reports. CHOP has been studied extensively in NHL, and was used as the comparator arm in a Japanese ATLL study that is discussed in more detail later.[34] Two studies exist that show the efficacy of CHOEP in T-cell lymphomas, but these studies did not include patients with ATLL.[35,36] Evidence for EPOCH is primarily extrapolated, but a recent small study showed a RR of 67% for a regimen combining EPOCH with bortezomib and raltegravir.[37] In addition, 2 patients achieved a durable CR (12 and 18 months) with the use of hyperCVAD.[38]

The most robust ATLL data come from the Japanese Clinical Oncology Group (JCOG).[39] The group's earliest studies in the 1970s and 1980s used CHOP-like regimens that resulted in poor outcomes.[40,41] More aggressive regimens slightly improved the CR rate, but median survival was still abysmal.[42] More recently, JCOG researchers developed an intensive regimen known as VCAP-AMP-VECP (vincristine, cyclophosphamide, doxorubicin, and prednisone [VCAP], doxorubicin, ranimustine, and prednisone [AMP], and vindesine, etoposide, carboplatin, and prednisone [VCEP]), or LSG15.[43] This regimen became the standard of care for aggressive ATLL in Japan after it was compared with CHOP-14 in a randomized phase II trial.[34] In this trial, LSG15 showed a CR rate of 40% compared with a CR rate of 21% in the CHOP-14 group. The OS and progression-free survival (PFS) rates seemed to favor the LSG15 group, but the difference was not significant. This benefit came at the cost of excessive toxicity, including 3 treatment-related deaths (2 patients died of sepsis and 1 of interstitial pneumonitis) in the LSG15 arm. Note that, in the initial phase II trial, the CR rate was better for the lymphomatous type (66.7%) versus the acute type (19.6%).[43] This regimen contains several agents that are not available in the United States (ranimustine and vindesine) and, along with the excessive toxicity, this has precluded the use of LSG15 in the United States.

Targeted and Novel Therapies

Anti–CC chemokine receptor 4 therapy

Recent research has focused on the role of novel, targeted agents, either alone or in combination with chemotherapy. The first such agent is mogamulizumab, which is a defucosylated, humanized anti–CC chemokine receptor 4 (CCR4) monoclonal antibody.[44] Chemokines are responsible for inducing directed migration and tissue localization of various types of leukocytes, including lymphocytes. CCR4 is a chemokine involved in T-helper 2 (Th2) regulation, and has been shown to be highly expressed in ATLL.[45] One study showed that CCR4 was expressed in 88.3% of ATLL cases, and that this expression was associated with a poorer prognosis.[46] Mogamulizumab was evaluated in a phase II study including 27 CCR-positive patients with aggressive, relapsed ATLL.[44] Mogamulizumab was given at a dose of 1.0 mg/kg intravenous weekly for 8 weeks, and the study found a median PFS of 5.2 months, and a median OS of 13.7 months. Common adverse events were cytopenias, fever, rash, chills, and 1 case of erythema multiforme. These results led to a randomized phase II study comparing mogamulizumab in combination with the LSG15 regimen versus LSG15 alone in newly diagnosed patients with aggressive ATLL.[47] The primary end point in this study was the CR rate, which was 52% in the combination arm and 33% in the LSG15-alone arm. The median PFS for the mogamulizumab with LSG15 group was 8.5 months versus 6.3 months in the LSG15-alone arm. Median OS was not reached in either arm after 413 and 502 days of follow-up, respectively. Importantly, a recent study found an increased risk of severe and corticosteroid-refractory graft-versus-host disease, nonrelapse mortality, and overall mortality in patients treated with mogamulizumab before allogeneic transplant.[48] For this reason, mogamulizumab should be used cautiously in transplant-eligible patients.

Antibody therapy

Another novel agent is brentuximab vedotin (BV), which is an antibody-drug conjugate that combines an anti-CD30 monoclonal antibody with the microtubule disrupting agent, monomethyl auristatin E (MMAE).[49] This agent binds CD30, and is then internalized and transported to lysosomes where the MMAE is released from CD30. MMAE then binds tubulin and causes cell-cycle arrest. This agent was initially studied in, and has been approved for, Hodgkin lymphoma and anaplastic large cell lymphoma, both of which universally express CD30.[50,51] In addition, BV has been shown to induce responses in a range of other lymphomas that variably express CD30, including peripheral T-cell lymphoma (PTCL) not otherwise specified, angioimmunoblastic T-cell lymphoma, cutaneous T-cell lymphoma, and diffuse large B-cell lymphoma.[52–54]

Interest in BV for the treatment of ATLL is based on the fact that ATLL has been shown to express CD30. As mentioned previously, a study published in 2013 showed that 22.1% of ATLL cases were CD30 positive.[26] It is notable that the cutoff value for CD30 expression in this study was fairly high at 30%, and BV may have an effect in ATLL cases with lower levels of CD30 expression. There has been 1 prospective BV trial that included patients with ATLL: a phase I multicenter trial that evaluated the safety and efficacy of BV in CD30-positive PTCL.[55] Of the 39 patients in this study, 2 had ATLL. Both of these patients with ATLL were in the BV-CHP (cyclophosphamide, doxorubicin, and prednisone) group, and both experienced a CR. Specifically, 1 patient was stage IV with an IPI score of 3 and 25% CD30 expression. This patient had a PFS of 7.1 months. The other patient was stage IV with an IPI score of 5 and 98% CD30 expression. This patient had a PFS of 22.8 months. At present, a phase 3 trial is enrolling patients to compare BV-CHP with CHOP in the initial treatment of CD30-positive mature T-cell lymphomas, including patients with ATLL.[56]

Because CD25 (interleukin-2 receptor alpha chain) is universally expressed in ATLL, it is an obvious target for monoclonal antibody therapy. An anti-CD25 agent, daclizumab, which is used to prevent rejection in organ transplantation, has been evaluated in 2 ATLL clinical trials. One study evaluated daclizumab alone (8 mg/kg) in 34 patients and found no response in the 18 patients with aggressive ATLL.[57] There were 6 PRs in the 16 patients with chronic or smoldering ATLL. The second study evaluated a lower dose of daclizumab (1 mg/kg) in combination with standard CHOP chemotherapy.[58] This study included 15 patients with ATLL (11 acute type and 4 lymphomatous type), and 5 (33%) achieved a CR lasting more than 2 months. Three patients (20%) achieved a PR lasting at least 2 months. The median OS was 10 months. Taken together, the response to daclizumab was not as robust as was hoped, and use of this agent has not been widely adopted.

Immunomodulatory therapy

The immunomodulatory agent lenalidomide has been evaluated in ATLL.[59,60] Most recently, preliminary results from a phase II study were presented at the 2015 American Society of Hematology conference.[61] This study included aggressive (N = 22) and chronic unfavorable (N = 4) ATLL that had relapsed after at least 1 prior therapy. These patients received lenalidomide 25 mg daily continuously until disease progression or unacceptable toxicity. The CR and overall response rate (ORR) were higher in the lymphomatous type (29% and 57%) versus the acute type (20% and 33%). The median PFS was 3.8 months and the median OS was 20.3 months. Most of the side effects were hematologic, with 65% of patients requiring a dose reduction. It was noted that the patients on this trial had a long natural history of disease before enrolling on the trial, and may not be representative of most patients with ATLL seen in practice.

Allogeneic Stem Cell Transplantation

As mentioned earlier, the goal for all patients with aggressive ATLL is alloSCT in first remission. The best evidence for alloSCT is from the Japanese literature. A nationwide retrospective study in Japan found that, by 2012, more than 1000 patients had received alloSCT for ATLL.[16,62] Approximately 120 patients undergo alloSCT for ATLL in Japan yearly. In another retrospective study, patients who received an alloSCT from an HLA-matched donor had a 3-year OS of 41%, whereas those who received unrelated bone marrow had a 3-year OS of 39%.[63] There seems to be a graft-versus-leukemia effect in ATLL, as shown by a longer OS in patients with grade I/II acute graft-versus-host disease.[64] There does not seem to be a difference in OS between myeloablative conditioning (MAC) and reduced-intensity conditioning (RIC), although, in older patients, there was a trend toward superior OS with RIC.[65] Because of high transplant-related mortality with MAC, much of the recent research has focused on RIC.[66] A study evaluating long-term outcomes after RIC found that 10 of 29 patients survived for a median of 82 months with a 5-year OS of 34%.[67] Although not a perfect treatment, some patients can achieve long-term survival, which is not possible without alloSCT (see Tejaswini M. Dhawale, and Andrei R. Shustov's article, "Autologous and Allogeneic Hematopoietic Cell Transplantation in Peripheral T/NK-cell Lymphomas: A Histology-Specific Review," in this issue, for further discussion).

Treatment Recommendations

It is difficult to make a recommendation regarding the most appropriate regimen for treating aggressive ATLL given the limited available data. In addition, some of the therapeutic agents mentioned earlier are not currently available in the United States (eg, mogamulizumab, ranimustine, vindesine). For this reason, the importance of collaboration between institutions to refer eligible patients for clinical trials is paramount.

Despite the lack of data, it is clear that CHOP is inadequate therapy for aggressive ATLL. The addition of etoposide, as in CHOEP or dose-adjusted EPOCH, is a reasonable approach for first-line chemotherapy; the ultimate goal should be for allogeneic transplant in first remission. In the smoldering and chronic favorable subtypes, the authors recommend AZT/IFN as initial therapy.

Supportive Care

ATLL is a highly lethal disease because of both the aggressive leukemia/lymphoma and the myriad complications that accompany the disease. The major complications associated with ATLL are discussed below.

Infectious complications

Patients with ATLL are immunosuppressed from a dysfunctional T-lymphocyte population. In the seminal description of ATLL, Shimoyama[15] found that 27% of patients with acute-type ATLL had an infection at diagnosis. Infections included bacterial, fungal, parasitic, and viral pathogens. Our clinical practice includes prophylaxis for pneumocystis pneumonia with trimethoprim-sulfamethoxazole 3 times weekly and herpes simplex/zoster prophylaxis with acyclovir or valacyclovir. The authors have a low threshold for initiating antifungal therapy for thrush or candidal esophagitis. We reserve prophylactic antibiotic therapy for patients with an absolute neutrophil count less than 500 mcL. In this setting, we start levofloxacin 500 mg daily. Although these patients are at risk for invasive strongyloides infections, we manage this by screening patients with ATLL for strongyloides serology and stool parasites, and only initiating therapy if there is a positive result.

Metabolic complications

The profound hypercalcemia that often accompanies the acute type ATLL is nearly pathognomonic for this disease. Treatment is similar to the management for standard hypercalcemia, with aggressive intravenous hydration for volume expansion (with furosemide as needed), early bisphosphonate initiation, and close monitoring for cardiac arrhythmias. Most important is the rapid diagnosis and treatment of the ATLL, which is the only way to ensure that the calcium level responds for a sustainable period.

Central nervous system complications

Patients with aggressive ATLL are at high risk for CNS complications. All patients with aggressive ATLL should have brain imaging to assess for parenchymal involvement at diagnosis, as well as an LP to evaluate for leptomeningeal disease. The LP can be deferred to the first administration of intrathecal (IT) chemotherapy. Cerebrospinal fluid (CSF) should be sent for chemistry, cell count, cytology, and flow cytometry. If the CSF is negative, then all patients with aggressive ATLL should have prophylactic IT chemotherapy given with systemic treatment. At our institution, we prefer a combination of methotrexate, cytarabine, and hydrocortisone. CSF positive for ATLL involvement should prompt more aggressive IT therapy with twice-weekly administration until the CSF clears, followed by greater intervals to prevent relapse.

Tumor lysis syndrome

As in all aggressive hematologic malignancies, patients with ATLL are at risk for TLS. Early and aggressive intravenous hydration, along with allopurinol administration, is of the utmost importance. Because G6PD deficiency is common in men of African descent, the authors send for G6PD testing early in the presentation so that we have the option of using rasburicase for severe TLS. Prompt diagnosis and treatment of the underlying ATLL is paramount.

Future Directions

Future treatment modalities are likely to focus on agents that show response in T-cell lymphomas, such as the histone deacetylase inhibitors (vorinostat, panobinostat, and romidepsin), the aurora A kinase inhibitor alisertib, and the antimetabolite pralatrexate. In addition, agents showing efficacy in B-cell lymphomas may prove useful in T-cell lymphomas, and possibly ATLL. These agents include the phosphoinositide 3-kinase inhibitors, Bruton tyrosine kinase inhibitors, and the proteasome inhibitors. Another important group of novel therapies is the immune checkpoint inhibitors. Preliminary results were reported at American Society of Hematology (ASH) 2014 regarding the use of a programmed cell death protein 1 (PD-1) inhibitor, nivolumab, in relapsed lymphoid malignancies.[68] Although nivolumab had some activity in 5 cases of PTCL (PR, 40%), there were no complete or partial response in patients with other T-cell lymphomas.

A nascent treatment approach is the direct targeting of Tax via anti-Tax vaccines. This approach was studied in a recent pilot study in which 3 previously treated patients received an autologous dendritic cell vaccine with Tax peptides corresponding with a cytotoxic T-lymphocyte (CTL) epitope.[69] All patients had a Tax-specific CTL response, and 2 patients had a partial response at 8 weeks, which was maintained for at least 19 months. The third patient had stable disease at 8 weeks, then slowly progressed. Further research is needed to fully evaluate this therapeutic approach.

Due to its rarity and aggressiveness, ATLL is suboptimal for evaluation in clinical trials. Despite this, clinical trial data from the United States are desperately needed. In order to evaluate rare lymphomas, including ATLL, several Boston-area hospitals including, Boston University Medical Center, Dana-Farber Cancer Institute, Massachusetts General Hospital, and Beth Israel Deaconess Medical Center have joined with the University of North Carolina at Chapel Hill to form the Rare Lymphoma Working Group (RLWG). An ATLL project evaluating brentuximab vedotin with cyclophosphamide, doxorubicin, etoposide, and prednisone (BV-CHEP) is ongoing and will serve as the prototype for the working group. If successful, we can focus on other regimens for ATLL, as well as treatment approaches for other rare types of lymphoma.

CONCLUSION

Adult T-cell leukemia/lymphoma (ATLL) is a rare T-cell disorder that is etiologically linked to chronic infection with human T-cell lymphotropic virus type 1. ATLL is divided into four subtypes: acute, lymphomatous, chronic, and smoldering. Treatment strategies traditionally have focused on antiviral therapy with zidovudine and interferon-alpha, as well as combination chemotherapy. The current therapeutic approach in the United States is to give a CHOP-like regimen containing etoposide (either CHOEP or DA-EPOCH), but this is suboptimal. Novel therapeutic approaches include the use of antibody-drug conjugates (brentuximab vedotin), anti-CCR4 therapy, immunomodulatory therapy, and anti-TAX vaccines. Future research must focus on multi-institutional clinical trial participation because of the rarity of this deadly hematologic malignancy.

REFERENCES

1. Poiesz BJ, Ruscetti FW, Gazdar AF, et al. Detection and isolation of type C retrovirus particles from fresh and cultured lymphocytes of a patient with cutaneous T-cell lymphoma. Proc Natl Acad Sci U S A 1980;77(12):7415–9.
2. Poiesz BJ, Ruscetti FW, Reitz MS, et al. Isolation of a new type C retrovirus (HTLV) in primary uncultured cells of a patient with Sézary T-cell leukaemia. Nature 1981; 294:268–71.
3. Proietti FA, Carneiro-Proietti ABF, Catalan-Soares BC, et al. Global epidemiology of HTLV-1 infection and associated diseases. Oncogene 2005;24:6058–68.
4. Goncalves DU, Proietti FA, Ribas JGR, et al. Epidemiology, treatment, and prevention of human T-cell leukemia virus 1-associated diseases. Clin Microbiol Rev 2010;23(3):577–89.
5. Courouce AM, Pillonel J, Lemaire JM, et al. HTLV testing in blood transfusion. Vox Sang 1998;74:165–9.
6. Centers for Disease Control and Prevention. Human T-lymphotropic virus type I screening in volunteer blood donors – United States, 1989. MMWR Morb Mortal Wkly Rep 1990;39(50):915, 921–4.

7. International Agency for Research on Cancer. IARC monographs on the evaluation of carcinogenic risks to humans, volume 100B. Biological Agents. Lyon (France): IARC; 2012. Available at: http://monographs.iarc.fr/ENG/Monographs/vol100B.

8. Hino S, Katamine S, Miyata H, et al. Primary prevention of HTLV-1 in Japan. Leukemia 1997;11:57–9.

9. De Martel C, Ferlay J, Franceschi S, et al. Global burden of cancers attributable to infections in 2008: A review and synthetic analysis. Lancet Oncol 2012;13:607–15.

10. Yoshida N, Chihara D. Incidence of adult T-cell leukemia/lymphoma in nonendemic areas. Curr Treat Options Oncol 2015;16(7):1–8.

11. Fujikawa D, Nakagawa S, Hori M, et al. Polycomb-dependent epigenetic landscape in adult T-cell leukemia. Blood 2016;127:1790–802.

12. Bazarbachi A. Tax fingerprint in adult T-cell leukemia. Blood 2016;127:1737–8.

13. Bazerbachi A, Suarez F, Fields P, et al. How I treat adult T-cell leukemia/lymphoma. Blood 2011;118:1736–45.

14. Satou Y, Yasunaga J, Yoshida M, et al. HTLV-1 basic leucine zipper factor gene mRNA supports proliferation of adult T cell leukemia cells. Proc Natl Acad Sci U S A 2006;103:720–5.

15. Shimoyama M. Diagnostic criteria and classification of clinical subtypes of adult T-cell leukaemia-lymphoma. Br J Haematol 1991;79:428–37.

16. Utsunomiya A, Choi I, Chihara D, et al. Recent advances in the treatment of adult T-cell leukemia-lymphomas. Cancer Sci 2015;106(4):344–51.

17. Nosaka K, Miyamoto T, Sakai T, et al. Mechanism of hypercalcemia in adult T-cell leukemia: overexpression of receptor activator of nuclear factor kB ligand on adult T-cell leukemia cells. Blood 2002;99:634–40.

18. Nadella MVP, Dirksen WP, Nadella KS, et al. Transcriptional regulation of parathyroid hormone-related protein promoter P2 by NF-kB in adult T-cell leukemia/lymphoma. Leukemia 2007;21:1752–62.

19. Bellon M, Ko NL, Lee MJ, et al. Adult T-cell leukemia cells overexpress Wnt5a and promote osteoclast differentiation. Blood 2013;121:5045–54.

20. Ogata M, Ogata Y, Kohno K, et al. Eosinophilia associated with adult T-cell leukemia: role of interleukin 5 and granulocyte-macrophage colony-stimulating factor. Am J Hematol 1998;59:242–5.

21. Katsuya H, Ishitsuka K, Utsunomiya A, et al. Treatment and survival among 1594 patients with ATL. Blood 2015;126:2570–7.

22. Suzumiya J, Ohshima K, Tamura K, et al. The international prognostic index predicts outcome in aggressive adult T-cell leukemia/lymphoma: analysis of 126 patients from the international peripheral T-cell lymphoma project. Ann Oncol 2009;20:715–21.

23. Katsuya H, Yamanaka T, Ishitsuka K, et al. Prognostic index for acute- and lymphoma-type adult T-cell leukemia/lymphoma. J Clin Oncol 2012;30:1635–40.

24. Takasaki Y, Iwanaga M, Tsukasaki K, et al. Impact of visceral involvements and blood cell count abnormalities on survival in adult T-cell leukemia/lymphoma (ATLL). Leuk Res 2007;31:751–7.

25. Utsunomiya A, Ishida T, Inagaki A, et al. Clinical significance of a blood eosinophilia in adult T-cell leukemia/lymphoma: a blood eosinophilia is a significant unfavorable prognostic factor. Leuk Res 2007;31:915–20.

26. Campuzano-Zuluaga G, Pimentel A, Diaz LA, et al. CD30 expression is associated with decreased survival in patients with acute and unfavorable chronic types of adult T-cell leukemia-lymphoma. Blood 2013;122:4312.

27. Hermine O, Allard I, Levy V, et al. A prospective phase II clinical trial with the use of zidovudine and interferon-alpha in the acute and lymphoma forms of adult T-cell leukemia/lymphoma. Hematol J 2002;3:276–82.

28. Bazerbachi A, Plumelle Y, Ramos JC, et al. Meta-analysis on the use of zidovudine and interferon-alpha in adult T-cell leukemia/lymphoma showing improved survival in the leukemic subtypes. J Clin Oncol 2010;28:4177–83.

29. Hodson A, Crichton S, Montoto S, et al. Use of zidovudine and interferon alfa with chemotherapy improves survival in both acute and lymphoma subtypes of adult T-cell leukemia/lymphoma. J Clin Oncol 2011;29:4696–701.

30. Bazerbachi A, El-Sabban ME, Nasr R, et al. Arsenic trioxide and interferon-alpha synergize to induce cell cycle arrest and apoptosis in human T-cell lymphotropic virus type I-transformed cells. Blood 1999;93:278–83.

31. Hermine O, Dombret H, Poupon J, et al. Phase II trial of arsenic trioxide and alpha interferon in patients with relapsed/refractory adult T-cell leukemia/lymphoma. Hematol J 2004;5:130–4.

32. Kchour G, Tarhini M, Kooshyar MM, et al. Phase 2 study of the efficacy and safety of the combination of arsenic trioxide, interferon alpha, and zidovudine in newly diagnosed chronic adult T-cell leukemia/lymphoma (ATL). Blood 2009;113: 6528–32.

33. National Comprehensive Cancer Network. Non-Hodgkin's lymphomas (version 3.2016). Available at: https://www.nccn.org/professionals/physician_gls/pdf/nhl.pdf. Accessed May 13, 2016.

34. Tsukasaki K, Utsunomiya A, Fukuda H, et al. VCAP-AMP-VECP compared with biweekly CHOP for adult T-cell leukemia-lymphoma: Japan Clinical Oncology Group study (JCOG9801). J Clin Oncol 2007;25:5458–64.

35. Ellin F, Landstrom J, Jerkeman M, et al. Real-world data on prognostic factors and treatment in peripheral T-cell lymphomas: a study from the Swedish Lymphoma Registry. Blood 2014;124:1570–7.

36. Schmitz N, Trumper L, Ziepert M, et al. Treatment and prognosis of mature T-cell and NK-cell lymphoma: an analysis of patients with T-cell lymphoma treated in studies of the German High-Grade Non-Hodgkin Lymphoma Study Group. Blood 2010;116:3418–25.

37. Ratner L, Rauch D, Abel H, et al. Dose-adjusted EPOCH chemotherapy with bortezomib and raltegravir for human T-cell leukemia virus-associated adult T-cell leukemia lymphoma. Blood Cancer J 2016;6:e408.

38. Alduaij A, Butera JN, Treaba D, et al. Complete remission in two cases of adult T-cell leukemia/lymphoma treated with hyper-CVAD: a case report and review of the literature. Clin Lymphoma Myeloma Leuk 2010;16:76–81.

39. Tsukasaki K, Tobinai K, Hotta T, et al. Lymphoma study group of JCOG. Jpn J Clin Oncol 2012;42:85–95.

40. Shimoyama M, Ichimaru M, Yunoki K, et al. Final results of cooperative study of VEPA [vincristine, cyclophosphamide (Endoxan), prednisolone and Adriamycin] therapy in advanced adult non-Hodgkin's lymphoma: relation between T- or B-cell phenotype and response. Jpn J Clin Oncol 1982;12:227–37.

41. Shimoyama M, Ota K, Kikuchi M, et al. Chemotherapeutic results and prognostic factors of patients with advanced non-Hodgkin's lymphoma treated with VEPA or VEPA-M. J Clin Oncol 1988;6:128–41.

42. Tobinai K, Shimoyama M, Minato K, et al. Japan Clinical Oncology Group phase II trial of second-generation 'LSG4 protocol' in aggressive T- and B-lymphoma: a new predictive model for T- and B-lymphoma [abstract]. Proc - Am Soc Clin Oncol, Meet 1994;13:378a.

43. Yamada Y, Tomonaga M, Fukuda H, et al. A new G-CSF-supported combination chemotherapy, LSG15, for adult T-cell leukemia-lymphoma (ATL): Japan Clinical Oncology Group (JCOG) Study 9303. Br J Haematol 2001;113:375–82.

44. Ishida T, Joh T, Uike N, et al. Defucosylated anti-CCR4 monoclonal antibody (KW-0761) for relapsed adult T-cell leukemia-lymphoma: a multicenter phase II study. J Clin Oncol 2012;30:837–42.

45. Yoshie O, Fujisawa R, Nakayama T, et al. Frequent expression of CCR4 in adult T-cell leukemia and human T-cell leukemia virus type 1-transformed T cells. Blood 2002;99:1505–11.

46. Ishida T, Utsunomiya A, Iida S, et al. Clinical significance of CCR4 expression in adult T-cell leukemia/lymphoma: its close association with skin involvement and unfavorable outcome. Clin Cancer Res 2003;9:3625–34.

47. Ishida T, Jo T, Takemoto S, et al. Dose-intensified chemotherapy alone or in combination with mogamulizumab in newly diagnosed aggressive adult T-cell leukaemia-lymphoma: a randomized phase II study. Br J Haematol 2015;169: 672–82.

48. Fuji S, Inoue Y, Utsunomiya A, et al. Pretransplantation anti-CCR4 antibody mogamulizumab against adult T-cell leukemia/lymphoma is associated with significantly increased risks of severe and corticosteroid-refractory graft-versus-host disease, nonrelapse mortality, and overall mortality. J Clin Oncol 2016;34:1–8.

49. Younes A, Bartlett NL, Leonard JP, et al. Brentuximab vedotin (SGN-35) for relapsed CD30-positive lymphomas. N Engl J Med 2010;363:1812–21.

50. Younes A, Gopal AK, Smith SE, et al. Results of a pivotal phase II study of brentuximab vedotin for patients with relapsed or refractory Hodgkin's lymphoma. J Clin Oncol 2012;30:2183–9.

51. Pro B, Advani R, Brice P, et al. Brentuximab vedotin (SGN-35) in patients with relapsed or refractory systemic anaplastic large-cell lymphoma: results of a phase II study. J Clin Oncol 2012;30:2190–6.

52. Horwitz SM, Advani RH, Bartlett NL, et al. Objective responses in relapsed T-cell lymphomas with single-agent brentuximab vedotin. Blood 2014;123:3095–100.

53. Duvic M, Tetzlaff MT, Gangar P, et al. Results of a phase II trial of brentuximab vedotin for CD30+ cutaneous T-cell lymphoma and lymphomatoid papulosis. J Clin Oncol 2015;33:3759–65.

54. Jacobsen ED, Sharman JP, Oki Y, et al. Brentuximab vedotin demonstrates objective responses in a phase 2 study of relapsed/refractory DLBCL with variable CD30 expression. Blood 2015;125:1394–402.

55. Fanale MA, Horwitz SM, Forero-Torres A, et al. Brentuximab vedotin in the frontline treatment of patients with CD30+ peripheral T-cell lymphomas: results of a phase I study. J Clin Oncol 2014;32(28):3137–43.

56. O'Connor OA, Pro B, Illidge T, et al. Phase 3 trial of brentuximab vedotin and CHP versus CHOP in the frontline treatment of patients (pts) with CD30+ mature T-cell lymphomas (MTCL). J Clin Oncol 2014;32:5s (Suppl; abstr TPS8612).

57. Berkowitz JL, Janik JE, Stewart DM, et al. Safety, efficacy, and pharmacokinetics/pharmacodynamics of daclizumab (anti-CD25) in patients with adult T-cell leukemia/lymphoma. Clin Immunol 2014;155:176–87.

58. Ceesay MM, Matutes E, Taylor GP, et al. Phase II study on combination therapy with CHOP-Zenapax for HTLV-1 associated adult T-cell leukaemia/lymphoma (ATLL). Leuk Res 2012;36:857–61.

59. Ogura M, Imaizumi Y, Uike N, et al. Lenalidomide in relapsed adult T-cell leukaemia-lymphoma or peripheral T-cell lymphoma (ATLL-001): a phase 1, multicenter, dose-escalation study. Lancet Haematol 2016;3:e107–18.

60. Phillips AA, Giddings J, Lee SM, et al. Lenalidomide in patients with relapsed or refractory HTLV-1 related adult T-cell leukemia/lymphoma (ATLL). Int J Blood Res Disord 2015;2:1–3.

61. Fujiwara H, Ishida T, Nosaka K, et al. Multicenter phase II study of lenalidomide in patients with relapsed adult T-cell leukemia-lymphoma. Oral session presented at: 57th Annual Meeting & Exposition of the American Society of Hematology. Orlando (FL), December 5–8, 2015.

62. Hematopoietic Cell Transplantation in Japan. Annual report of nationwide survey 2013. Aichi, Japan: The Japanese Data Center for Hematopoietic Cell Transplantation/The Japan Society for Hematopoietic Cell Transplantation; 2014.

63. Hishizawa M, Kanda J, Utsunomiya A, et al. Transplantation of allogeneic hematopoietic stem cells for adult T-cell leukemia: a nationwide retrospective study. Blood 2011;116:1369–76.

64. Kanda J, Hishizawa M, Utsunomiya A, et al. Impact of graft-versus-host disease on outcomes after allogeneic hematopoietic cell transplantation for adult T-cell leukemia: a retrospective cohort study. Blood 2012;119:2141–8.

65. Ishida T, Hishizawa M, Kato K, et al. Allogeneic hematopoietic stem cell transplantation for adult T-cell leukemia lymphoma with special emphasis on preconditioning regimen: a nationwide retrospective study. Blood 2012;120:1734–41.

66. Okamura J, Utsunomiya A, Tanosaki R, et al. Allogeneic stem-cell transplantation with reduced conditioning intensity as a novel immunotherapy and antiviral therapy for adult T-cell leukemia/lymphoma. Blood 2005;105:4143–5.

67. Choi I, Tanosaki R, Uike N, et al. Long-term outcomes after hematopoietic SCT for adult T-cell leukemia/lymphoma: results of prospective trials. Bone Marrow Transplant 2011;46:116–8.

68. Lesokhin AM, Ansell SM, Armand P, et al. Preliminary results of a phase I study of nivolumab (BMS-936558) in patients with relapsed or refractory lymphoid malignancies. Oral session presented at: 56th ASH Annual Meeting and Exposition. San Francisco (CA), December 6–9, 2014.

69. Suehiro Y, Hasegawa A, Iino T, et al. Clinical outcomes of a novel therapeutic vaccine with Tax peptide-pulsed dendritic cells for adult T cell leukaemia/lymphoma in a pilot study. Br J Haematol 2015;169:356–67.

T-cell Prolymphocytic Leukemia

Amit Sud, MBChB, MRes, MRCP[a,b], Claire Dearden, BSc, MBBS, MD, FRCP, FRCPath[a,b],*

KEYWORDS

- T-cell prolymphocytic leukemia • T-cell • Leukemia • Alemtuzumab

KEY POINTS

- T-cell prolymphocytic leukemia is a rare and aggressive leukemia.
- The current therapeutic approach includes immunotherapy followed by a hematopoietic stem cell transplant in eligible cases.
- Genomic and molecular studies may increase our understanding of this disease, with the promise of novel therapeutic options.

INTRODUCTION

T-cell prolymphocytic leukemia (T-PLL) is a rare and aggressive T-cell malignancy first described by Catovsky and colleagues[1] more than 40 years ago. Although termed 'prolymphocytic,' the disease is characterized by the proliferation of post-thymic T-lymphocytes. T-PLL can be distinguished from other lymphoid diseases by the evaluation and integration of clinical features, morphology, immunopheno-typing, cyto-genetics, and molecular features. The current therapeutic approach re-lies on immunotherapy followed by a hematopoietic stem cell transplant (HSCT) in selected cases. Clinical outcomes are generally poor, although insights from genomic and molecular studies may increase our understanding of this disease, with the promise of additional effective therapeutic options.

EPIDEMIOLOGY

T-PLL accounts for 2% of mature lymphocytic leukemia in adults.[2] The median age at presentation is 61 years and there is a male predominance.[3] Three cases of children with T-PLL have been reported, although incomplete diagnostics were reported in

Disclosure Statement: A. Sud has no conflict of interest to declare. C. Dearden undertakes con-sultancy for Genzyme.
[a] Department of Haemato-Oncology, The Royal Marsden Biomedical Research Centre, London, UK; [b] Department of Haemato-Oncology, The Royal Marsden NHS Foundation Trust, Downs Road, Sutton, Surrey SM2 5PT, UK
* Corresponding author. Department of Haemato-Oncology, The Royal Marsden NHS Founda-tion Trust, Downs Road, Sutton, Surrey SM2 5PT, UK.
E-mail address: Claire.Dearden@rmh.nhs.uk

1 case.[4–6] Patients with ataxia telangiectasia are at increased risk of developing T-PLL (as well as other lymphoid malignancies) with a younger median age at presentation of approximately 31 years.[7] An individual with Nijmegen breakage syndrome developing T-PLL has been reported.[8] Aside from these findings, no other genetic or environmental risk factor has been robustly identified thus far.

CLINICAL FEATURES

Most patients with T-PLL present with a brief history of B symptoms, hepatosplenomegaly (splenomegaly is often massive) and a marked lymphocytosis (typically >100 × 10^9/l).[3] Lymphadenopathy, although present in a majority of patients, is rarely bulky. Anemia and thrombocytopenia are seen in up to one-half of patients.[3] Erythematous or nodular skin rashes involving the trunk or limbs, peripheral edema, and pleuroperitoneal effusions may be seen in up to one-quarter of patients with T-PLL.[9] T-PLL may also involve the face, where it manifests as purpura and edema, often in a periorbital distribution.[10,11] Central nervous system involvement is rare. A minority of patients have no symptoms at diagnosis. This 'indolent' phase can persist for a variable length of time, and can be as long as years. Disease progression may be rapid when it occurs.

LABORATORY DIAGNOSIS

The diagnosis of T-PLL relies on an integrated evaluation of clinical features, peripheral blood, morphology, immunophenotyping, bone marrow, cytogenetics, and molecular tests.

Morphology

The 'typical' morphology observed in 75% of cases consists of medium sized lymphoid cells with partial chromatin condensation, a visible nucleolus, and a round or oval nucleus (**Fig. 1**).[2,9] A slight basophilic cytoplasm is present, often with protrusions and an absence of granules. A 'small cell variant' is seen in 20% of cases. These small cells possess condensed chromatin with a small nucleolus (observed only by electron microscopy). Finally, the 'cerebriform (Sézary cell–like) variant' is seen in

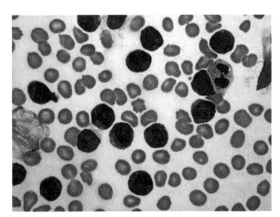

Fig. 1. Peripheral blood smear from a patient with T-prolymphocytic leukemia demonstrating a 'typical' morphology. The T-prolymphocytic leukemia cells are medium sized lymphoid cells with partial chromatin condensation and a visible nucleolus. The cytoplasm is basophilic with protrusions and an absence of granules.

5% of patients in which the morphology resembles the Sézary cells seen in the Sézary syndrome/mycosis fungoides. The bone marrow is infiltrated in an interstitial pattern by cells with a similar morphology to that seen in the peripheral blood. Skin biopsy of affected areas demonstrates a wide cytomorphologic spectrum similar to that observed in the peripheral blood with a perivascular or diffuse dermal infiltrate, sometimes with accompanying hemorrhage.[10,11] These findings are distinct from mycosis fungoides in which atypical small to medium sized T-cells (with characteristic 'cerebriform' nuclei) infiltrate the epidermis and upper dermis, form Pautrier's microabscesses with Langerhans cells, and accumulate along the basal layer of the epidermis (termed 'string of pearls').[12] The spleen demonstrates an atrophied white pulp with dense lymphoid infiltrates in the red pulp that invade the capsule. Lymph node involvement is diffuse, often with prominent high-endothelial venules.

Immunophenotype

Flow cytometry confirms a post-thymic T-cell population (TDT⁻, CD1A⁻, CD5⁺, CD2⁺, CD7⁺).[2] The majority of cases are CD4⁺/CD8⁻. Dual CD4⁺/CD8⁺ cells occur in approximately 25% of cases (this is unique to the postthymic T-cell malignancies) and only a minority of cases express a CD4⁻/CD8⁺ phenotype. CD52 is expressed strongly. Cytoplasmic CD3 is always present, but the membrane expression may be weak or negative. Natural killer cell and cytoplasmic granule markers are consistently negative. Typically CD7 expression is strong, whereas CD25 may be negative, thus helping to distinguish T-PLL from adult T-cell leukemia and the Sézary syndrome. T-PLL patients are also negative for human T-cell leukemia virus type 1.

Molecular Genetics

T-cell receptor genes are rearranged and are identical, confirming a clonal expansion of T-cells. Although cytogenetic and mutational analysis does not alter management, the identification of abnormalities can aid diagnosis as well as provide insight into the pathogenesis of T-PLL.

The most frequently observed group of cytogenetic abnormalities involve chromosome 14 (90%). These may take the form of inv(14), t(14;14)(q11;q32), which involve the TCL1A and TCL1B locus and t(X;14)(q28;q11) involving a homolog of TCL1, MTCP1 (mature T cell proliferation 1 gene), which is located on the X chromosome.[13] Transgenic mouse models have confirmed the oncogenic roles of TCL1 and MTCP1,[14,15] and functional work identifies TCL1 as an Akt kinase coactivator, promoting cell survival and proliferation.[16] Cytogenetic abnormalities involving chromosome 8 are the next most frequently observed (idic(8p11), t(8;8) and trisomy 8q).[17,18] Other recurrent abnormalities seen with conventional techniques include loss of 11q23 (ATM inactivation) together with additional losses (22q, 13q, 6q, 9p, 12p, 17p) and gains (22q and 6p).[17,18] 12p13 deletion, which probably occurs in up to one-half of T-PLL cases, is thought to contribute to the pathogenesis of T-PLL by causing haploinsufficiency of CDKN1B.[19] With the advent of high-throughput sequencing, additional mutations in T-PLL have been identified. These include highly recurrent, largely exclusive, gain-of-function mutations involving IL2RG, JAK1/3, and STAT5B, which lead to constitutive STAT5 signaling (**Fig. 2**).[20–22] Deleterious mutations in EZH2, FBXW10, and CHEK2 may further contribute to the pathogenesis of T-PLL through their roles in DNA repair, epigenetic transcriptional regulation, and proteasome degradation pathways.[20] Further genomic analysis, including sequential tumor sequencing, may define driver mutations and also the clonal architecture of T-PLL. Understanding the functional consequence of these mutations is essential in furthering our understanding of T-PLL and developing novel therapeutics.[20]

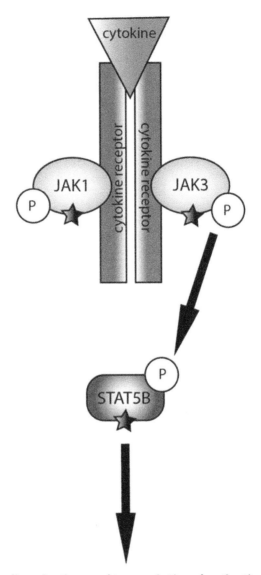

dimerization and transcriptional activation

Fig. 2. A pathway diagram illustrates the interaction of JAK1, JAK3, and STAT5B during cytokine activation. Cytokine binding results in JAK autophosphorylaton, leading to STAT recruitment and activation through tyrosine phosphorylation. Activated STAT proteins then dimerize and translocate to the nucleus to regulate transcription of numerous genes involved in differentiation, proliferation, and survival. Mutated components of the JAK1–JAK3–STAT5B pathway are highlighted (*star*). Mutations have also been described in IL2RG, which is a cytokine receptor. P, phosphate group, covalently bound to a protein.

TREATMENT

Owing to the rarity of T-PLL, few published data exist regarding treatment. No randomized clinical trials have been conducted. The following recommendations are based on best available evidence and personal experience.

Watch and Wait

Not all patients diagnosed with T-PLL require treatment immediately. Chemo-immunotherapy can be associated with significant toxicity and, aside from HSCT, current chemoimmunotherapy regimens in T-PLL are not curative. Furthermore, some patients present with an 'indolent phase' of the disease. Although disease progression occurs eventually, patients can be monitored for years before requiring intervention. Close monitoring (eg, blood count and clinical examination at regular intervals) is required because disease progression can be rapid and fatal. A pretreatment lymphocyte doubling time of less than 8.5 months has been shown to be associated with a worse outcome,[23] although an absolute lymphocyte count with lymphocyte doubling time should be taken into consideration when deciding on treatment initiation. Indications for treatment include B symptoms; symptomatic anemia or thrombocytopenia; disease infiltration in the skin, lungs, or central nervous system; and progressive disease demonstrated by an increasing lymphocytosis or rapidly enlarging spleen, liver, or lymph nodes.

First-Line Therapy

Treatment is initiated with the aim of attaining a complete response (CR) and patients should be offered a clinical trial when available. There is a limited response to conventional treatment regimens such as alkylating agents or anthracyclines, with a median overall survival (OS) of 7 months in historical series.[3] In the absence of a clinical trial, patients should be offered an alemtuzumab (anti-CD52) regimen. This was used initially more than 2 decades ago and was first used owing to the strong CD52 expression on treatment-naïve T-PLL cells. Studies suggest an overall response rate (ORR) of greater than 80% in the first-line setting and in 50% to 76% of relapsed-refractory cases (**Table 1**).[24–27] Although progression-free survival (PFS) is longer when compared with other therapies (>1 year in responders), relapse invariably occurs and there are few long-term survivors, with a median OS from treatment of less than 2 years. For this reason, eligible patients should be considered for consolidation therapies such as HSCT. The results of alemtuzumab therapy compare favorably with outcomes reported with the use of purine analogues in which ORR are less than 50% and remission durations are less than 1 year.[28–30] Single-agent pentostatin has shown the greatest efficacy of all purine analogues in T-PLL,[28] although no randomized, controlled trials have directly compared single agent pentostatin and alemtuzumab. The use of pentostatin is discussed further in relapsed/refractory disease. Small, prospective studies have evaluated the use of alemtuzumab in combination with chemotherapy agents. For example, Hopfinger and colleagues[31] reported a prospective, multicenter, phase II trial investigating the use of fludarabine, mitoxantrone, and cyclophosphamide induction followed by alemtuzumab in 16 treatment-naïve patients and 9 previously treated patients. The ORR to fludarabine, mitoxantrone, and cyclophosphamide therapy was 68%, increasing to 92% after the addition of alemtuzumab. The median OS and PFS were 17.1 months and 11.9 months, respectively. Alemtuzumab increases an individual's susceptibility to opportunistic infections. Patients should, therefore, be on appropriate antibacterial and antiviral prophylaxis and under-go serologic testing for cytomegalovirus (CMV), herpes simplex virus, and hepatitis B and C before the commencement of treatment. In individuals who are seropositive for CMV before commencing alemtuzumab, serial CMV viral load should be monitored for the early detection and management of CMV reactivation. Owing to the risk of infertility with chemotherapy and HSCT, men and women should receive appropriate counseling and options for fertility preservation before commencing any treatment. Intravenous

Table 1
Treatment trials in T-PLL (>10 patients)

Regimen	Number of Patients	CR (%)	ORR (%)	MPFS Months	MS Months	Reference
Alemtuzumab (IV)	39 pretreated	60	76	7	10	Dearden,[41] 2012
Alemtuzumab (IV)	32 untreated	81	91	—	—	Dearden et al,[32] 2011
Bendamustine	9 pretreated 6 untreated	20	53	5	8.7	Herbaux et al,[38] 2015
FMC, then alemtuzumab (IV)	9 pretreated 16 untreated	24 (FMC) 48 (alemtuzumab)	92 for all 25 patients 68 after FMC 95 in 21 patients receiving alemtuzumab	11.5	17.1	Hopfinger et al,[31] 2013
Pentostatin + alemtuzumab (IV)	13 (pretreated + untreated)	62	69	7.8	10.2	Ravandi et al,[37] 2009

Abbreviations: CR, complete remission; FMC, fludarabine, mitoxantrone, and cyclophosphamide; IV, intravenous; MPFS, median progression-free survival; MS, median overall survival; ORR, overall response rate; T-PLL, T-cell prolymphocytic leukemia.

administration of alemtuzumab is more effective than subcutaneous administration.[32] Infusion reactions are common with alemtuzumab and measures should be used to reduce the severity and occurrence of infusional reactions. One month after the completion of therapy, response to treatment should be measured by history, physical examination, full blood count, bone marrow aspirate and biopsy, and computed tomography of the chest, abdomen, and pelvis. Response is defined using the criteria created for disease assessment in chronic lymphocytic leukemia.

Postremission Therapy

Approximately 80% of patients achieve a CR after alemtuzumab treatment. However, without additional therapy, a majority of patients relapse within 2 years. HSCT is used to consolidate responses in eligible patients. A number of studies have investigated the use of HSCT in T-PLL and suggest that OS can be improved and in a minority of cases can achieve a cure (**Table 2**).[33–36] The main challenges to contend with are the treatment-related mortality (TRM) and risk of relapse. A retrospective study by Guillaume and colleagues[35] reported 27 patients undergoing allogeneic HSCT (14 of who were in CR at time of HSCT). The relapse rate at 3 years was 47%, with a TRM of 31% and an OS of 36%. The European Group for Blood and Marrow Transplantation Registry had 41 patients with T-PLL who had received an allogeneic HCT.[34] The 3-year OS was 21% with TRM and relapse rates of 41% (although nearly one half of the patients had refractory disease at the time of transplantation). We reported a similar TRM rate and lower 3-year relapse rate from a smaller cohort of patients, although a greater proportion of patients in our study were in CR, highlighting the importance of disease status at time of HSCT.[33] Although the number of patients is small, we also demonstrated similar OS in patients who received an autologous SCT compared with those who received an allogenic SCT.[33] Although not offering a cure, given the lower risk of treatment-related toxicity, autologous SCT may be an option for less fit patients. Relapse after HSCT is usually within 2 years, but can occur late. Given the increasing use of reduced-intensity conditioning and matched unrelated donors, as well as improvements in supportive care, more patients are eligible for HSCT, and the data that exist currently regarding HSCT may not be applicable to prospective cohorts of T-PLL patients.

Therapy for Relapsed and Refractory Disease

Few data exist regarding the treatment of relapsed or refractory disease. Approximately one half of the patients who relapse after a previous response to alemtuzumab can achieve a second disease remission with further alemtuzumab therapy, although this is usually of shorter duration. Flow cytometry should be repeated as T-PLL cells can lose CD52 expression.

Patients who fail to achieve a remission with single-agent alemtuzumab should have pentostatin added to the treatment regimen. Although no randomized trials have compared single-agent therapy with combination therapy, pentostatin has demonstrated efficacy as a single agent in a small, retrospective study. The ORR was 45%, independent of previous treatment with a median PFS and OS of 6 and 9 months, respectively.[28] A phase II study evaluated combination alemtuzumab with pentostatin in 13 patients with newly diagnosed or relapsed or refractory T-PLL. The ORR was 69% with a median OS and PFS of 10.2 and 7.8 months, respectively.[37] Despite adequate prophylaxis, common side effects included infection (including CMV reactivation) as well as neutropenia, thrombocytopenia, anemia, and nausea.

Other treatment options include nelarabine or bendamustine, although durable remissions with these therapies are uncommon.[30] Herbaux and colleagues[38] reported

Table 2
Allogeneic stem cell transplant in T-cell prolymphocytic leukemia

Number of Patients	Median Age in Years (Range)	Disease Status at Transplant	TRM at 3 y (%)	Relapse Rate at 3 y (%)	Median OS (mo)	3 Y OS (%)	Reference
13	51 (39–61)	10 CR, 1 PR	31	33	33	62	Krishnan et al,[33] 2010
41	51 (24–71)	11 CR, 12 PR	41	41	—	21	Wiktor-Jedrzejczak et al,[34] 2012
27	54 (36–65)	14 CR	31	47	—	36	Guillaume et al,[35] 2015

Abbreviations: CR, complete remission; OS, overall survival; PR, partial remission; TRM, transplant-related mortality.

15 patients with T-PLL treated with bendamustine, 7 of whom had failed front-line therapy with alemtuzumab. The ORR was 53% (20% CR), median PFS of 5 months and OS of 8.7 months, independent of prior exposure to alemtuzumab. The treatment of patients with relapsed or refractory disease is currently suboptimal. Effective novel therapies are needed to improve the outcome for these patients.

Novel Therapies

New approaches aim to use our expanding knowledge of T-PLL to target pathways involved in disease pathogenesis and resistance. Given the high frequency of mutations observed, and the perturbed signaling pathways, small molecule inhibitors targeting JAK-STAT pathway represents a therapeutic strategy available for patients. Pimozide, a STAT5 inhibitor, has been shown to induce apoptosis in primary T-PLL cells.[20] Histone-deacetlyase inhibitors in combination with hypomethylating agents aim to act synergistically to increase the expression of silenced tumor suppressor genes. The combination of cladribine and alemtuzumab with or without a histone-deacetlyase inhibitor can overcome alemtuzumab resistance and induce the expression of other molecules liable to targeting with additional agents.[39] Cells with inactive ATM demonstrate impaired DNA double-strand break repair capabilities. Poly (ADP-ribose) polymerase inhibition imposes the requirement for DNA double strand break repair capabilities and therefore selectively sensitize ATM-deficient tumor cells to killing.[40] Finally, chimeric antigen receptor natural killer cells targeting CD7 may represent a novel therapeutic avenue not yet explored.

SUMMARY

T-PLL is a rare lymphoid malignancy with an aggressive clinical course and poor prognosis. Careful evaluation of clinical features and laboratory tests are necessary to make an accurate diagnosis and ensure appropriate prognostication and treatment. Current therapy relies on alemtuzumab followed by an HSCT in eligible patients achieving a CR. In patients with relapsed or refractory disease, pentostatin can be added. Clinical outcomes are generally poor, although our increased understanding of the biology of T-PLL offers the promise of additional effective therapeutic options.

REFERENCES

1. Catovsky D, Galetto J, Okos A, et al. Prolymphocytic leukaemia of B and T cell type. Lancet 1973;2(7823):232–4.
2. Swerdlow S, Campo E, Harris N. World Health Organization classification of tumours of haematopoietic and lymphoid tissues. Lyon (France): IARC Press; 2008.
3. Matutes E, Brito-Babapulle V, Swansbury J, et al. Clinical and laboratory features of 78 cases of T-prolymphocytic leukemia. Blood 1991;78(12):3269–74.
4. Bellone M, Svensson AM, Zaslav AL, et al. Pediatric T-cell prolymphocytic leukemia with an isolated 12(p13) deletion and aberrant CD117 expression. Exp Hematol Oncol 2012;1(1):7.
5. Mitton B, Coutre S, Willert J, et al. A pediatric case of T-cell prolymphocytic leukemia. Pediatr Blood Cancer 2015;62(6):1061–2.
6. Moser AM, Quider AA, Groen JA, et al. A gamma/delta T-cell receptor prolymphocytic leukemia and CD4-/CD8- double-negative immunophenotype in a pediatric patient. J Pediatr Hematol Oncol 2015;37(4):e218–219.
7. Suarez F, Mahlaoui N, Canioni D, et al. Incidence, presentation, and prognosis of malignancies in ataxia-telangiectasia: a report from the French National Registry of Primary Immune Deficiencies. J Clin Oncol 2015;33(2):202–8.

8. Michallet AS, Lesca G, Radford-Weiss I, et al. T-cell prolymphocytic leukemia with autoimmune manifestations in Nijmegen breakage syndrome. Ann Hematol 2003; 82(8):515–7.

9. Ravandi F, O'Brien S. Chronic lymphoid leukemias other than chronic lymphocytic leukemia: diagnosis and treatment. Mayo Clin Proc 2005;80(12):1660–74.

10. Magro CM, Morrison CD, Heerema N, et al. T-cell prolymphocytic leukemia: an aggressive T cell malignancy with frequent cutaneous tropism. J Am Acad Dermatol 2006;55(3):467–77.

11. Herling M, Valbuena JR, Jones D, et al. Skin involvement in T-cell prolymphocytic leukemia. J Am Acad Dermatol 2007;57(3):533–4.

12. Song SX, Willemze R, Swerdlow SH, et al. Mycosis fungoides. Report of the 2011 Society for Hematopathology/European Association for Haematopathology Workshop. Am J Clin Pathol 2013;139(4):466–90.

13. Maljaei SH, Brito-Babapulle V, Hiorns LR, et al. Abnormalities of chromosomes 8, 11, 14, and X in T-prolymphocytic leukemia studied by fluorescence in situ hybridization. Cancer Genet Cytogenet 1998;103(2):110–6.

14. Gritti C, Dastot H, Soulier J, et al. Transgenic mice for MTCP1 Develop T-Cell Prolymphocytic Leukemia. Blood 1998;92(2):368–73.

15. Virgilio L, Lazzeri C, Bichi R, et al. Deregulated expression of TCL1 causes T cell leukemia in mice. Proc Natl Acad Sci U S A 1998;95(7):3885–9.

16. Laine J, Kunstle G, Obata T, et al. The protooncogene TCL1 is an Akt kinase coactivator. Mol Cell 2000;6(2):395–407.

17. Costa D, Queralt R, Aymerich M, et al. High levels of chromosomal imbalances in typical and small-cell variants of T-cell prolymphocytic leukemia. Cancer Genet Cytogenet 2003;147(1):36–43.

18. Soulier J, Pierron G, Vecchione D, et al. A complex pattern of recurrent chromosomal losses and gains in T-cell prolymphocytic leukemia. Genes Chromosomes Cancer 2001;31(3):248–54.

19. Le Toriellec E, Despouy G, Pierron G, et al. Haploinsufficiency of CDKN1B contributes to leukemogenesis in T-cell prolymphocytic leukemia. Blood 2008; 111(4):2321–8.

20. Kiel MJ, Velusamy T, Rolland D, et al. Integrated genomic sequencing reveals mutational landscape of T-cell prolymphocytic leukemia. Blood 2014;124(9): 1460–72.

21. Bellanger D, Jacquemin V, Chopin M, et al. Recurrent JAK1 and JAK3 somatic mutations in T-cell prolymphocytic leukemia. Leukemia 2014;28(2):417–9.

22. Lopez C, Bergmann AK, Paul U, et al. Genes encoding members of the JAK-STAT pathway or epigenetic regulators are recurrently mutated in T-cell prolymphocytic leukaemia. Br J Haematol 2016;173(2):265–73.

23. Herling M, Patel KA, Teitell MA, et al. High TCL1 expression and intact T-cell receptor signaling define a hyperproliferative subset of T-cell prolymphocytic leukemia. Blood 2008;111(1):328–37.

24. Pawson R, Dyer MJ, Barge R, et al. Treatment of T-cell prolymphocytic leukemia with human CD52 antibody. J Clin Oncol 1997;15(7):2667–72.

25. Ferrajoli A, O'Brien SM, Cortes JE, et al. Phase II study of alemtuzumab in chronic lymphoproliferative disorders. Cancer 2003;98(4):773–8.

26. Keating MJ, Cazin B, Coutré S, et al. Campath-1H treatment of T-cell prolymphocytic leukemia in patients for whom at least one prior chemotherapy regimen has failed. J Clin Oncol 2002;20(1):205–13.

27. Dearden CE, Matutes E, Cazin B, et al. High remission rate in T-cell prolymphocytic leukemia with CAMPATH-1H. Blood 2001;98(6):1721–6.

28. Mercieca J, Matutes E, Dearden C, et al. The role of pentostatin in the treatment of T-cell malignancies: analysis of response rate in 145 patients according to disease subtype. J Clin Oncol 1994;12(12):2588–93.
29. Kantarjian HM, Childs C, O'Brien S, et al. Efficacy of fludarabine, a new adenine nucleoside analogue, in patients with prolymphocytic leukemia and the prolymphocytoid variant of chronic lymphocytic leukemia. Am J Med 1991;90(2):223–8.
30. Gandhi V, Tam C, O'Brien S, et al. Phase I trial of nelarabine in indolent leukemias. J Clin Oncol 2008;26(7):1098–105.
31. Hopfinger G, Busch R, Pflug N, et al. Sequential chemoimmunotherapy of fludarabine, mitoxantrone, and cyclophosphamide induction followed by alemtuzumab consolidation is effective in T-cell prolymphocytic leukemia. Cancer 2013; 119(12):2258–67.
32. Dearden CE, Khot A, Else M, et al. Alemtuzumab therapy in T-cell prolymphocytic leukemia: comparing efficacy in a series treated intravenously and a study piloting the subcutaneous route. Blood 2011;118(22):5799–802.
33. Krishnan B, Else M, Tjonnfjord GE, et al. Stem cell transplantation after alemtuzumab in T-cell prolymphocytic leukaemia results in longer survival than after alemtuzumab alone: a multicentre retrospective study. Br J Haematol 2010;149(6): 907–10.
34. Wiktor-Jedrzejczak W, Dearden C, de Wreede L, et al. Hematopoietic stem cell transplantation in T-prolymphocytic leukemia: a retrospective study from the European Group for Blood and Marrow Transplantation and the Royal Marsden Consortium. Leukemia 2012;26(5):972–6.
35. Guillaume T, Beguin Y, Tabrizi R, et al. Allogeneic hematopoietic stem cell transplantation for T-prolymphocytic leukemia: a report from the French Society for Stem Cell Transplantation (SFGM-TC). Eur J Haematol 2015;94(3):265–9.
36. Kalaycio ME, Kukreja M, Woolfrey AE, et al. Allogeneic hematopoietic cell transplant for prolymphocytic leukemia. Biol Blood Marrow Transplant 2010;16(4): 543–7.
37. Ravandi F, Aribi A, O'Brien S, et al. Phase II study of alemtuzumab in combination with pentostatin in patients with T-cell neoplasms. J Clin Oncol 2009;27(32): 5425–30.
38. Herbaux C, Genet P, Bouabdallah K, et al. Bendamustine is effective in T-cell prolymphocytic leukaemia. Br J Haematol 2015;168(6):916–9.
39. Hasanali ZS, Saroya BS, Stuart A, et al. Epigenetic therapy overcomes treatment resistance in T-cell prolymphocytic leukemia. Sci Transl Med 2015;7(293): 293ra102.
40. Weston VJ, Oldreive CE, Skowronska A, et al. The PARP inhibitor olaparib induces significant killing of ATM-deficient lymphoid tumor cells in vitro and in vivo. Blood 2010;116(22):4578–87.
41. Dearden C. How I treat prolymphocytic leukemia. Blood 2012;120(3):538–51.

Uncommon Variants of T-Cell Lymphomas

Neha Mehta-Shah, MD[a], Steven Horwitz, MD[b],*

KEYWORDS

- Peripheral T-cell lymphomas • Non-Hodgkin lymphoma
- Angioimmunoblastic T-cell lymphoma

KEY POINTS

- Peripheral T-cell lymphomas represent 10% to 15% of non-Hodgkin lymphomas and comprise more than 20 different entities.
- Treatment of very rare T-cell lymphomas can be challenging because there are no large or randomized studies to guide clinical decision making and treatment paradigms are often based on small series or imperfect data.
- Although a strict algorithm cannot be written with certainty, through the literature that exists and clinical experience, themes and principles of approaches do emerge that when coupled with clinical judgment allow reasonable and logical decisions.

INTRODUCTION

As discussed in the prior sections, peripheral T-cell lymphomas (PTCLs) represent 10% to 15% of non-Hodgkin lymphomas (NHLs) and comprise more than 20 different entities. Given the uncommon occurrence of this heterogenous group of disorders, many of the current treatment strategies are borrowed from approaches used in aggressive B-cell lymphomas, phase 2 studies, and retrospective case series. The most common entities: PTCL, not otherwise specified (NOS), angioimmunoblastic T-cell lymphoma (AITL), and ALK-negative anaplastic large cell lymphoma (ALCL), account for more than 60% of cases. Therefore, most of the existing data is derived from these subsets. In the rarer entities, there is a greater paucity of data to guide therapy. In this section, some of the rarest T-cell lymphomas are focused on: enteropathy-associated T-cell lymphoma (EATL), monomorphic epitheliotropic intestinal T-cell lymphoma (MEITL), hepatosplenic T-cell lymphoma (HSTCL), and subcutaneous

Disclosure Statement: N. Mehta-Shah has no conflicts to disclose. Her fellowship is supported by CTSA UL1TR00457 and administered by the Clinical and Translational Science Center at Weill Cornell Medical Center and MSKCC. S. Horwitz has nothing to disclose.
[a] Department of Medicine, Memorial Sloan Kettering Cancer Center, 1233 York Avenue, New York, NY 10022, USA; [b] Department of Medicine, Memorial Sloan Kettering Cancer Center, Weill-Cornell Medical College, 1233 York Avenue, New York, NY 10022, USA
* Corresponding author.
E-mail address: horwitzs@mskcc.org

panniculitis-like T-cell lymphoma (SPTL). The existing data are reviewed regarding diagnosis and initial management of these diseases with an emphasis on how treatment strategies in these diseases may differ from the more common subtypes of T-cell lymphoma.

ENTEROPATHY-ASSOCIATED T-CELL LYMPHOMA AND MONOMORPHIC EPITHELIOTROPIC INTESTINAL T-CELL LYMPHOMA

EATL and MEITL are mature T-cell lymphomas that may present anywhere within the gastrointestinal tract but most commonly in the jejunum or ileum. Before the most recent version of the World Health Organization (WHO)'s classification of lymphoid neoplasms, EATL was referred to as EATL type I and MEITL was referred to as EATL type II.[1] Therefore, most of the literature to date has not differentiated EATL from MEITL. It is now better understood that these diseases have different histology, epidemiology, and mutational profile.

EATL and MEITL combined account for 6% to 9% of all PTCL in North America and Europe. Of these cases, approximately 10% to 20% are MEITL.[1–3] However, in Hispanic and Asian populations, there is a relative increase in the incidence of MEITL compared with EATL.[2,4] For example, in Asia, EATL and MEITL collectively make up only 2% of all PTCL, but up to 78% of cases are MEITL.[2]

A history of celiac disease is known to be a risk factor for the development of EATL, but is not associated with MEITL.[2,5] Previous reports suggest that up to 2% of patients with celiac disease eventually develop EATL, although that may be an overestimate given the high prevalence of celiac disease.[6] Those who have refractory celiac disease not responsive to a gluten-free diet are at highest risk of the development of EATL. Occasionally, a diagnosis of EATL may be the presenting feature of celiac disease.

In addition to their clinical presentation, EATL and MEITL are primarily distinguished based on their histologic and immunophenotypic features.[2] EATL is characteristically CD3+ and CD4−, CD8−, and CD56−, often with some expression of CD30. MEITL typically is CD3+, CD4−, CD8+ and shows a cytotoxic phenotype including common expression of CD56 and CD8$\gamma\delta$.[1,7,8] It has long been understood that EATL has been associated with HLA-DQ2 and DQ8 haplotypes.[9] More recently, the genomic landscape of MEITL has been investigated and demonstrates that most cases carry mutations in the JAK-STAT and G-coupled protein signaling pathways. One study identified that patients had mutations in STAT5 (63% of cases), JAK3 (35% of cases), and GNAI1 (24% of cases).[10] The characteristics of these diseases are summarized in **Table 1**.

Retrospective series of patients with EATL report a poor prognosis with median survival of 7 to 10 months.[2,11,12] Although there are limited data, there is a belief that MEITL carries a poorer prognosis.[13] Among patients with EATL, a history of celiac disease carries a slightly more unfavorable prognosis compared with those who have not had a history of celiac disease.[2]

Many patients with EATL present with acute abdominal symptoms often requiring urgent or emergent surgical procedures to arrive at the diagnosis resulting in a high fraction of patients beginning therapy with poor performance status or too ill to receive chemotherapy.[14] This was reflected in a series from the United Kingdom where 9/31 (29%) patients were either too sick to receive chemotherapy or died of complications of the first cycle of chemotherapy, mostly from bleeding or infection.[11] The importance of tumor burden and performance status in prognosis is further confirmed by the International T-cell lymphoma Project (ITCP) where poor performance status and high tumor burden correlated with a significantly worse outcome.[2] In the ITCP, 20% of

Table 1
Summary of the histopathologic characteristics

T-Cell Lymphoma Subtype	Clinical Presentation	Typical Histologic Features
EATL	• Most commonly present in gastrointestinal tract • Associated with celiac disease	Positive for CD3, often with some expression of CD30 Negative for CD4, CD8, and CD56
MEITL	• Most commonly present in gastrointestinal tract • Not associated with celiac disease	Positive for CD3, CD8, CD56, and CD8$\gamma\delta$ Negative for CD4
HSTCL	• Associated with history of immunosuppression • More common in young men • Most commonly present with disease involving spleen, liver and bone marrow	Positive for CD3 Negative for CD4 and CD8, express an γ/δ phenotype but α/β cases described—often shows isochromosome 7q
SPTL	Presents with regressing and remitting subcutaneous nodules	Positive for CD8 and CD56, express an α/β phenotype
Cutaneous gamma/delta T-cell lymphoma	Presents with ulcerating skin lesions and can be associated with HLH	Positive for CD8 and CD56, express a γ/δ phenotype
Chronic active EBV infection	• Present with vesiculopapular eruptions in sun-exposed areas • Associated with fevers, weight loss, hepatosplenomegaly without HLH	Positive for EBER and often polyclonal or oligoclonal
Systemic EBV-positive T-cell lymphoma of childhood	• Associated with fevers, weight loss, hepatosplenomegaly without HLH • Associated with HLH	Positive for CD3, TIA-1, EBER, CD8, and CD56
Primary cutaneous CD4+ small/medium T-cell lymphoproliferative disorder	• Associated with papules or nodules in skin • Carries indolent course	Positive for CD4, PD1, CXCL-13, BCL6
Primary cutaneous acral CD8+ T-cell lymphoma	Presents as cutaneous papules affecting the ear	Positive for monomorphic CD8

patients who received anthracycline-containing chemotherapy were alive and failure free at 2 years, whereas none of the patients who could not receive such therapy were alive without progression at 1 year. When critically evaluating the literature, it is important to recognize that the subset of patients who are too unfit to receive chemotherapy skew the outcomes of this patient population.

There is a suggestion that more intensive treatment approaches can lead to better outcomes in these diseases. The European Society for Blood and Marrow Transplantation (EBMT) reported results on 44 subjects who received autologous stem cell transplant (ASCT) as a consolidation (n = 31) or salvage (n = 13) therapy. Among those who had adequate response and performance status to pursue ASCT in first complete remission (CR) or partial remission, 66% of patients were alive at 4 years.[15] The largest prospective multicenter trial of an intensified approach is the Nordic study, wherein patients with major subtypes of PTCL were treated with cyclophosphamide, doxorubicin, vincristine, and prednisone (CHOP) with etoposide (CHOEP) followed by ASCT. Among the 160 subjects treated, 21 had EATL. On an intent-to-treat basis, those with EATL fared similarly to those with PTCL-NOS and AITL with a 5-year progression-free survival (PFS) and overall survival (OS) of 38% and 48%, respectively. The Scotland and Newcastle Lymphoma Group piloted an intensive upfront regimen. After one cycle of CHOP, patients with de novo EATL who were able to tolerate high-dose treatment as determined by a multidisciplinary consensus received IVE (ifosfamide, epirubicin, etoposide) alternating with methotrexate followed by ASCT (IVE/MTX-ASCT).[14] When the IVE/MTX-ASCT patients were compared with historical controls, they had similar median age of 56 years versus 57 years, and similar impaired performance status (Eastern Cooperative Oncology Group 2–4) of 77% versus 88%. When compared with the control patients who received an anthracycline-containing regimen, patients treated with IVE/MTX-ASCT had a higher overall response rate (ORR) (69% vs 42%), higher 5-year PFS (52% vs 22%), and higher 5-year OS (60% vs 22%). Although not always specified, the aforementioned studies were conducted in Europe where it is likely most patients would be classified as having EATL and not MEITL.

Although the data are limited, it seems that EATL type II carries a poorer prognosis.[13] Given that EATL type II shares histopathologic features with NK/T-cell lymphomas and other cytotoxic T-cell lymphomas, alternate strategies such as L-asparaginase–containing regimens have been attempted.[13] However, the incorporation of L-asparaginase is not clearly superior to other regimens, although the published experience is small.

It is important to note that there are 2 indolent lymphoproliferative processes of the gastrointestinal tract that should be distinguished from EATL or MEITL: indolent T-cell lymphoproliferative disease of the gastrointestinal tract and NK enteropathy.[16] Although neither of these disorders typically requires or responds well to systemic therapy, they almost always follow an indolent course.

HEPATOSPLENIC T-CELL LYMPHOMA

HSTCL is a very rare lymphoma, representing 2% to 3% of all T-cell lymphomas. Patients typically present with disease infiltrating the spleen, liver, and bone marrow in addition to cytopenias, B symptoms, and an elevated lactate dehydrogenase.[17] In most cases, the malignant cells carry a cytotoxic gamma/delta phenotype; however, an alpha/beta phenotype has been reported.[18] Immunohistochemistry is positive for CD3 and is usually negative for CD4 and CD8.[19] Clonal rearrangement of the T-cell receptor-γ (TCR-γ) gene is usually present, and many cases show an isochromosome 7q [I(7)(q10)].[20] HSTCL most commonly occurs in young men and is strongly associated with immunosuppression such as occurs with tumor necrosis factor-α inhibitors or thiopurine drugs, which are used in the treatment of inflammatory bowel disease or immunosuppression following solid organ transplant[21,22] (see **Table 1**).

HSTCL carries an aggressive course with a median survival of 16 months.[23] There is no single standard therapy for HTSCL, and the optimal initial therapy is not clearly defined. In initial reports, most subjects received CHOP with poor results. In a series of 21 patients, 19 were treated with a CHOP-like regimen, and of these, none were alive at 4 years from diagnosis.[23] The only 2 surviving patients were induced with a cisplatin-ara-c–based regimen followed by ASCT. Given the poor outcomes with CHOP-based therapy, the authors adopted a strategy of a non-CHOP induction, replacing it with either ifosfamide, carboplatin, etoposide (ICE) or ifosfamide, etoposide, cytarabine with intrathecal methotrexate (IVAC), followed promptly by hematopoietic stem cell transplant (HSCT), either allogeneic or autologous, in first CR.[24] With this approach, the authors have demonstrated a 63% OS among those treated with ICE or IVAC as initial therapy with the goal of HSCT in first CR. Although this represents a small series, the results are promising when compared with other published treatment strategies.[25] Furthermore, the EBMT has recently published that, among 18 patients with HSTCL who were consolidated with an allogeneic stem cell transplant, the 3-year PFS was 48% compared with 29% for those who received consolidation with an autologous transplant.[26]

Because many of these patients diagnosed with HSTCL are young, a dose-intensified approach is usually feasible. In the authors' experience, regimens such as ICE or IVAC for 3 or 4 cycles followed by stem cell transplantation (with a preference for allogeneic over autologous when possible) have resulted in most of their patients surviving. However, given the rare nature of this disorder and a paucity of literature, no standard approach currently exists.

As the understanding of HSCTL improves, it is hoped that there will be a role of targeted therapies in the management of these patients. Recent whole exome sequencing efforts have shown that most cases of HSTCL have mutations in chromatin-modifying genes, such as SETD2, INO80, and ARID1B. Mutations in the JAK-STAT and phophoinositol 3 kinase genes were also seen in a minority of cases.[27]

It is important to note that a variant of large granular lymphocytic leukemia (LGL) with aggressive behavior can be mistaken for HSTCL.[28] Although LGL typically expresses an α/β TCR, there may be clinical overlap between these entities, and distinguishing them with certainty may be challenging and not always achievable. Especially when considering high-dose therapy and consolidation with transplant, it is important to confirm the diagnosis of HSTCL to the extent possible.

SUBCUTANEOUS PANNICULITIS-LIKE T-CELL LYMPHOMA AND CUTANEOUS GAMMA/DELTA T-CELL LYMPHOMA

SPTCL is a rare primary cutaneous T-cell lymphoma (CTCL) that makes up less than 1% of T-cell lymphomas.[29] SPTCL presents with subcutaneous nodules that may regress and remit.[30–32] The lesions consist of atypical lymphoid cells expressing CD8 and CD56 that rim individual adipocytes with associated reactive histiocytes often associated with coagulation necrosis. Histologically, the cells express an α/β phenotype. The γ/δ-expressing phenotype of this disease is now classified as cutaneous gamma/delta T-cell lymphoma and tends to carry a more aggressive clinical course[18,32] (see **Table 1**).

Therapy for SPTCL remains controversial. SPTCL usually follows an indolent course and carries a favorable prognosis, particularly when hemophagocytic lymphohistiocytosis (HLH) is not present. Therefore, one approach has been to treat these similarly to other CTCLs, as discussed in other sections of this issue. Although patients may respond to combination chemotherapy, the duration of response is often short and CRs are rare.[33,34] There are reports of successful allogeneic stem cell transplantation[35–37] and prolonged remissions with combination chemotherapy followed by an ASCT.[38] However, the rarity of this disease and the infrequent need for aggressive therapy hamper the understanding of the utility of such approaches. Importantly, as is true of many indolent lymphomas, relapses are frequent and do not often correlate with poor survival. Milder approaches include single-agent bexarotene, which has significant clinical activity with an ORR of 82%, including complete responses in one series.[39] Other systemic agents as used for CTCL, such as oral methotrexate and histone deacetylase inhibitors, have activity. Anecdotal responses to glucocorticoids, interferon-α, zidovudine, and cyclosporine also have been reported.[40–44] The use of denileukin diftitox in 2 patients has been reported with evidence of activity.[45]

In contrast to STPCL, cutaneous gamma/delta T-cell lymphoma usually presents with ulcerating skin lesions and is more frequently associated with HLH. In the largest multicenter retrospective series of this disorder, the median survival was 31 months, but others have cited medium survivals of approximately 1 year.[46,47] More recently, as the ability to perform gamma staining by immunohistochemistry has become more reliable, it has been observed that there may be a less aggressive form of cutaneous gamma/delta T-cell lymphoma that has histologic features of SPTCL.[4,48,49]

Given the poor prognosis, aggressiveness, and poor responsiveness to conventional-dose treatments, many prefer to manage these patients with aggressive cutaneous gamma/delta lymphomas patients similarly to other cytotoxic T-cell lymphomas (eg, HSTCL).

It has been the authors' approach to treat those with SPTCL or clinically indolent cutaneous gamma-delta T-cell lymphoma with therapies that may be less aggressive but more tolerable for long periods of time (eg, bexarotene or methotrexate). In select cases, observation alone may be appropriate. This strategy more closely follows the authors' approach for CTCL as opposed to how they approach those with aggressive systemic PTCL. In patients who are physically fit who are being treated with curative intent and show an aggressive disease course (short duration of response on milder therapies, presence of HLH), one can consider combination chemotherapy with consolidation with an allogeneic transplant. Similarly, in patients with cutaneous gamma/delta T-cell lymphoma, one may consider combination chemotherapy followed by an allogeneic transplant as outcomes are poor with milder therapies.

CHRONIC ACTIVE EPSTEIN-BARR VIRUS INFECTION AND SYSTEMIC EPSTEIN-BARR VIRUS–POSITIVE T-CELL LYMPHOMA OF CHILDHOOD

Chronic active Epstein-Barr virus infection (CAEBV) and systemic Epstein-Barr virus (EBV)-positive T-cell lymphoma of childhood are entities recently revised in the most recent WHO classification.[1] CAEBV that carries an NK/T-cell phenotype can present as what was previously referred to as hydroa vacciniforme-like lymphoma. CAEBV is an EBV–associated lymphoproliferative disorder with malignant potential.[18] This disorder predominantly occurs in childhood and is seen most in Central and South America and Asia.[50] Although most patients present with vesiculopapular eruptions in sun-exposed areas often involving the face, these can develop into ulceration.[51] Although skin involvement is common, it has been reported without cutaneous manifestations.[52] In the acute phase, the disorder is associated with fevers, weight loss, and hepatosplenomegaly, and rarely, HLH.[50] In most cases, patients report a marked hypersensitivity to insect bites. In contrast, systemic EBV+ T-cell lymphoma of childhood is often associated with hemophagocytic syndrome and carries a fulminant clinical course.[1,53]

Histopathologically, the disease is represented by an NK- or T-cell infiltrate extending from the epidermis to subcutis, associated with necrosis, angiocentricity, and angioinvasion. Immunohistochemistry is positive for TIA-1, CD3, and EBER in situ hybridization, although most cases exhibit expression of CD8 or CD56. T-cell gene rearrangement studies show a monoclonal population that is particularly helpful in confirming this diagnosis. CD30 expression is seen more commonly in the NK pheno-type of this disease[50,54] (see **Table 1**).

As this disease is very rare, the understanding of this disease is primarily through case series. The literature demonstrates that patients with the CAEBV can have a re-lapsing remitting course with therapy such as thalidomide, steroids, chloroquine, cyclosporine, intravenous immunoglobulin, or a combination thereof.[50,52] CHOP-based combination chemotherapy has been given but with transient benefit. A small fraction of patients progress to have systemic involvement, and prognosis of these pa-tients is poor. Another series from Korea demonstrated that patients with systemic disease, particularly HLH, carried poorer prognosis.[53] In patients with true systemic EBV+ T-cell lymphoma, allogenic transplant appears to be a potentially curative strategy.[52]

PRIMARY CUTANEOUS CD4+ SMALL/MEDIUM T-CELL LYMPHOPROLIFERATIVE DISORDER (CD4+ SMALL-MEDIUM PLEOMORPHIC T-CELL LYMPHOMA)/PRIMARY CUTANEOUS ACRAL CD8+ T-CELL LYMPHOMA

Previously known as primary cutaneous CD4+ small-medium pleomorphic T-cell lym-phoma (CD4+ SMPTCL), primary cutaneous CD4+ SMPTCL is an indolent lympho-proliferative process often presenting as solitary papule or nodule, usually located on the head and neck.[55] Trunk and extremities can be involved, and a multifocal pre-sentation has been occasionally associated with a more aggressive course with sys-temic involvement. No surface markers are predictive of an aggressive course, including Ki-67 index.[56]

Histologically, the lesions are characterized by dense dermal infiltrate of small- to medium-sized atypical lymphocytes (CD4+/CD8+) without significant epidermotrop-ism.[57] Immunohistochemistry reveals expression of T-follicular helper cell markers (PD-1, CXCL-13, and BCL-6) by the lymphocytic infiltrate in CD4+ SMPTCL, which can aid in diagnosis in cases with a polymorphous infiltrate along with a dominant T-cell clone.[57] The malignant potential of this disorder has been debated, leading to its renaming in the most recent WHO classification[56,58] (see **Table 1**).

Similarly, primary cutaneous acral CD8+ T-cell lymphoma is newly recognized in the WHO classification as a clonal CD8+ T-cell lymphoma characterized by cuta-neous acral lesions affecting the ear.

Data suggest excellent prognosis in patients with both of these disorders and dura-ble response to skin-directed treatment modalities.[56,58–64] Treatment options include local excision, topical/intralesional steroids, and local radiation. The rates of remission are high irrespective of the treatment modality used, and the relapse rates are low. Pa-tients with multifocal progressive disease and/or symptoms suggestive of systemic involvement must be evaluated with staging studies such as computed tomography, PET scan, bone marrow biopsy, and flow cytometry of the peripheral blood to exclude PTCL, NOS.[56]

SUMMARY

Treatment of these very rare T-cell lymphomas can be challenging because there are no large or randomized studies to guide clinical decision making, and treatment paradigms are often based on small series or imperfect data. Although a strict algo-rithm cannot be written with certainty, through the literature that exists and clinical experience, themes and principles of approaches do emerge that when coupled with clinical judgment, allow reasonable and logical decisions.

REFERENCES

1. Swerdlow SH, Campo E, Pileri SA, et al. The 2016 revision of the World Health Organization classification of lymphoid neoplasms. Blood 2016;127(20):2375–90.
2. Delabie J, Holte H, Vose JM, et al. Enteropathy-associated T-cell lymphoma: clinical and histological findings from the international peripheral T-cell lymphoma project. Blood 2011;118(1):148–55.
3. Foukas PG, de Leval L. Recent advances in intestinal lymphomas. Histopathology 2015;66(1):112–36.
4. Garcia-Herrera A, Song JY, Chuang SS, et al. Nonhepatosplenic gammadelta T-cell lymphomas represent a spectrum of aggressive cytotoxic T-cell lymphomas with a mainly extranodal presentation. Am J Surg Pathol 2011;35(8):1214–25.
5. Di Sabatino A, Biagi F, Gobbi PG, et al. How I treat enteropathy-associated T-cell lymphoma. Blood 2012;119(11):2458–68.
6. Rubio-Tapia A, Ludvigsson JF, Brantner TL, et al. The prevalence of celiac disease in the United States. Am J Gastroenterol 2012;107(10):1538–44 [quiz: 1537, 1545].
7. Deleeuw RJ, Zettl A, Klinker E, et al. Whole-genome analysis and HLA genotyping of enteropathy-type T-cell lymphoma reveals 2 distinct lymphoma subtypes. Gastroenterology 2007;132(5):1902–11.
8. Chan JK, Chan AC, Cheuk W, et al. Type II enteropathy-associated T-cell lymphoma: a distinct aggressive lymphoma with frequent γδ T-cell receptor expression. Am J Surg Pathol 2011;35(10):1557–69.
9. Howell WM, Leung ST, Jones DB, et al. HLA-DRB, -DQA, and -DQB polymorphism in celiac disease and enteropathy-associated T-cell lymphoma. Common features and additional risk factors for malignancy. Hum Immunol 1995;43(1):29–37.
10. Nairismagi ML, Tan J, Lim JQ, et al. JAK-STAT and G-protein-coupled receptor signaling pathways are frequently altered in epitheliotropic intestinal T-cell lymphoma. Leukemia 2016;30(6):1311–9.
11. Gale J, Simmonds PD, Mead GM, et al. Enteropathy-type intestinal T-cell lymphoma: clinical features and treatment of 31 patients in a single center. J Clin Oncol 2000;18(4):795–803.
12. Tan SY, Chuang SS, Tang T, et al. Type II EATL (epitheliotropic intestinal T-cell lymphoma): a neoplasm of intra-epithelial T-cells with predominant CD8alphaalpha phenotype. Leukemia 2013;27(8):1688–96.
13. Tse E, Gill H, Loong F, et al. Type II enteropathy-associated T-cell lymphoma: a multicenter analysis from the Asia Lymphoma Study Group. Am J Hematol 2012;87(7):663–8.
14. Sieniawski M, Angamuthu N, Boyd K, et al. Evaluation of enteropathy-associated T-cell lymphoma comparing standard therapies with a novel regimen including autologous stem cell transplantation. Blood 2010;115(18):3664–70.
15. Jantunen E, Boumendil A, Finel H, et al. Autologous stem cell transplantation for enteropathy-associated T-cell lymphoma: a retrospective study by the EBMT. Blood 2013;121(13):2529–32.
16. Perry AM, Warnke RA, Hu Q, et al. Indolent T-cell lymphoproliferative disease of the gastrointestinal tract. Blood 2013;122(22):3599–606.
17. Vose JM. Peripheral T-cell non-Hodgkin's lymphoma. Hematol Oncol Clin North Am 2008;22(5):997–1005.
18. Swerdlow S, Campo E, Harris NL, et al. WHO classification of tumours of haematopoietic and lymphoid tissues. Lyon (France): International Agency for Research on Cancer; 2008.

19. Farcet JP, Gaulard P, Marolleau JP, et al. Hepatosplenic T-cell lymphoma: sinusal/sinusoidal localization of malignant cells expressing the T-cell receptor gamma delta. Blood 1990;75(11):2213–9.
20. Kanavaros P, Farcet JP, Gaulard P, et al. Recombinative events of the T cell antigen receptor delta gene in peripheral T cell lymphomas. J Clin Invest 1991;87(2):666–72.
21. Clarke CA, Morton LM, Lynch C, et al. Risk of lymphoma subtypes after solid organ transplantation in the United States. Br J Cancer 2013;109(1):280–8.
22. Mason M, Siegel CA. Do inflammatory bowel disease therapies cause cancer? Inflamm Bowel Dis 2013;19(6):1306–21.
23. Belhadj K, Reyes F, Farcet JP, et al. Hepatosplenic gammadelta T-cell lymphoma is a rare clinicopathologic entity with poor outcome: report on a series of 21 patients. Blood 2003;102(13):4261–9.
24. Voss MH, Lunning MA, Maragulia JC, et al. Intensive induction chemotherapy followed by early high-dose therapy and hematopoietic stem cell transplantation results in improved outcome for patients with hepatosplenic T-cell lymphoma: a single institution experience. Clin Lymphoma Myeloma Leuk 2013;13(1):8–14.
25. Falchook GS, Vega F, Dang NH, et al. Hepatosplenic gamma-delta T-cell lymphoma: clinicopathological features and treatment. Ann Oncol 2009;20(6):1080–5.
26. Tanase A, Schmitz N, Stein H, et al. Allogeneic and autologous stem cell transplantation for hepatosplenic T-cell lymphoma: a retrospective study of the EBMT Lymphoma Working Party. Leukemia 2015;29(3):686–8.
27. Aronson LI, Davenport EL, Mirabella F, et al. Understanding the interplay between the proteasome pathway and autophagy in response to dual PI3K/mTOR inhibition in myeloma cells is essential for their effective clinical application. Leukemia 2013;27(12):2397–403.
28. Ok CY, Yin CC, Yabe M, et al. Lymphoma with features intermediate between aggressive T-large granular lymphocytic leukemia and hepatosplenic T-cell lymphoma: a diagnostic dilemma? Clin Lymphoma Myeloma Leuk 2014;14(3):e95–100.
29. Gallardo F, Pujol RM. Subcutaneous panniculitic-like T-cell lymphoma and other primary cutaneous lymphomas with prominent subcutaneous tissue involvement. Dermatol Clin 2008;26(4):529–40, viii.
30. Takeshita M, Okamura S, Oshiro Y, et al. Clinicopathologic differences between 22 cases of CD56-negative and CD56-positive subcutaneous panniculitis-like lymphoma in Japan. Hum Pathol 2004;35(2):231–9.
31. Paulli M, Berti E. Cutaneous T-cell lymphomas (including rare subtypes). Current concepts. II. Haematologica 2004;89(11):1372–88.
32. Willemze R, Hodak E, Zinzani PL, et al. Primary cutaneous lymphomas: ESMO Clinical Practice Guidelines for diagnosis, treatment and follow-up. Ann Oncol 2013;24(Suppl 6):vi149–54.
33. Go RS, Wester SM. Immunophenotypic and molecular features, clinical outcomes, treatments, and prognostic factors associated with subcutaneous panniculitis-like T-cell lymphoma: a systematic analysis of 156 patients reported in the literature. Cancer 2004;101(6):1404–13.
34. Matsue K, Itoh M, Tsukuda K, et al. Successful treatment of cytophagic histiocytic panniculitis with modified CHOP-E. Cyclophosphamide, adriamycin, vincristine, predonisone, and etoposide. Am J Clin Oncol 1994;17(6):470–4.

35. Perez-Persona E, Mateos-Mazon JJ, Lopez-Villar O, et al. Complete remission of subcutaneous panniculitic T-cell lymphoma after allogeneic transplantation. Bone Marrow Transplant 2006;38(12):821–2.

36. Ichii M, Hatanaka K, Imakita M, et al. Successful treatment of refractory subcutaneous panniculitis-like T-cell lymphoma with allogeneic peripheral blood stem cell transplantation from HLA-mismatched sibling donor. Leuk Lymphoma 2006; 47(10):2250–2.

37. Yuan L, Sun L, Bo J, et al. Durable remission in a patient with refractory subcutaneous panniculitis-like T-cell lymphoma relapse after allogeneic hematopoietic stem cell transplantation through withdrawal of cyclosporine. Ann Transplant 2011;16(3):135–8.

38. Mukai HY, Okoshi Y, Shimizu S, et al. Successful treatment of a patient with subcutaneous panniculitis-like T-cell lymphoma with high-dose chemotherapy and total body irradiation. Eur J Haematol 2003;70(6):413–6.

39. Mehta N, Wayne AS, Kim YH, et al. Bexarotene is active against subcutaneous panniculitis-like T-cell lymphoma in adult and pediatric populations. Clin Lymphoma Myeloma Leuk 2012;12(1):20–5.

40. Wang CY, Su WP, Kurtin PJ. Subcutaneous panniculitic T-cell lymphoma. Int J Dermatol 1996;35(1):1–8.

41. Papenfuss JS, Aoun P, Bierman PJ, et al. Subcutaneous panniculitis-like T-cell lymphoma: presentation of 2 cases and observations. Clin Lymphoma 2002; 3(3):175–80.

42. Springinsfeld G, Guillaume JC, Boeckler P, et al. Two cases of subcutaneous panniculitis-like T-cell lymphoma (CD4- CD8+ CD56-). Ann Dermatol Venereol 2009;136(3):264–8 [in French].

43. Jung HR, Yun SY, Choi JH, et al. Cyclosporine in relapsed subcutaneous panniculitis-like T-cell lymphoma after autologous hematopoietic stem cell transplantation. Cancer Res Treat 2011;43(4):255–9.

44. Lee WS, Hwang JH, Kim MJ, et al. Cyclosporine a as a primary treatment for panniculitis-like T cell lymphoma: a case with a long-term remission. Cancer Res Treat 2014;46(3):312–6.

45. Hathaway T, Subtil A, Kuo P, et al. Efficacy of denileukin diftitox in subcutaneous panniculitis-like T-cell lymphoma. Clin Lymphoma Myeloma 2007;7(8):541–5.

46. Guitart J, Weisenburger DD, Subtil A, et al. Cutaneous gammadelta T-cell lymphomas: a spectrum of presentations with overlap with other cytotoxic lymphomas. Am J Surg Pathol 2012;36(11):1656–65.

47. Toro JR, Liewehr DJ, Pabby N, et al. Gamma-delta T-cell phenotype is associated with significantly decreased survival in cutaneous T-cell lymphoma. Blood 2003; 101(9):3407–12.

48. Takahashi Y, Takata K, Kato S, et al. Clinicopathological analysis of 17 primary cutaneous T-cell lymphoma of the gammadelta phenotype from Japan. Cancer Sci 2014;105(7):912–23.

49. Magro CM, Wang X. Indolent primary cutaneous gamma/delta T-cell lymphoma localized to the subcutaneous panniculus and its association with atypical lymphocytic lobular panniculitis. Am J Clin Pathol 2012;138(1):50–6.

50. Quintanilla-Martinez L, Ridaura C, Nagl F, et al. Hydroa vacciniforme-like lymphoma: a chronic EBV+ lymphoproliferative disorder with risk to develop a systemic lymphoma. Blood 2013;122(18):3101–10.

51. Sangueza M, Plaza JA. Hydroa vacciniforme-like cutaneous T-cell lymphoma: clinicopathologic and immunohistochemical study of 12 cases. J Am Acad Dermatol 2013;69(1):112–9.

52. Kimura H, Ito Y, Kawabe S, et al. EBV-associated T/NK-cell lymphoproliferative diseases in nonimmunocompromised hosts: prospective analysis of 108 cases. Blood 2012;119(3):673–86.
53. Paik JH, Choe JY, Kim H, et al. Clinicopathological categorization of Epstein-Barr virus-positive T/NK-cell lymphoproliferative disease: an analysis of 42 cases with an emphasis on prognostic implications. Leuk Lymphoma 2017;58:53–63.
54. Nava VE, Jaffe ES. The pathology of NK-cell lymphomas and leukemias. Adv Anat Pathol 2005;12(1):27–34.
55. Beltraminelli H, Müllegger R, Cerroni L. Indolent CD8+ lymphoid proliferation of the ear: a phenotypic variant of the small-medium pleomorphic cutaneous T-cell lymphoma? J Cutan Pathol 2010;37(1):81–4.
56. James E, Sokhn JG, Gibson JF, et al. CD4+ primary cutaneous small/medium-sized pleomorphic T-cell lymphoma: a retrospective case series and review of literature. Leuk Lymphoma 2015;56(4):951–7.
57. Rodriguez Pinilla SM, Roncador G, Rodriguez-Peralto JL, et al. Primary cutaneous CD4+ small/medium-sized pleomorphic T-cell lymphoma expresses follicular T-cell markers. Am J Surg Pathol 2009;33(1):81–90.
58. Beltraminelli H, Leinweber B, Kerl H, et al. Primary cutaneous CD4+ small-/medium-sized pleomorphic T-cell lymphoma: a cutaneous nodular proliferation of pleomorphic T lymphocytes of undetermined significance? A study of 136 cases. Am J Dermatopathol 2009;31(4):317–22.
59. Swick BL, Baum CL, Venkat AP, et al. Indolent CD8+ lymphoid proliferation of the ear: report of two cases and review of the literature. J Cutan Pathol 2011;38(2):209–15.
60. Bekkenk MW, Vermeer MH, Jansen PM, et al. Peripheral T-cell lymphomas unspecified presenting in the skin: analysis of prognostic factors in a group of 82 patients. Blood 2003;102(6):2213–9.
61. Grogg KL, Jung S, Erickson LA, et al. Primary cutaneous CD4-positive small/medium-sized pleomorphic T-cell lymphoma: a clonal T-cell lymphoproliferative disorder with indolent behavior. Mod Pathol 2008;21(6):708–15.
62. Williams VL, Torres-Cabala C, Duvic M. Primary cutaneous small- to medium-sized CD4+ pleomorphic T-cell lymphoma: a retrospective case series and review of the provisional cutaneous lymphoma category. Am J Clin Dermatol 2011;12(6):389–401.
63. Baum CL, Link BK, Neppalli VT, et al. Reappraisal of the provisional entity primary cutaneous CD4+ small/medium pleomorphic T-cell lymphoma: a series of 10 adult and pediatric patients and review of the literature. J Am Acad Dermatol 2011;65(4):739–48.
64. Suchak R, O'Connor S, McNamara C, et al. Indolent CD8-positive lymphoid proliferation on the face: part of the spectrum of primary cutaneous small-/medium-sized pleomorphic T-cell lymphoma or a distinct entity? J Cutan Pathol 2010;37(9):977–81.

Mycosis Fungoides and Sezary Syndrome

Francine M. Foss, MD[a],*, Michael Girardi, MD[b]

KEYWORDS

- Mycosis fungoides • Sezary syndrome • T-cell lymphoma • Immunotherapy
- Allogeneic stem cell transplantation

KEY POINTS

- Mycosis fungoides (MF) and the Sezary syndrome represent a heterogenous group of presentations and is incurable for the majority of patients.
- The disease can be difficult to diagnose in its earliest stages because it may mimic a number of benign skin disorders.
- The International Society of Cutaneous Lymphoma has established criteria for diagnosis of early stage MF.
- In its advanced stages the disease is in incurable and patients are often treated with a multimodality approach with skin-directed and systemic agents.

Mycosis fungoides (MF) and the Sezary syndrome (SS) are the most common forms of cutaneous T-cell lymphoma. The World Health Organization and European Organization for Research and Treatment of Cancer classification of primary cutaneous lymphomas distinguishes MF and SS from other types of cutaneous T-cell lymphomas[1] (**Box 1**). The overall incidence of MF/SS according to the Surveillance, Epidemiology, and End Results registry is approximately 4 per 1 million. According to a recent review of Surveillance, Epidemiology, and End Results data, 1713 patients were diagnosed with MF from 2004 to 2008.[2] The mean age for patients at the time of diagnosis is between 40 and 60 years of age, but the disease has been reported in children. MF is more common in males, and is seen more frequently in African Americans relative to Caucasians. The disease presents at a younger age in non-Caucasians and is more likely to present in an advanced stage in African Americans.[2]

The etiology of MF/SS is not well-understood, but there has been consideration of a potential association with conditions leading to chronic antigenic stimulation or

The authors have nothing to disclose.
[a] Hematology and Bone Marrow Transplantation, Yale University School of Medicine, 333 Cedar Street, New Haven, CT 06510, USA; [b] Department of Dermatology, Yale University School of Medicine, New Haven, CT 06510, USA
* Corresponding author.
E-mail address: Francine.foss@yale.edu

Hematol Oncol Clin N Am 31 (2017) 297–315
http://dx.doi.org/10.1016/j.hoc.2016.11.008
0889-8588/17/© 2016 Elsevier Inc. All rights reserved.

hemonc.theclinics.com

Box 1
World Health Organization–European Organization for Research and Treatment of Cancer classification of cutaneous lymphomas with primary cutaneous manifestations

Cutaneous T-cell and NK cell lymphomas
  MF
  MF variants and subtypes
    Folliculotropic MF
    Pagetoid reticulosis
    Granulomatous slack skin
  Sezary syndrome
  Adult T-cell leukemia/lymphoma
  Primary cutaneous CD30$^+$ lymphoproliferative disorders
    Primary cutaneous anaplastic large cell lymphoma
    Lymphomatoid papulosis
  Subcutaneous panniculitis-like T-cell lymphoma
  Extranodal NK/T-cell lymphoma, nasal type
  Primary cutaneous peripheral T-cell lymphoma, unspecified
    Primary cutaneous aggressive epidermotropic CD8$^+$ T-cell lymphoma (provisional)
  Cutaneous γ/δ T-cell lymphoma (provisional)
  Primary cutaneous CD4$^+$ small/medium-sized pleomorphic T-cell lymphoma (provisional)

Cutaneous B-cell lymphomas
  Primary cutaneous marginal zone B-cell lymphoma
  Primary cutaneous follicle center lymphoma
  Primary cutaneous diffuse large B-cell lymphoma, leg type
  Primary cutaneous diffuse large B-cell lymphoma, other
    Intravascular large B-cell lymphoma

Precursor hematologic neoplasm
  CD4$^+$/CD56$^+$ hematodermic neoplasm (blastic NK-cell lymphoma)

Abbreviations: MF, mycosis fungoides; NK, natural killer.
  Data from Willemze R, Jaffe ES, Burg G, et al. WHO-EORTC classification for cutaneous lymphomas. Blood 2005;105:3768–85.

---

pesticide and chemical exposure.[3] Although there is no known geographic clustering and no evidence of maternal transmission of the disease, MF/SS has been reported in a small number of families.

ETIOLOGY AND BIOLOGY OF MYCOSIS FUNGOIDES AND THE SEZARY SYNDROME

The malignant T cell in MF/SS is derived from a mature CD4$^+$ CD45RO$^+$ memory T cells that express adhesion molecules such as CCR4 and CLA. The circulating malignant Sezary cells have a different phenotype in that they express CCR7 and L-selectin.[4] Skin homing is characteristic of Sezary cells and epidermotropism, is a characteristic feature of the disease, along with Pautrier's microabscesses, which are intraepidermal collections of malignant cells. Immunohistochemistry of the infiltrating malignant T lymphocytes often shows diminished expression or loss of common T-cell antigens, such as CD7, CD5, CD26, or CD2 and dim expression of CD3. Immunosuppression with aberrant T-cell presentation, cutaneous anergy, and increased susceptibility to bacterial and opportunistic infections is a characteristic of the disease.[5,6]

Although there is not a classic chromosomal translocation in MF and SS, significant chromosomal instability has been noted. Losses on 1p, 10q, 13q, and 17p and gains of 4, 17q, and 18 have been identified.[7,8] Genetic instability has been characterized by significant copy number alterations.[9] Studies have shown a high prevalence of deletions or translocations involving a gene, *NAV3*, at 12q2, which has helicaselike activity.[10] Chromosomal amplification of JunB at 19p12 has also been identified in MF/SS and may be related to the T helper 2 cytokine profile characteristic of Sezary cells.[7] Amplification in 21 and deletion in 42 regions were identified, with significant amplifications of 8q (MYC) and 17q (STAT3) and deletions of 17p (TP53) and 10 (PTEN, FAS).[9] These specific gene alterations have been confirmed and extended by more recent next-generation sequencing, which has further implicated other copy number deletions (ZEB1, ARID1A, DNMT3A, CDKN2A, FAS, ATM, CTCF), copy number additions (STAT5B, PRKCQ), and somatic mutations (NFKB2, CD28, RHOA), among others.[11]

CLINICAL DIAGNOSIS AND STAGING OF MYCOSIS FUNGOIDES AND THE SEZARY SYNDROME

The diagnosis of MF/SS is made based on consideration of both clinical and histopathologic criteria. Although most patients present with skin patches and plaques that resemble eczema, psoriasis, or other benign skin disorders, patients with more advanced disease can present with cutaneous tumors or nodules or diffuse skin erythema with or without exfoliation (**Fig. 1**). The disease is often found in non–sun-exposed areas (bathing trunk distribution) and lesions may be hyperpigmented or hypopigmented, or may ulcerate. Tumors are typically greater than 1 cm in size with evidence of depth or vertical growth. Erythroderma can be patchy or diffuse and can be associated with cracking or fissuring of the palms and soles.[12] Because early stage disease can be confused with benign dermatoses, the International Society for Cutaneous Lymphoma has defined the criteria for diagnosis, which include immunohistochemistry, presence of epidermitropism or cellular atypia, clinical distribution of lesions, and T-cell receptor clonality (T-cell receptor rearrangement [TCRR]; **Table 1**).[13] The presence of TCRR in a skin lesion is not pathognomic for T-cell lymphoma and can be found in

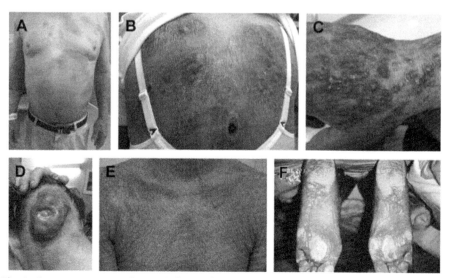

Fig. 1. Cutaneous stages of mycosis fungoides and Sezary syndrome. (*A*) Cutaneous plaques. (*B*) Ulcerated plaques. (*C*) Cutaneous tumors. (*D*) Large cell transformation. (*E*) Erythroderma. (*F*) Hyperkeratosis of soles of the feet.

Table 1
International Society for Cutaneous Lymphomas algorithm for the diagnosis of early stage mycosis fungoides

Criteria	Major (2 Points)	Minor (1 Point)
Clinical		
Persistent and/or progressive patches and plaques plus	Any 2	Any 1
1. Non–sun-exposed location		
2. Size/shape variation		
3. Poikiloderma		
Histopathologic		
Superficial lymphoid infiltrate plus	Both	Either
1. Epidermotropism		
2. Atypia		
Molecular/biological		
Clonal TCR gene rearrangement		Present
Immunopathologic		
1. CD2, CD3, CD5 in <59% of T cells		Any 1
2. CD7 in <10% of T cells		
3. Epidermal discordance from expression of CD2, CD3, CD5, and CD7 on dermal T cells		

Abbreviation: TCR, T-cell receptor.
Data from Pimpinelli N, Olsen EA, Santucci M, et al. Defining early mycosis fungoides. J Am Acad Dermatol 2005;53:1053–63.

parapsoriasis, lymphomatoid papulosis, and pityriasis lichenoides; likewise, the absence of TCRR using the most common assay for gamma rearrangements of the T-cell receptor does not rule out the disease.[14] Although most patients present with patches and plaques, a subset of patients may present with cutaneous tumors (*tumor d'emblée*).

The SS is defined as erythroderma along with the presence of at least 1000 circulating Sezary cells/mm.[12] Diagnosis of SS in the skin biopsy can be challenging, because epidermotropism may not be present. The CD4/CD8 ratio is often greater than 10. The phenotype of the malignant SS is typically aberrant with expression of CLA and CCR4 and loss of CD7 and CD26.[15] Clonality of the malignant population is often seen, but is not pathognomonic of SS and can be seen in up to 5% of patients with benign dermatoses that have characteristic erythroderma.[16] Clonality can be assessed by molecular studies or by flow cytometry using T-cell receptor-Vβ usage analysis, which we found to be more sensitive.[17] Cytogenetic studies have revealed translocations and deletions, often implicating 1p, 10q, 14q, and 15q, in conjunction with clonal evolution and chromosomal instability.[7]

Patients with the SS often report significant skin discomfort in the form of itching or pain and often develop infections related to the loss of cutaneous integrity. Hyperkeratosis of the palms and soles occurs with more advanced disease. Extensive skin infiltration can be associated with skin edema, and/or hypoalbuminemia owing to insensible fluid loss secondary to impaired skin integument. Lymphadenopathy and bone marrow involvement are relatively common in SS. Owing to the high risk of infections from resident skin organisms such as *Staphylococcus aureus*, permanent enteral indwelling catheters are not advised in these patients.

STAGING AND PROGNOSTIC FEATURES OF MYCOSIS FUNGOIDES AND THE SEZARY SYNDROME

The staging system for MF includes assessment of skin, blood, and internal organs.[18] Skin involvement is classified based on the type of lesions and extent (see **Fig. 1**). T1 and T2 lesions are classified as patches or plaques involving less than or more than 10% of the skin surface, respectively. T3 disease includes at least 1 cutaneous tumor. T4 level disease is classified as erythroderma. Lymph node stage is based on histopathologic involvement of the node in question. The LN2 node demonstrates atypical lymphocytes in 3 to 6 cell clusters, and LN3 nodes demonstrate larger aggregates of atypical lymphocytes with possible expansion of the parafollicular zone. Nodal architecture is often preserved.[19] The LN4 node is effaced by tumor cells and TCRR is noted in approximately 50% of patients with LN3, but is not associated usually with LN2 histology.[20] Bone marrow involvement is of prognostic importance, with cytologically atypical lymphoid aggregates and infiltrative disease linked to decreased survival.[21] Marrow involvement has been associated with blood and more progressive lymph node involvement.[22–25] Blood involvement has been defined more precisely in a revised International Society for Cutaneous Lymphoma staging system (**Table 2**).[26] Significant blood involvement (B2) is defined as the presence of a dominant clone in the blood along with greater than 1000 Sezary cells/μL or an expanded CD4/CD8 ratio of 10 or greater. Patients with B2 disease have been shown to have an inferior outcome compared with those with no or minimal (B1) blood involvement.[27]

The most important prognostic factors in MF/SS are the type and extent of cutaneous involvement and the presence of viscera disease.[23,25] Patients with patch/plaque disease involving less than 10% of their skin have a prognosis equivalent to those with similar age-, sex-, and race-matched controls.[28] The 10-year disease-specific survival for those patients with extensive patches or plaques is 83%. Those individuals with tumors or with pathologically proven lymph node involvement have survivals of 42% or 20%, respectively. Patients with effaced lymph nodes or the demonstration of large cell transformation have a poor prognosis.[22,29] Additional poor prognostic factors include blood involvement and loss of the T-cell markers CD5 and CD7.[30] The prognostic factors important in advanced disease were studied in 1275 patients. Stage IV disease, age greater than 60, elevated lactate dehydrogenase, and large cell transformation were independent poor prognostic factors in this retrospective review.[31]

CLINICAL ASSESSMENT OF MYCOSIS FUNGOIDES AND THE SEZARY SYNDROME

The clinical evaluation of patients with MF/SS includes assessment of the type and extent of skin involvement, presence of palpable nodes, imaging studies to evaluate for visceral disease, and examination of the peripheral blood by flow cytometry and molecular analysis for presence of circulating Sezary cells. The Modified Skin Weighted Assessment Tool may be useful for the measurement and quantitation of skin involvement. This tool divides the body surface into areas that are assigned a value based on the percent of total body surface area represented plus a 'weight' for the variety of skin involvement (patch, plaque, tumor).[32] The skin score is characterized by a sum. Skin biopsies should be examined for presence of large cell transformation as well as for immunophenotype and presence of T-cell receptors. Peripheral blood should be examined by flow cytometry to assess for the presence of SS and should be assessed for clonality by molecular testing for TCRR or by the flow cytometry panel for the T-cell receptor Vβ family of antigens.[17] The antigens typically used in flow cytometry include the common T-cell antigens CD4, CD8, CD7, CD3, CD45R0, and CD26.

Table 2
Staging systems for MF

MF Cooperative Group 1979			
Stage	T	N	M
IA	1	0	0
IB	2	0	0
IIA	1–2	1	0
IIB	3	0, 1	0
III	4	0, 1	0
IVA	1–4	2–3	0
IVB	1–4	2–3	1

ISCL Group 2007[a]				
Stage	T	N	M	B
IA	1	0	0	0, 1
IB	2	0	0	0, 1
II	1–2	1–2	0	0, 1
IIB	3	0–2	0	0, 1
III	4	0–2	0	0–1
IIIA	4	0–2	0	0
IIIB	4	0–2	0	1
IVA$_1$	1–4	0–2	0	2
IVA$_2$	1–4	3	0	0–2
IVA$_3$		0–3	1	0–2

Abbreviations: B0, <5% of lymphocytes are atypical; B1, greater than 5% of lymphocytes are atypical; B2, >1000 Sezary cells/mm^3 with positive clone; ISCL, International Society of Cutaneous Lymphoma; MF, mycosis fungoides; N1, LN 0 to 2; N2, LN 3; N3, LN 4; T1 patches or plaques, <10% bovine serum albumin (BSA); T2 patches or plaques, >10% BSA; T3, cutaneous tumors; T4, erythroderma.

[a] Proposed modifications to the staging system by the ISCL.

Data from [MF Cooperative Group 1979] Stadler R, Otte HG, Luger T, et al. Prospective randomized multicenter clinical trial on the use of interferon -2a plus acitretin versus interferon -2a plus PUVA in patients with cutaneous T-cell lymphoma stages I and II. Blood 1998;92:3578–81; and *Adapted from* [ISCL Group 2007] Olsen E, Vonderheid E, Piminelli N, et al. Revisions to the staging and classification of mycosis fungoides and Sezary syndrome: a proposal of the International Society for Cutaneous Lymphomas (ISCL) and the cutaneous lymphoma task force of the European organization of Research and treatment of Cancer (EORTC). Blood 2007;110:1713–22.

Imaging studies (computed tomography scan or MRI) are recommended as part of initial staging in all patients except those with limited (T1) skin involvement. PET may also be considered especially in patients with tumor stage disease or adenopathy.[33,34] Lymph node biopsy should be performed in patients with nodes 1.5 cm or larger, or for clinically suspicious nodes such as those that may be highly PET avid. A bone marrow biopsy should be performed in patients with SS and in those with compromised hematologic function. Biopsies of visceral organs such as liver should be considered as indicated clinically.

THERAPEUTIC APPROACHES FOR MYCOSIS FUNGOIDES AND THE SEZARY SYNDROME

The treatment algorithms for MF/SS are directed at both skin manifestations and systemic disease. Palliation of symptoms such as skin itching and skin breakdown from ulcerating lesions or erythroderma are often driving factors because disease palliation is a major goal for most patients. Except in its earliest stages, the disease is incurable short of allogeneic stem cell transplantation, and most patients require multiple therapies over the course of years to manage their disease. Long-term morbidity from therapies remains a focus for younger patients. With early-stage disease confined to the skin (patch or plaque disease), outcomes are excellent with skin-directed therapies. In contrast, tumor stage disease, extensive plaque stage disease that is refractory to topical therapy, and nodal or visceral disease often require a multimodality approach. Because most patients are immunocompromised by their disease, initial therapies are often biological or immunomodulatory, and aggressive and immunosuppressive chemotherapies are avoided (**Box 2**).

SKIN-DIRECTED THERAPIES

The majority of patients with MF/SS receive a multitude of skin-directed therapies with or without systemic agents. Skin-directed therapies include electron beam radiotherapy, ultraviolet light therapy, topical chemotherapy such as bexarotene, carmustine, or nitrogen mustard, and other topical immunomodulatory agents, including steroids and imiuqimod. Skin-directed therapies exert their effects by inducing apoptosis or interfering with cytokine and chemokines in the skin microenvironment.[35]

Topical nitrogen mustard formulated in an aqueous or ointment base has been used for many years in MF/SS. Recently, a gel-based formulation of mechlorethamine (Valchlor, Actelion Pharmaceuticals, Allschwill, Switzerland) was approved by the US Food and Drug Administration (FDA) based on a comparator study showing a 50% to 60% overall response rate in early stage (stage IA-IIA) MF patients.[36,37] The long-term effects of nitrogen mustard include basal and squamous cell carcinomas and hyperpigmentation and hypopigmentation. Bexarotene gel is an RXR retinoid that was approved for the treatment of the cutaneous manifestations of MF based on an overall response rate of 28% in stage I or IIA MF patients who were refractory or intolerant to prior treatment.[38] A major side effect included irritant dermatitis. In many cases, topical bexarotene gel is used in conjunction with topical steroids in an effort to decrease local skin inflammation.

Phototherapy in the form of ultraviolet A light with oral methoxypsoralen (PUVA) and narrow band ultraviolet B light are highly effective to induce skin clearing. The intensity of the light and frequency of administration are adjusted based on patient response and tolerance of the regimen. Maintenance treatment is often required to maintain clinical control of disease. Narrow-band ultraviolet B light therapy has a lower risk of secondary skin neoplasms.[39] Patients receive therapy several times a week to establish remission. Frequency is then often decreased over time depending on clinical results.

Both PUVA and ultraviolet B light therapy are often used in combination with biological agents, including interferons (IFN) alpha or gamma, as well as retinoids.[40] A randomized controlled trial evaluated the comparison of PUVA (2–5 times weekly) plus IFN alpha (9 MU 3 times weekly) with IFN alpha plus an retinoic acid receptor retinoid (acitretin; 25–50 mg/d).[41] In 82 patients with stage I or II level of disease, complete response rates were 70% in the PUVA/IFN group in contrast with 38% in the IFN/acitretin group with a time to response of 18.6 weeks in the PUVA/IFN group. Patients may respond faster when a combination therapeutic approach is used.

Total skin electron beam (TSEB) therapy requires the use of electrons typically ranging in energy between 4 and 7 MeV directed at the skin surface.[42] Structures below the deep dermis are moderately spared because the majority of the dose is

---

Box 2
Treatment approaches for MF/SS based on NCCN

Stage IA

Skin-directed therapy

Topical steroids

Topical retinoids

Topical nitrogen mustard or carmustine

Topical imiquimod

Local radiotherapy (EB or orthovoltage)

Excimer laser

Stage IB-IIA

Skin-directed therapy ± immunomodulatory agents or single agents

Total skin electron beam therapy for extensive involvement

Interferon alfa or gamma

Oral retinoids

Methotrexate (low dose)

HDAC inhibitors-vorinostat, romidepsin

Denileukin difititox

Other agents (see below), clinical trials

Stage IIB

Local XRT or other skin-directed therapies plus immunomodulatory or other systemic therapies

Immunomodulatory/biologic agents (HDAC, interferons, oral retinoids)

Chemotherapies: methotrexate, gemcitabine, liposomal doxorubicin, pralatrexate

Etoposide, penostatin, other agents, clinical trials

Consider allogeneic stem cell transplant

Stage III

Total body topical therapy topical mustard or carmustine, PUVA, total skin electron beam irradiation

Immunomodulatory therapy such as photopheresis, interferon, retinoids or combinations, alemtuzumab, other antibodies

Denileukin diftitox

HDAC inhibitors: vorinostat, romidepsin

Methotrexate, pentostatin

Clinical trials

Consider allogeneic stem cell transplantation

Stage IV

Skin-directed therapies and immunomodulatory therapies

Clinical trials: Single-agent chemotherapies: HDAC inhibitors, pralatrexate, methotrexate, pentostatin, gemcitabine, liposomal doxorubicin, bortezomib, alemtuzumab, cyclophosphamide, chlorambucil and prednisone

Multiagent chemotherapy (EPOCH, others)

Allogeneic stem cell transplantation

Abbreviations: EB, external beam; EPOCH, etoposide, vincristine, doxorubicin, bolus cyclophosphamide, and oral prednisone; HDAC, histone deacetylase; MF, mycosis fungoides; NCCN, National Comprehensive Cancer Network; PUVA, ultraviolet A light with oral methoxypsoralen; SS, Sezary syndrome; XRT, x-ray therapy.

deposited in the in the first 1 cm of tissue, and less than 5% is delivered beyond 2 cm depth. Historically, the dose prescribed to the skin has been in the range of 30 to 36 Gy, but more recently a dose of 12 Gy has become more standard, given improved tolerance and impressive response rates.[43] Blood, superficial lymph nodes, and supporting structure tissues receive 20% to 40% of the skin surface dose.

TSEB therapy is effective for patients with diffuse cutaneous involvement with plaques, tumors, or erythroderma.[44] Clinical complete responses range from 70% to 98% for early stage (T1, T2) patients, with 5-year disease-free and overall survival rates of 50% to 65% and 80% to 90%, respectively. Patients with cutaneous tumors involving less than 10% of the total skin surface do better with TSEB therapy than those with more extensive tumor involvement. Patients with erythrodermic MF (stage T4) treated with TSEB therapy (32–40 Gy), have a reported complete remission rate of 70% with 5-year progression-free, cause-specific, and overall survivals of 26%, 52%, and 38%, respectively.[44] The side effects of TSEB include hyperhidrosis, xerosis, alopecia, and desquamation of skin, as well as changes in the nails. Cumulative exposure to potentially mutagenic skin therapies such as topical mechlorethamine, PUVA, or TSEB increase the risk for secondary skin cancers.[45,46] Second or third courses of TSEB can be administered at reduced doses compared with the initial higher dose course and may be effective for relapsed disease.[47,48] Adjuvant therapies used after TSEB to consolidate response have included PUVA, topical mechlorethamine, and photopheresis.[49–51]

SYSTEMIC APPROACHES FOR MYCOSIS FUNGOIDES AND THE SEZARY SYNDROME
Immunomodulatory Therapies

IFN alpha is the first biological agent that was used in MF/SS and was found to be effective for many patients with responses ranging from 40% to 80%.[52] The dose of IFN is 3 to 9 million units 3 to 7 times a week with doses escalated as tolerated and as needed to control disease symptoms. The side effects of IFN include constitutional symptoms and bone marrow suppression. Gamma IFN has likewise shown activity.[53,54] Intermediate dose interleukin (IL)-2 and IL-12 have shown activity in phase II studies but are not currently in use.[55,56]

Extracorporeal photochemotherapy

Extracorporeal photopheresis (ECP) involves the ex vivo exposure of a peripheral blood mononuclear cell fraction to ultraviolet A light in the presence of methoxypsoralen, a DNA-damaging agent. The ECP process induces apoptosis in circulating Sezary cells and modulates antigen presentation to immune activation.[57,58] ECP is administered for 2 consecutive days monthly but alternative schedules have included 2 days every 2 weeks or weekly. Response to ECP is greatest in patients with blood involvement; response rates of 31% to 86% have been reported.[59,60] Immune-based adjuvant therapies have been combined with ECP.[61,62] In 1 study, patients with stages III and IV MF/SS were treated either with ECP alone or ECP in combination with IFN alfa, bexarotene, or granulocyte monocyte colony-stimulating factor. The overall response rate was higher in favor of combination therapy compared with ECP alone (57% vs 40%).[59]

Retinoids

A number of retinoids have shown activity in MF/SS, including acetretin and 13-cis retinoic acid.[63] Bexaroxtene (Targretin, Valeant Pharmaceuticals, Laval, Quebec, Canada) is an orally bioavailable RXR selective retinoid that is FDA approved for the treatment of MF/SS. Bexarotene has pleotropic activity in malignant cells and can alter T–cell trafficking via downregulation of CCR4 and E-selectin.[64] The response rate to oral bexarotene was 54% in early-stage and 45% in advanced-stage MF/SS patients. Pruritus decreased significantly in the treated patients and favorably impacted overall improvement in quality of life.[65,66] Bexarotene toxicity includes elevations in serum lipids and cholesterol, and suppression of thyroid function with decrease in thyroid-stimulating hormone. Although the approved dose of bexarotene is 300 mg/m^2 based on clinical trial data, treatment is often initiated at a lower dose while the effects of the drug on lipids and thyroid function are be assessed and supplemental agents such as atorvastatin and synthroid are incorporated. The dose is then escalated as tolerated. Bexarotene has been used in combination with a number of other agents, including IFN alfa-2b and PUVA.[67]

Histone deacetylate inhibitors

Histone deacetylase inhibitors have pleotropic effects to modulate expression of genes as well as cellular proteins, which are acetylated. The histone deacetylase inhibitor romidepsin was administered at a dose of 14 mg/m^2 given intravenously on days 1, 8, and 15 of a 21-day cycle in 2 phase II trials.[68] The response rate was 35% in patients who had either relapsed or had refractory disease.[68,69] The most frequent adverse events associated with romidepsin were nausea, constitutional symptoms, thrombocytopenia, and reversible ST-T wave changes on electrocardiography.

Vorinostat (Zolinza [Merck & Co. Kenilworth, NJ]; suberoylanilide hydroxamic acid), an orally bioavailable histone deacetylase inhibitor, is also FDA approved for the treatment of MF/SS based on a phase II trial with a response rate of 29% in relapsed/refractory patients.[70] The approved dose of vorinostat is 400 mg/d, but patients may require dose reduction for toxicity and symptoms such as nausea and diarrhea.

Denileukin diftitox

Denileukin diftitox is a fusion protein that includes the IL-2 gene joined to the active and membrane-translocating domains of the diphtheria toxin. The drug was FDA approved for relapsed and refractory MF/SS, but has been taken off the market.[71] A randomized, placebo-controlled, phase III trial comparing denileukin diftitox at dose levels of 9 μg/kg, 18 μg/kg, and placebo showed response rates of 37%, 46%, and 15%, respectively, in patients with stages I through III disease.[72] A modified version of denileukin difititox, E7777, is currently in clinical trials for MF/SS.

Monoclonal antibodies

Alemtuzumab, a humanized anti-CD52 antibody, has activity in MF/SS. Studies of low-dose alemtuzumab (10 mg subcutaneously administered 3 times per week) resulted in 2 complete responses and 4 partial responses among 10 patients with minimal immunosuppression.[73,74] Zanolimumab, which targets the CD4 receptor, is also promising with a 44% response rate in a trial of 49 patients with biopsy-proven CD4$^+$ MF/SS.[75]

The chemokine receptor, CCR4, is a novel target on MF/SS and has led to the development of mogamulizumab (KW-0761), a humanized anti-CCR4 antibody.[76] The overall response rate for mogamaluzimab in a phase II trial of relapsed/refractory MF/SS patients was 37% (29% in MF, 47% in SS).[77] A randomized trial comparing magamulizumab with vorinostat has been completed and analysis is underway.[78]

The expression of CD30 has been demonstrated on cases of both transformed and nontransformed MF/SS.[79] This has led to the use of brentuximab vedotin, a CD30-targeted antibody conjugated to an auristatin, an antitubulin agent in MF/SS. A phase II trial of 48 patients with CD30$^+$ T-cell lymphomas of the skin, including lymphomatoid papulosis, primary cutaneous anaplastic large cell lymphoma, and MF, showed an overall response rate of 71%, with 35% complete response.[80] Another study that correlated response with the level of expression of CD30 showed little chance of response in patients whose biopsies showed less than 5% CD30 expression. Brentuximab vedotin has a compendium listing in the National Comprehensive Cancer Network guidelines for the treatment of MF.[81]

Cytotoxic Chemotherapy for Mycosis Fungoides and the Sezary Syndrome

Combination chemotherapy regimens has shown efficacy in patients with advanced MF/SS, but response durations have been short. EPOCH (etoposide, vincristine, doxorubicin, bolus cyclophosphamide, and oral prednisone) has been shown to have an overall response rate of 80% with 27% complete response and median response duration of 8 months.[82] Myelosuppression related to multiagent chemotherapy regimens and the availability of novel agents has led to the preferential use of single-agent therapies except in patients who are refractory or who present with extensive adenopathy and/or visceral involvement or require immediate and aggressive palliation.

Pentostatin has been used in a phase I/II trial at doses of 3 to 5 mg/m^2 per day for 3 days through a 21-day schedule in 42 patients with cutaneous T-cell lymphoma, resulting in a response rate of 56%.[83] Grade 3/4 neutropenia was noted in 21% of patients and prophylactic trimethoprim and antiviral therapies were incorporated in an effort to prevent opportunistic infections. Other purine analogs, such as fludarabine and cladribine, have shown some activity in MF/SS.[84,85]

Gemcitabine has demonstrated impressive clinical activity in advanced and refractory disease. Overall response rates of 70% have been reported with the use of gemcitabine administered on days 1, 8, and 15 of a 28-day schedule at doses of 1000 to 1200 mg/m^2.[86] In a study of chemotherapy-naïve patients treated with 1200 mg/m^2, the response rate was 75%, with a complete response rate of 22%.[87] Skin flare can be seen after the initiation of gemcitabine in patients with extensive skin involvement.

Liposomal doxorubicin has also shown activity in MF/SS with a response rate of 80%.[88] An European Organization for Research and Treatment of Cancer study including 49 patients with stage IIB, IVA, or IVB MF reported complete response in 3 patients and a partial response in 11. The median duration of response was 6 months with a median time to progression of 7 months.[89] Although liposomal doxorubicin was associated with infusion-related events, it was well-tolerated with no grade 3 or 4 adverse events. The combination of gemcitabine plus liposomal doxorubicin has been highly effective in advanced MF/SS with an overall response rate of 65%.[90]

Pralatrexate is a novel folate antagonist that has been shown in vitro to be more potent than methotrexate.[91] The FDA approved pralatrexate for the treatment of aggressive T-cell lymphomas and transformed MF.[92] In an open-label phase 1/II clinical trial of pralatrexate at escalating doses in 54 patients with MF/SS who failed at least 1 systemic therapy, the response rate was 41%. Grade 3/4 adverse events included mucositis and leukopenia. The recommended dose for MF/SS from this trial is 15 mg/m^2 administered weekly for 3 weeks on a 4-week cycle. All patients must receive vitamin B_{12} and folate supplementation. For those patients with MF and large cell transformation, the overall response rate to pralatrexate at the higher dose of 30 mg/m^2 weekly for 6 weeks on a 7-week cycle was 25%.[93]

Lenalidomide is an immunomodulatory agent that affects T-cell and natural killer cell activation and the tumor microenvironment. A phase II study of lenalidomide in MF/SS showed an overall response rate of 28% with no complete responses in heavily pretreated patients. Adverse events included both fatigue and bone marrow suppression. The microenvironment impact of the drug revealed increases in CD8$^+$ and FoxP3$^+$ cells.[94] Lenalidomide is being combined with a number of agents, including romidepsin, and trials have shown tolerability of this combination.

The Role of Allogeneic Stem Cell Transplantation in Mycosis Fungoides and the Sezary Syndrome

Early studies with ablative allogeneic stem cell transplantation demonstrated a graft-versus-tumor effect in patients with advanced and refractory MF/SS.[95] Allogenic transplantation may be a cure for patients with advanced and refractory MF/SS. Reduced intensity regimens are most commonly used. Paralkar and colleagues[96] reported data using reduced intensity conditioning regimens in 12 patients with refractory cutaneous T-cell lymphoma and demonstration of a complete remission rate of 50%, and median response duration of 22 months. In a retrospective bone marrow transplant registry (Center for International Blood and Marrow Transplant Research) analysis of allogeneic transplant for MF and SS, 129 patients were identified, and median time from diagnosis to transplantation was 30 months (range, 4–206). A total of 64% of patients underwent reduced intensity conditioning regimens. The risk of disease progression was 50% (95% confidence interval, 41%–60%) at 1 year and 61% (95% confidence interval, 50%–71%) at 5 years. The 5-year overall survival was 32%.[97] MD Anderson reported their results with 19 MF/SS patients with the addition of an intensification for skin involvement in the form of reduced dose of TSEB irradiation before a reduced intensity conditioning regimen. Of 18 patients treated who engrafted, 12 had acute graft-versus-host disease, and 12 had chronic graft-versus-host disease. The complete response rate was 58%; 8 patients relapsed and 5 responded to either reduction in immunosuppression or donor lymphocyte infusion.[98] Based on this study, most institutions incorporate skin irradiation as part of the conditioning regimen for patients with MF/SS undergoing allogeneic transplantation.

SUMMARY

MF/SS represents a heterogenous group of presentations and is incurable for the majority of patients. The disease can be difficult to diagnose in its earliest stages because it may mimic a number of benign skin disorders. The International Society for Cutaneous Lymphomas has established criteria for diagnosis of early stage MF. In its advanced stages the disease is incurable and patients are often treated with a multimodality approach with skin-directed and systemic agents:

- Treatment of MF/SS depends the clinical stage and disease manifestations, such as type of skin lesions, extent of skin involvement, degree of pruritus, and presence of blood or nodal involvement.
- Owing to poor skin integument, infections are frequent and are the major cause of death in patients with advanced stage disease.
- Most patients require skin-directed therapies during the entire course of their disease.

- Cumulative, overlapping toxicities of therapy limit duration and intensity of long-term use of many agents and must be taken into consideration as therapies are implemented.
- Disease palliation is of significant benefit to patients and disease stability on therapy is a goal for many patients.
- Novel, effective therapies without typical cytotoxic profiles have shown promise as has allogeneic bone marrow transplantation as a curative option.
- Pharmacoeconomic considerations are a factor for many patients on long-term therapy and may impact treatment decisions.

REFERENCES

1. Willemze R, Jaffe ES, Burg G, et al. WHO-EORTC classification for cutaneous lymphomas. Blood 2005;105:3768–85.
2. Wilson LD, Hinds GA, Yu JB. Age, race, sex, stage, and incidence of cutaneous lymphoma. Clin Lymphoma Myeloma Leuk 2012;12:291–6.
3. Wohl Y, Tur E. Environmental risk factors for mycosis fungoides. Curr Probl Dermatol 2007;35:52–64.
4. Campbell JJ, Clark RA, Watanabe R, et al. Sezary syndrome and mycosis fungoides arise from distinct T-cell subsets: a biologic rationale for their distinct clinical behaviors. Blood 2010;116:767–71.
5. Axelrod PI, Lorber B, Vonderheid EC. Infections complicating mycosis fungoides and Sezary syndrome. JAMA 1992;267:1354–8.
6. Yawalkar N, Ferenczi K, Jones DA, et al. Profound loss of T-cell receptor repertoire complexity in cutaneous T-cell lymphoma. Blood 2003;102:4059–66.
7. Mao X, Orchard G, Lillington DM, et al. Genetic alterations in primary cutaneous CD30+ anaplastic large cell lymphoma. Genes Chromosomes Cancer 2003;37:176–85.
8. Scarisbrick JJ, Woolford AJ, Russell-Jones R, et al. Loss of heterozygosity on 10q and microsatellite instability in advanced stages of primary cutaneous T-cell lymphoma and possible association with homozygous deletion of PTEN. Blood 2000;95:2937–42.
9. Lin YL, Pasero P. Interference between DNA replication and transcription as a cause of genomic instability. Curr Genomics 2012;13:65–73.
10. Karenko L, Hahtola S, Paivinen S, et al. Primary cutaneous T-cell lymphomas show a deletion or translocation affecting NAV3, the human UNC-53 homologue. Cancer Res 2005;65:8101–10.
11. Choi J, Goh G, Walradt T, et al. Genomic landscape of cutaneous T cell lymphoma. Nat Genet 2015;47:1011–9.
12. Vonderheid EC, Bernengo MG, Burg G, et al. Update on erythrodermic cutaneous T-cell lymphoma: report of the International Society for Cutaneous Lymphomas. J Am Acad Dermatol 2002;46:95–106.
13. Pimpinelli N, Olsen EA, Santucci M, et al. Defining early mycosis fungoides. J Am Acad Dermatol 2005;53:1053–63.
14. Wood GS, Tung RM, Haeffner AC, et al. Detection of clonal T-cell receptor gamma gene rearrangements in early mycosis fungoides/Sezary syndrome by polymerase chain reaction and denaturing gradient gel electrophoresis (PCR/DGGE). J Invest Dermatol 1994;103:34–41.
15. Olsen EA, Rook AH, Zic J, et al. Sezary syndrome: immunopathogenesis, literature review of therapeutic options, and recommendations for therapy by the

United States Cutaneous Lymphoma Consortium (USCLC). J Am Acad Dermatol 2011;64:352–404.

16. Duangurai K, Piamphongsant T, Himmungnan T. Sezary cell count in exfoliative dermatitis. Int J Dermatol 1988;27:248–52.

17. Gibson JF, Huang J, Liu KJ, et al. Cutaneous T-cell lymphoma (CTCL): current practices in blood assessment and the utility of T-cell receptor (TCR)-Vbeta chain restriction. J Am Acad Dermatol 2016;74:870–7.

18. Bunn PA Jr, Lamberg SI. Report of the Committee on Staging and Classification of Cutaneous T-Cell Lymphomas. Cancer Treat Rep 1979;63:725–8.

19. Sausville EA, Worsham GF, Matthews MJ, et al. Histologic assessment of lymph nodes in mycosis fungoides/Sezary syndrome (cutaneous T-cell lymphoma): clinical correlations and prognostic import of a new classification system. Hum Pathol 1985;16:1098–109.

20. Lynch JW Jr, Linoilla I, Sausville EA, et al. Prognostic implications of evaluation for lymph node involvement by T-cell antigen receptor gene rearrangement in mycosis fungoides. Blood 1992;79:3293–9.

21. Graham SJ, Sharpe RW, Steinberg SM, et al. Prognostic implications of a bone marrow histopathologic classification system in mycosis fungoides and the Sezary syndrome. Cancer 1993;72:726–34.

22. Diamandidou E, Colome-Grimmer M, Fayad L, et al. Transformation of mycosis fungoides/Sezary syndrome: clinical characteristics and prognosis. Blood 1998; 92:1150–9.

23. Sausville EA, Eddy JL, Makuch RW, et al. Histopathologic staging at initial diagnosis of mycosis fungoides and the Sezary syndrome. Definition of three distinctive prognostic groups. Ann Intern Med 1988;109:372–82.

24. Salhany KE, Greer JP, Cousar JB, et al. Marrow involvement in cutaneous T-cell lymphoma. A clinicopathologic study of 60 cases. Am J Clin Pathol 1989;92:747–54.

25. Toro JR, Stoll HL Jr, Stomper PC, et al. Prognostic factors and evaluation of mycosis fungoides and Sezary syndrome. J Am Acad Dermatol 1997;37:58–67.

26. Olsen E, Vonderheid E, Pimpinelli N, et al. Revisions to the staging and classification of mycosis fungoides and Sezary syndrome: a proposal of the International Society for Cutaneous Lymphomas (ISCL) and the cutaneous lymphoma task force of the European Organization of Research and Treatment of Cancer (EORTC). Blood 2007;110:1713–22.

27. Agar NS, Wedgeworth E, Crichton S, et al. Survival outcomes and prognostic factors in mycosis fungoides/Sezary syndrome: validation of the revised International Society for Cutaneous Lymphomas/European Organisation for Research and Treatment of Cancer staging proposal. J Clin Oncol 2010;28:4730–9.

28. Kim YH, Bishop K, Varghese A, et al. Prognostic factors in erythrodermic mycosis fungoides and the Sezary syndrome. Arch Dermatol 1995;131:1003–8.

29. Dmitrovsky E, Matthews MJ, Bunn PA, et al. Cytologic transformation in cutaneous T cell lymphoma: a clinicopathologic entity associated with poor prognosis. J Clin Oncol 1987;5:208–15.

30. Olsen EA, Whittaker S, Kim YH, et al. Clinical end points and response criteria in mycosis fungoides and Sezary syndrome: a consensus statement of the International Society for Cutaneous Lymphomas, the United States Cutaneous Lymphoma Consortium, and the Cutaneous Lymphoma Task Force of the European Organisation for Research and Treatment of Cancer. J Clin Oncol 2011;29:2598–607.

31. Scarisbrick JJ, Prince HM, Vermeer MH, et al. Cutaneous lymphoma international consortium study of outcome in advanced stages of mycosis fungoides and Sezary syndrome: effect of specific prognostic markers on survival and development of a prognostic model. J Clin Oncol 2015;33:3766–73.

32. Stevens SR, Ke MS, Parry EJ, et al. Quantifying skin disease burden in mycosis fungoides-type cutaneous T-cell lymphomas: the severity-weighted assessment tool (SWAT). Arch Dermatol 2002;138:42–8.

33. Kumar R, Xiu Y, Zhuang HM, et al. 18F-fluorodeoxyglucose-positron emission tomography in evaluation of primary cutaneous lymphoma. Br J Dermatol 2006; 155:357–63.

34. Tsai EY, Taur A, Espinosa L, et al. Staging accuracy in mycosis fungoides and Sezary syndrome using integrated positron emission tomography and computed tomography. Arch Dermatol 2006;142:577–84.

35. Dewey WC, Ling CC, Meyn RE. Radiation-induced apoptosis: relevance to radiotherapy. Int J Radiat Oncol Biol Phys 1995;33:781–96.

36. In brief: mechlorethamine gel (Valchlor) for cutaneous T-cell lymphoma. Med Lett Drugs Ther 2015;57(1467):e66.

37. Talpur R, Venkatarajan S, Duvic M. Mechlorethamine gel for the topical treatment of stage IA and IB mycosis fungoides-type cutaneous T-cell lymphoma. Expert Rev Clin Pharmacol 2014;7:591–7.

38. Breneman D, Duvic M, Kuzel T, et al. Phase 1 and 2 trial of bexarotene gel for skin-directed treatment of patients with cutaneous T-cell lymphoma. Arch Dermatol 2002;138:325–32.

39. Brazzelli V, Antoninetti M, Palazzini S, et al. Narrow-band ultraviolet therapy in early-stage mycosis fungoides: study on 20 patients. Photodermatol Photoimmunol Photomed 2007;23:229–33.

40. Kuzel TM, Roenigk HH Jr, Samuelson E, et al. Effectiveness of interferon alfa-2a combined with phototherapy for mycosis fungoides and the Sezary syndrome. J Clin Oncol 1995;13:257–63.

41. Stadler R, Otte HG, Luger T, et al. Prospective randomized multicenter clinical trial on the use of interferon -2a plus acitretin versus interferon -2a plus PUVA in patients with cutaneous T-cell lymphoma stages I and II. Blood 1998;92: 3578–81.

42. Jones GW, Kacinski BM, Wilson LD, et al. Total skin electron radiation in the management of mycosis fungoides: consensus of the European Organization for Research and Treatment of Cancer (EORTC) Cutaneous Lymphoma Project Group. J Am Acad Dermatol 2002;47:364–70.

43. Harrison C, Young J, Navi D, et al. Revisiting low-dose total skin electron beam therapy in mycosis fungoides. Int J Radiat Oncol Biol Phys 2011;81:e651–7.

44. Jones GW, Rosenthal D, Wilson LD. Total skin electron radiation for patients with erythrodermic cutaneous T-cell lymphoma (mycosis fungoides and the Sezary syndrome). Cancer 1999;85:1985–95.

45. Jones G, Wilson LD, Fox-Goguen L. Total skin electron beam radiotherapy for patients who have mycosis fungoides. Hematol Oncol Clin North Am 2003;17: 1421–34.

46. Licata AG, Wilson LD, Braverman IM, et al. Malignant melanoma and other second cutaneous malignancies in cutaneous T-cell lymphoma. The influence of additional therapy after total skin electron beam radiation. Arch Dermatol 1995; 131:432–5.

47. Becker M, Hoppe RT, Knox SJ. Multiple courses of high-dose total skin electron beam therapy in the management of mycosis fungoides. Int J Radiat Oncol Biol Phys 1995;32:1445–9.
48. Wilson LD, Quiros PA, Kolenik SA, et al. Additional courses of total skin electron beam therapy in the treatment of patients with recurrent cutaneous T-cell lymphoma. J Am Acad Dermatol 1996;35:69–73.
49. Chinn DM, Chow S, Kim YH, et al. Total skin electron beam therapy with or without adjuvant topical nitrogen mustard or nitrogen mustard alone as initial treatment of T2 and T3 mycosis fungoides. Int J Radiat Oncol Biol Phys 1999;43:951–8.
50. Quiros PA, Jones GW, Kacinski BM, et al. Total skin electron beam therapy followed by adjuvant psoralen/ultraviolet-A light in the management of patients with T1 and T2 cutaneous T-cell lymphoma (mycosis fungoides). Int J Radiat Oncol Biol Phys 1997;38:1027–35.
51. Wilson LD, Licata AL, Braverman IM, et al. Systemic chemotherapy and extracorporeal photochemotherapy for T3 and T4 cutaneous T-cell lymphoma patients who have achieved a complete response to total skin electron beam therapy. Int J Radiat Oncol Biol Phys 1995;32:987–95.
52. Olsen EA, Bunn PA. Interferon in the treatment of cutaneous T-cell lymphoma. Hematol Oncol Clin North Am 1995;9:1089–107.
53. Hino R, Shimauchi T, Tokura Y. Treatment with IFN-gamma increases serum levels of Th1 chemokines and decreases those of Th2 chemokines in patients with mycosis fungoides. J Dermatol Sci 2005;38:189–95.
54. Kaplan EH, Rosen ST, Norris DB, et al. Phase II study of recombinant human interferon gamma for treatment of cutaneous T-cell lymphoma. J Natl Cancer Inst 1990;82:208–12.
55. Duvic M, Sherman ML, Wood GS, et al. A phase II open-label study of recombinant human interleukin-12 in patients with stage IA, IB, or IIA mycosis fungoides. J Am Acad Dermatol 2006;55:807–13.
56. Querfeld C, Rosen ST, Guitart J, et al. Phase II trial of subcutaneous injections of human recombinant interleukin-2 for the treatment of mycosis fungoides and Sezary syndrome. J Am Acad Dermatol 2007;56:580–3.
57. Berger C, Hoffmann K, Vasquez JG, et al. Rapid generation of maturationally synchronized human dendritic cells: contribution to the clinical efficacy of extracorporeal photochemotherapy. Blood 2010;116:4838–47.
58. Girardi M, Berger C, Hanlon D, et al. Efficient tumor antigen loading of dendritic antigen presenting cells by transimmunization. Technol Cancer Res Treat 2002;1:65–9.
59. Duvic M, Chiao N, Talpur R. Extracorporeal photopheresis for the treatment of cutaneous T-cell lymphoma. J Cutan Med Surg 2003;7:3–7.
60. Knobler R, Duvic M, Querfeld C, et al. Long-term follow-up and survival of cutaneous T-cell lymphoma patients treated with extracorporeal photopheresis. Photodermatol Photoimmunol Photomed 2012;28:250–7.
61. Bisaccia E, Gonzalez J, Palangio M, et al. Extracorporeal photochemotherapy alone or with adjuvant therapy in the treatment of cutaneous T-cell lymphoma: a 9-year retrospective study at a single institution. J Am Acad Dermatol 2000;43:263–71.
62. Suchin KR, Cucchiara AJ, Gottleib SL, et al. Treatment of cutaneous T-cell lymphoma with combined immunomodulatory therapy: a 14-year experience at a single institution. Arch Dermatol 2002;138:1054–60.
63. Huen AO, Kim EJ. The role of systemic retinoids in the treatment of cutaneous T-cell lymphoma. Dermatol Clin 2015;33:715–29.

64. Richardson SK, Newton SB, Bach TL, et al. Bexarotene blunts malignant T-cell chemotaxis in Sezary syndrome: reduction of chemokine receptor 4-positive lymphocytes and decreased chemotaxis to thymus and activation-regulated chemokine. Am J Hematol 2007;82:792–7.

65. Duvic M, Hymes K, Heald P, et al. Bexarotene is effective and safe for treatment of refractory advanced-stage cutaneous T-cell lymphoma: multinational phase II-III trial results. J Clin Oncol 2001;19:2456–71.

66. Duvic M, Martin AG, Kim Y, et al. Phase 2 and 3 clinical trial of oral bexarotene (Targretin capsules) for the treatment of refractory or persistent early-stage cutaneous T-cell lymphoma. Arch Dermatol 2001;137:581–93.

67. Straus DJ, Duvic M, Kuzel T, et al. Results of a phase II trial of oral bexarotene (Targretin) combined with interferon alfa-2b (Intron-A) for patients with cutaneous T-cell lymphoma. Cancer 2007;109:1799–803.

68. Piekarz RL, Frye R, Turner M, et al. Phase II multi-institutional trial of the histone deacetylase inhibitor romidepsin as monotherapy for patients with cutaneous T-cell lymphoma. J Clin Oncol 2009;27:5410–7.

69. Whittaker SJ, Demierre MF, Kim EJ, et al. Final results from a multicenter, international, pivotal study of romidepsin in refractory cutaneous T-cell lymphoma. J Clin Oncol 2010;28:4485–91.

70. Olsen EA, Kim YH, Kuzel TM, et al. Phase IIb multicenter trial of vorinostat in patients with persistent, progressive, or treatment refractory cutaneous T-cell lymphoma. J Clin Oncol 2007;25:3109–15.

71. Olsen E, Duvic M, Frankel A, et al. Pivotal phase III trial of two dose levels of denileukin diftitox for the treatment of cutaneous T-cell lymphoma. J Clin Oncol 2001;19:376–88.

72. Prince HM, Duvic M, Martin A, et al. Phase III placebo-controlled trial of denileukin diftitox for patients with cutaneous T-cell lymphoma. J Clin Oncol 2010;28:1870–7.

73. Kennedy GA, Seymour JF, Wolf M, et al. Treatment of patients with advanced mycosis fungoides and Sezary syndrome with alemtuzumab. Eur J Haematol 2003;71:250–6.

74. Lundin J, Hagberg H, Repp R, et al. Phase 2 study of alemtuzumab (anti-CD52 monoclonal antibody) in patients with advanced mycosis fungoides/Sezary syndrome. Blood 2003;101:4267–72.

75. Rider DA, Havenith CE, de Ridder R, et al. A human CD4 monoclonal antibody for the treatment of T-cell lymphoma combines inhibition of T-cell signaling by a dual mechanism with potent Fc-dependent effector activity. Cancer Res 2007;67:9945–53.

76. Ishida T, Inagaki H, Utsunomiya A, et al. CXC chemokine receptor 3 and CC chemokine receptor 4 expression in T-cell and NK-cell lymphomas with special reference to clinicopathological significance for peripheral T-cell lymphoma, unspecified. Clin Cancer Res 2004;10:5494–500.

77. Duvic M, Pinter-Brown LC, Foss FM, et al. Phase 1/2 study of mogamulizumab, a defucosylated anti-CCR4 antibody, in previously treated patients with cutaneous T-cell lymphoma. Blood 2015;125:1883–9.

78. Horwitz SM, Kim YH, Foss F, et al. Identification of an active, well-tolerated dose of pralatrexate in patients with relapsed or refractory cutaneous T-cell lymphoma. Blood 2012;119:4115–22.

79. Edinger JT, Clark BZ, Pucevich BE, et al. CD30 expression and proliferative fraction in nontransformed mycosis fungoides. Am J Surg Pathol 2009;33:1860–8.

80. Duvic M, Tetzlaff MT, Gangar P, et al. Results of a phase II trial of brentuximab Vedotin for CD30+ cutaneous T-cell lymphoma and lymphomatoid papulosis. J Clin Oncol 2015;33:3759–65.

81. Kim YH, Tavallaee M, Sundram U, et al. Phase II investigator-initiated study of brentuximab vedotin in mycosis fungoides and Sezary syndrome with variable CD30 expression level: a multi-institution collaborative project. J Clin Oncol 2015;33:3750–8.

82. Akpek G, Koh HK, Bogen S, et al. Chemotherapy with etoposide, vincristine, doxorubicin, bolus cyclophosphamide, and oral prednisone in patients with refractory cutaneous T-cell lymphoma. Cancer 1999;86:1368–76.

83. Kurzrock R, Pilat S, Duvic M. Pentostatin therapy of T-cell lymphomas with cutaneous manifestations. J Clin Oncol 1999;17:3117–21.

84. Trautinger F, Schwarzmeier J, Honigsmann H, et al. Low-dose 2-chlorodeoxyadenosine for the treatment of mycosis fungoides. Arch Dermatol 1999;135:1279–80.

85. Von Hoff DD, Dahlberg S, Hartstock RJ, et al. Activity of fludarabine monophosphate in patients with advanced mycosis fungoides: a Southwest Oncology Group study. J Natl Cancer Inst 1990;82:1353–5.

86. Zinzani PL, Baliva G, Magagnoli M, et al. Gemcitabine treatment in pretreated cutaneous T-cell lymphoma: experience in 44 patients. J Clin Oncol 2000;18: 2603–6.

87. Marchi E, Alinari L, Tani M, et al. Gemcitabine as frontline treatment for cutaneous T-cell lymphoma: phase II study of 32 patients. Cancer 2005;104:2437–41.

88. Quereux G, Marques S, Nguyen JM, et al. Prospective multicenter study of pegylated liposomal doxorubicin treatment in patients with advanced or refractory mycosis fungoides or Sezary syndrome. Arch Dermatol 2008;144:727–33.

89. Dummer R, Quaglino P, Becker JC, et al. Prospective international multicenter phase II trial of intravenous pegylated liposomal doxorubicin monochemotherapy in patients with stage IIB, IVA, or IVB advanced mycosis fungoides: final results from EORTC 21012. J Clin Oncol 2012;30:4091–7.

90. Horwitz SM, Olsen EA, Duvic M, et al. Review of the treatment of mycosis fungoides and Sezary syndrome: a stage-based approach. J Natl Compr Canc Netw 2008;6:436–42.

91. Izbicka E, Diaz A, Streeper R, et al. Distinct mechanistic activity profile of pralatrexate in comparison to other antifolates in in vitro and in vivo models of human cancers. Cancer Chemother Pharmacol 2009;64:993–9.

92. O'Connor OA, Pro B, Pinter-Brown L, et al. Pralatrexate in patients with relapsed or refractory peripheral T-cell lymphoma: results from the pivotal PROPEL study. J Clin Oncol 2011;29:1182–9.

93. Foss F, Horwitz SM, Coiffier B, et al. Pralatrexate is an effective treatment for relapsed or refractory transformed mycosis fungoides: a subgroup efficacy analysis from the PROPEL study. Clin Lymphoma Myeloma Leuk 2012;12:238–43.

94. Querfeld C, Rosen ST, Guitart J, et al. Results of an open-label multicenter phase 2 trial of lenalidomide monotherapy in refractory mycosis fungoides and Sezary syndrome. Blood 2014;123:1159–66.

95. Molina A, Zain J, Arber DA, et al. Durable clinical, cytogenetic, and molecular remissions after allogeneic hematopoietic cell transplantation for refractory Sezary syndrome and mycosis fungoides. J Clin Oncol 2005;23:6163–71.

96. Paralkar VR, Nasta SD, Morrissey K, et al. Allogeneic hematopoietic SCT for primary cutaneous T cell lymphomas. Bone Marrow Transplant 2012;47:940–5.

97. Lechowicz MJ, Lazarus HM, Carreras J, et al. Allogeneic hematopoietic cell transplantation for mycosis fungoides and Sezary syndrome. Bone Marrow Transplant 2014;49:1360–5.
98. Duvic M, Donato M, Dabaja B, et al. Total skin electron beam and non-myeloablative allogeneic hematopoietic stem-cell transplantation in advanced mycosis fungoides and Sezary syndrome. J Clin Oncol 2010;28:2365–72.

CD30⁺ Lymphoproliferative Disorders of the Skin

Maxwell B. Sauder, MD, FRCPC, John T. O'Malley, MD, PhD,
Nicole R. LeBoeuf, MD, MPH*

KEYWORDS

- CD30⁺ • Cutaneous lymphoproliferative disorders • Lymphomatoid papulosis
- Primary cutaneous anaplastic large cell lymphoma
- Secondary cutaneous anaplastic large cell lymphoma

KEY POINTS

- Primary cutaneous CD30⁺ lymphoproliferative disorders encompass a spectrum of benign to malignant phenotypes including lymphomatoid papulosis (LyP), primary cutaneous anaplastic large cell lymphoma (pcALCL) and borderline cases.
- LyP is characterized by recurrent crops of several to hundreds of red to violaceous papulonodules measuring up to 20mm, usually on the trunk and extremities, while pcALCL presents with a solitary or localized red to violaceous nodulotumor greater than 20mm that may occur anywhere on the body.
- Patients with LyP are at increased risk of secondary malignancy, most often mycosis fungoides or ALCL, may be diagnosed before, during or after the diagnosis of LyP and should undergo ongoing surveillance.
- Patients presenting with cutaneous ALCL should be worked-up to ensure it is primary cutaneous and not secondary cutaneous involvement of systemic ALCL.
- LyP is benign, limited to the skin and self-resolving with a 5-year survival rate of 100%, while pcALCL is usually limited to the skin and responsive to directed therapies, with a 5-year survival of over 95%; aggressive systemic or multi-agent chemotherapeutic regimens should be avoided.

INTRODUCTION

Cluster of differentiation 30 (CD30), a 120-kDa type I transmembrane glycoprotein of the tumor necrosis factor receptor superfamily member 8 (TNFRSF8) gene and previously known as Ki-1 antigen, is a cell surface cytokine receptor present on activated T and B cells. Upon T-cell activation, CD28 and other costimulatory receptors, including

Disclosure Statement: The authors have nothing to disclose.
Department of Dermatology, The Center for Cutaneous Oncology, Dana Farber Cancer Institute, Brigham and Women's Hospital, Harvard Medical School, 450 Brookline Avenue, Boston, MA 02115, USA
* Corresponding author.
E-mail address: nleboeuf@partners.org

Hematol Oncol Clin N Am 31 (2017) 317–334
http://dx.doi.org/10.1016/j.hoc.2016.11.006
0889-8588/17/© 2017 Elsevier Inc. All rights reserved.

CD30, are upregulated. CD30 expression requires CD28 or interleukin-4 receptor signaling and, when CD30 is activated, downstream signaling augments T-cell proliferation at low levels and regulates T-cell survival.[1,2]

CD30 interacts with CD30 ligand (CD30L, CD153, TNFSF8), a 40-kDa type II membrane-associated glycoprotein belonging to the TNF family[1,2] that is expressed on activated T cells, primarily CD4 T cells of both T helper 1 and 2 (Th1 and Th2) phenotypes, as well as on a subset of accessory cells[1,3,4] and B cells.[5,6] CD30 signaling ultimately leads to nuclear factor-κB activation through both TNFR-associated factor 2-dependent and TNFR-associated factor 2-independent pathways that can inhibit effector cell activity, promote apoptosis, or promote survival depending on the cell type and different intracellular signaling pathways activated.[7–9] For example, ligation of CD30 signals can downregulate the cytotoxic effector molecules Fas ligand, perforin, and granzyme B, and inhibit cytotoxicity.[4] CD30 signaling also promotes apoptosis by strongly inhibiting the expression of the oncogene c-myc and upregulating Fas (TNFRSF6), death receptor 3 (TNFRSF25), and TNF-related apoptosis-inducing ligand (TNFSF10, TRAIL).[10] In addition to increasing the cell's susceptibility to apoptosis, CD30 signaling strongly upregulates chemokine receptor 7, a homing molecule that enhances the cell's ability to home to lymphoid organs. A variety of causes have been implicated in the induction of CD30 expression in human cutaneous reactive and neoplastic lymphocytic processes including infectious, exogenous, inflammatory, and lymphoproliferative disorders (LPD; **Table 1**).

CD30 is expressed in a subset of B-cell lymphoid malignancies (approximately 20%) and T-cell lymphoid malignancies (30%), including the most common CD30+ lymphoid malignancies, Hodgkin's lymphoma, and systemic anaplastic large cell lymphoma.[11–13] However, there is a subset of non-Hodgkin's lymphoma where the disease process is contained within the skin with no other evidence of blood or lymph node involvement. This article focuses on the diagnosis, clinical presentation, and management of these primary cutaneous CD30+ LPD.

Primary cutaneous CD30+ LPD comprise a spectrum of conditions with similar histologic and molecular features, but different clinical presentations. According to the World Health Organization and European Organization for Research and Treatment classifications, this group accounts for 20% of all cutaneous lymphomas, second most common cutaneous T-cell lymphomas behind mycosis fungoides (MF).[14] The primary cutaneous CD30+ LPD include lymphomatoid papulosis (LyP), primary cutaneous anaplastic large cell lymphoma (pcALCL), and borderline or indeterminate cases.

Both pcALCL and LyP can be thought of as a clinical spectrum where indeterminate cases may have clinical and histologic features of either (**Fig. 1**). Patients with LyP may have a coexisting secondary lymphoma, including pcALCL; therefore, both conditions may exist simultaneously in an individual patient. Indeterminate cases tend to develop clinical features of either LyP or pcALCL over time. Historical diagnoses that may capture the full spectrum of CD30+ LPD include regressing atypical histiocytosis or indolent primary cutaneous Hodgkin lymphoma.[15]

LYMPHOMATOID PAPULOSIS
Epidemiology

Macaulay[16] first described LyP in 1968, aptly referring to the recurring self-healing eruption as clinically benign but histologically malignant. LyP is the most common CD30+ LPD, more common than pcALCL. Best estimates suggest that there are approximately 1.2 to 1.9 cases per million persons of LyP in the United States.[17] It presents in men more often than women with an average age of onset of 35 to 45 years[18]

Table 1
CD30⁺ lymphocytic disorders

Neoplastic	Lymphomatoid papulosis
	Primary cutaneous anaplastic large cell lymphoma
	Systemic cutaneous anaplastic large cell lymphoma
	Mycosis fungoides or Sezary syndrome with CD30⁺ large cell transformation
	Cutaneous Hodgkin's disease
	CD30⁺ large B-cell lymphoma
	EBV⁺ hydroa vacciniforme-like T-cell lymphoma
	HTLV-1 associated adult T-cell lymphoma/leukemia
	Eruptive keratoacantomas
Exogeneous	Drug-induced reactive lymphoid hyperplasia[44–49]
	Insect bite reaction[50]
	Scabies infestation[51]
Infection associated	EBV[52]
	HTLV-1/2
	Mycobacteria[53]
	Herpes simplex virus[53]
	Human immunodeficiency virus[54]
	Other infections: leishmaniasis, syphilis, varicella zoster virus, molluscum contagiosum virus, and parapox virus[46]
Inflammatory conditions	Pityriasis lichenoides
	○ Pityriasis lichenoides et varioliformis acuta
	○ Pityriasis lichenoides chronica
	Eruption of lymphocyte recovery[55]
	Atopic dermatitis[56]

Abbreviations: EBV, Epstein–Barr virus; HTLV1, human T-cell lymphotropic virus type 1.
  Adapted from LeBoeuf NR, McDermott S, Harris NL. Case records of the Massachusetts General Hospital. Case 5-2015. A 69-year-old woman with recurrent skin lesions after treatment for lymphoma. N Engl J Med 2015;372(7):653; and Werner B, Massone C, Kerl H, Cerroni L. Large CD30-positive cells in benign, atypical lymphoid infiltrates of the skin. J Cutan Pathol 2008;35:1100–7.

(**Table 2**). The etiology of LyP is not known, although hypotheses implicating reactive phenomena inducing overexpression of CD30 have been proposed.

Prognosis

The 5-year survival of patients with LyP is close to 100%, despite the increased risk of secondary malignancy that may be diagnosed before, during, or after the diagnosis of LyP.[14] This secondary malignancy risk can affect 5% to 30% of LyP patients,[19–22] although several larger retrospective series indicated that the incidence of a secondary malignancy may actually be closer to 40% to 60%.[23,24] MF and ALCL are the first and second most commonly associated malignancies, respectively, accounting for more than 90% of secondary malignancies in one series.[24] The majority of the secondary cases of MF are early stage, either IA or IB. Other secondary hematologic

Fig. 1. Primary cutaneous CD30⁺ lymphoproliferative disorders clinical spectrum. LyP, lymphomatoid papulosis; pcALCL, primary cutaneous anaplastic large cell lymphoma.

Table 2
Epidemiology of LyP and pcALCL

	LyP	pcALCL
Percent of primary cutaneous lymphomas	12	8
5-year survival (%)	100	>95
Incidence	1.2–1.9 cases per 1,000,000	Unknown
M:F ratio	1.4:1	3:1
Median age at diagnosis (y)	45.5	60
Age range (y)	4–88	16–89

Abbreviations: LyP, lymphomatoid papulosis; pcALCL, primary cutaneous anaplastic large cell lymphoma.
    Data from Refs.[14,20,59,60]

malignancies that have been reported to occur with LyP are listed in **Table 3**. Male sex and advanced age are risk factors associated with a greater risk of a secondary LPD; additional factors are noted in **Box 1**.

Presentation

Clinically, LyP is characterized by recurrent crops of red to violaceous papules and nodules measuring up to 20 mm, but typically 3 to 10 mm in diameter (**Table 4**). Patients often present with lesions in various stages owing to the recurrent and successive crops of papules and nodules, with hyperpigmented macules and varioliform scars in the background (**Fig. 2**). The number of lesions can range from a few to hundreds at a time. Lesions typically are generalized, with the majority on the trunk and extremities. Localized presentations of crops within regional areas or in agminated plaques have also been described.[25,26] Approximately one-half of all patients are asymptomatic, whereas others experience pruritus and/or pain secondary to ulceration, crusting, and central necrosis.[27] LyP is not associated with systemic symptoms. The resolving lesions often display postinflammatory hypopigmented or hyperpigmented macules. Necrotic lesions may leave varioliform scars, usually smaller than the original papules. Typically, lesions spontaneously resolve within 1 to 4 months,[28] most often between 2 and 8 weeks. The self-healing nature of LyP is a critical clinical pearl required for making the diagnosis, particularly in the face of a concerning pathology report. It is hypothesized that the feature of resolution may be associated with

Table 3
Secondary malignancies associated with lymphomatoid papulosis

Most common (>90% of cases)	Mycosis fungoides, stage IA or IB > later stage Anaplastic large cell lymphoma, primary cutaneous > nodal Hodgkin's disease
Rare reports (<10% of cases)	Chronic lymphocytic leukemia Acute myeloid leukemia B-cell lymphoma T-cell large granular lymphocytic leukemia Multiple myeloma Myelodysplastic syndrome

Data from de Souza A, el-Azhary RA, Camilleri MJ, et al. In search of prognostic indicators for lymphomatoid papulosis: a retrospective study of 123 patients. J Am Acad Dermatol 2012;66(6):928–37; and Wieser I, Tetzlaff MT, Torres Cabala CA, et al. Primary cutaneous CD30(+) lymphoproliferative disorders. J Dtsch Dermatol Ges 2016;14(8):767–82.

> **Box 1**
> **Risk factors for developing a secondary malignancy with LyP**
>
> Male sex (2.5–2.8 times more likely)[23]
>
> History of EBV either clinical or serologic (4.8 times more likely)[23]
>
> Histologic subtypes B (OR, 2.66) and C (OR, 2.83)[24]
>
> LyP with clonal T-cell receptor gene rearrangement (OR, 5.7–7.55)[22]
>
> Advanced age (OR, 1.05 per year)[57]
>
> *Abbreviations:* EBV, Epstein–Barr virus; LyP, lymphomatoid papulosis; OR, odds ratio.

CD30L expression on the neoplastic cells, causing the CD30 expressing cells to undergo apoptosis either through CD30–CD30L inhibition of neoplastic cell growth and/or increased sensitivity of the neoplastic cells to Fas-FasL–mediated apoptosis.[8] Patients with LyP may develop recurrent crops over several months or for decades, with cases reported to last more than 40 years.[18]

Differential Diagnosis

With histologic evidence of a CD30⁺ infiltrate, all entities in **Table 1** should be considered. Coupled with a clinical presentation of recurrent self-resolving crops of papulonodules, the main differential diagnoses include:

1. Pityriasis lichenoides
2. Borderline CD30⁺ LPD
3. Cutaneous anaplastic large cell lymphoma
4. Reactive lymphoid hyperplasia (lymphocytoma cutis) secondary to:
   a. Arthropod assault
   b. Scabies
   c. Medications
   d. Herpes simplex virus
   e. Varicella zoster virus

Pathology

When considering LyP, a skin biopsy is recommended for histologic and immunohistochemical evaluation to classify the cellular subtypes and rule out infectious entities. DNA should be sent for T-cell gene rearrangement polymerase chain reaction to assess for clonality.

> **Table 4**
> **Clinical features of LyP and pcALCL**
>
> | | LyP | pcALCL |
> | --- | --- | --- |
> | Size (mm) | 5–10 | >20 |
> | Number of lesions | Several to hundreds | Solitary or localized |
> | Distribution | Trunk and limbs | Anywhere |
> | Duration of lesions (wk) | 3–8 | >12 |
> | Self-resolving (%) | 100 | 28 (0–44) |
> | Extracutaneous disease (%) | 0 | 13 (0–24) |
>
> *Abbreviations:* LyP, lymphomatoid papulosis; pcALCL, primary cutaneous anaplastic large cell lymphoma.
> *Data from* Refs.[14,18,39]

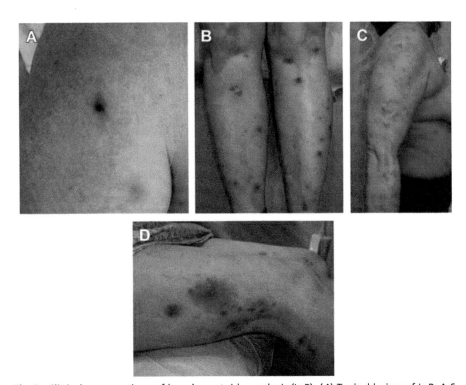

Fig. 2. Clinical presentations of lymphomatoid papulosis (LyP). (*A*) Typical lesion of LyP: A 6-mm violaceous papule with a necrotic center. (*B, C*) Crops of LyP in various stages of evolution. (*D*) Inflamed lesion of LyP, with a surrounding crop of more typical lesions.

There are currently 5 generally accepted histologic subtypes of LyP (A-E), as well as a recently proposed sixth subtype (F; **Table 5**). CD30[+] T-cell lymphocytes are the hallmark of all histologic types of LyP, although type B has variable positivity, reported to range from 0% to 77% of the infiltrate.[29] Subtypes may occur concurrently within the same biopsy or within different specimens taken from the same patient. Other rare pathologic variants include a γ/δ type[30] and an LyP with 6p25.3 rearrangement.[31] The significance of the γ/δ variant is unknown. The 6p25.3 type is described as biphasic with small to medium lymphocytes in the epidermis and larger pleomorphic lymphocytes in the dermis. Clinically, this variant presents in older individuals (mean, 75 years of age) and has a higher male predominance (3:1 male:female ratio). Otherwise, the course follows the same natural history of all other variants of LyP.

The clinical significance of the histologic subtypes remains unclear, with rare exceptions. As noted, type B can be CD30 negative and histologically resemble MF. In this setting, the clinical morphology and behavior is then required to distinguish the 2 entities and render a diagnosis of LyP. Additionally, subtypes B and C have been shown to be associated with a greater risk of secondary malignancy.[24]

Immunohistochemistry is required to characterize the infiltrate (**Table 6**). The majority of LyP cases are CD4[+] and CD45RO[+]; however, type D, type E and LyP in children are CD4[−] CD8[+].[30] CD45RO helps to differentiate LyP type D from aggressive epidermotropic CD8[+] cutaneous T-cell lymphomas with the former being CD45RO[+] and the latter being CD45RO[−].[14]

Table 5
Histologic morphologies of LyP

Type	Percent of Cases	Histologically Mimics	Description
A	47–82	Hodgkin lymphoma Transformed MF	Large Reed-Sternberg–like atypical lymphocytes Wedge-shaped heterogeneous infiltrate with lymphocytes, neutrophils, eosinophils and histiocytes
B	4–17	MF	Epidermotropic bandlike infiltrate Small irregular lymphocytes Cerebriform nuclei
C	7–22	ALCL	Sheets or clustered infiltrate Large atypical lymphocytes Few inflammatory cells
D	~8	Primary cutaneous aggressive CD8+ cytotoxic TCL PLC/PLEVA Pagetoid reticulosis Cutaneous gamma/delta TCL	Epidermotrophic infiltrate CD8+ Small to medium atypical lymphocytes
E	~0.6	Angiocentric Extranodal NK/T-cell lymphoma, nasal type Cutaneous gamma/delta TCL ALCL variant with angiocentric and/or angiodestructive growth	Small- to medium-sized lymphocytes Angiocentric: CD8+ infiltrating walls of small to medium-sized vessels Vasculitis: fibrin, thromboses and extravasation of red blood cells
F[58]	5–10	Folliculotropic Folliculotropic MF Pseudolymphoma Connective tissue diseases	Perifollicular infiltrate Medium to large lymphoid cells Follicular mucinosis Neutrophils within infundibula
Mixed	4–9		More than 1 histologic type in the same patient or lesion

Abbreviations: ALCL, anaplastic large cell lymphoma; LyP, lymphomatoid papulosis; MF, mycosis fungoides; NK, natural killer; pcALCL, primary cutaneous anaplastic large cell lymphoma; PLC/PLEVA, pityriasis lichenoides chronica/pityriasis lichenoides et varioliformis; TCL, T-cell lymphoma.
Data from Refs.[20,24,30,58,61]

T-cell receptor (TCR) gene rearrangement demonstrates clonality in 40% to 100% of cases of LyP, despite its benignity.[30] The significance of the clonality in the risk of developing a secondary malignancy remains to be determined. The majority of cases have α/β TCR clones with few reports of γ/δ TCR clonality, particularly in type D LyP.[32]

Table 6
Immunohistochemical profile of LyP and ALCL

	LyP	pcALCL	scALCL
Clonality	40%–100%	>90%	~90%
CD30	+ (type B, variably)	>75% + (required for diagnosis)	+
CD56	~10%	12%–75%	+ (worst prognosis)
Bcl-2	−	30%	+
Cytotoxic molecules: TIA-1, granzyme B or perforin	+	~50%	+
ALK	−	Rare	50%
Cutaneous lymphocyte antigen	+	Variable	−
Epithelial membrane antigen	−	−	+
t(2;5) (pq23;q35) translocation	−	<10%	70%–75%

Abbreviations: LyP, lymphomatoid papulosis; pcALCL, primary cutaneous anaplastic large cell lymphoma; TIA-1, T-cell intercellular antigen 1.
   Data from Refs.[30,62,63]

Workup

The evaluation of a patient with a suspected or biopsy confirmed case of CD30$^+$ LPD is outlined in **Fig. 3** and **Table 7**. Despite being a disorder visible on examination, definitive diagnosis is often delayed by 1 to 3 years.[33] In most cases, a diagnosis of LyP can be rendered based on history and thorough dermatologic physical

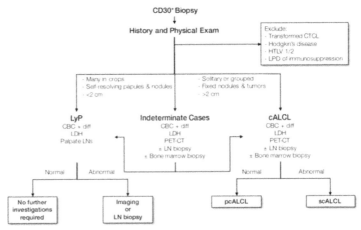

Fig. 3. Diagnosis algorithm for primary cutaneous CD30$^+$ lymphoproliferative disorders (LPD). CBC, complete blood count; CT, computed tomography; CTCL, cutaneous T-cell lymphoma; diff, differential; HTLV, human T-cell lymphotropic virus; LDH, lactate dehydrogenase; LN, lymph node; LyP, lymphomatoid papulosis; pcALCL, primary cutaneous anaplastic large cell lymphoma; scALCL, secondary cutaneous anaplastic large cell lymphoma.

Table 7 CD30⁺ workup	LyP	pcALCL	scALCL
History			
Spontaneous regression	✔	✔	✗
Previous lymphoid neoplasms (MF, nodal ALCL, or Hodgkin lymphoma)	✔	✗	✔
Immunosuppression	✗	✗	✗
B symptoms	✗	✗	✔
Physical examination			
Solitary lesion	✗	✔	✔
Many lesions	✔	✗	✔
Enlarged lymph nodes	✗	✗	✔
Hepatosplenomegaly	✗	✗	✔
Laboratory investigations			
Abnormal CBC with differential	✗	✗	✔
Abnormal LDH	✗	✗	✔
Serology for HTLV-1/2	✗	✗	✗
Other investigations			
Contrast enhanced CT ± PET of the chest, abdomen, and pelvis or whole body integrated PET-CT	✗	✔	✔
Bone marrow aspirate or biopsy	✗	Only if radiologic evidence of extracutaneous disease	✔
Lymph node biopsy	✗	If >1.5 cm palpable or evidence on imaging	✔

Abbreviations: ACLC, anaplastic large cell lymphoma; CBC, complete blood count; CT, computed tomography; HTLV, human T-cell lymphotropic virus types 1/2; LDH, lactate dehydrogenase; LyP, lymphomatoid papulosis; MF, mycosis fungoides; pcALCL, primary cutaneous anaplastic large cell lymphoma; TIA-1, T-cell intercellular antigen 1.

Adapted from Kempf W, Pfaltz K, Vermeer MH, et al. EORTC, ISCL, and USCLC consensus recommendations for the treatment of primary cutaneous CD30-positive lymphoproliferative disorders: lymphomatoid papulosis and primary cutaneous anaplastic large-cell lymphoma. Blood 2011;118:4024.

examination alone, with a biopsy providing diagnostic confirmation. For accuracy of diagnosis and to exclude those entities described in the differential diagnosis, the following investigations are recommended:

1. Skin biopsy, including immunohistochemical and TCR gene rearrangement
2. Complete blood count with differential
3. Lactate dehydrogenase
4. Serology for Human T-cell lymphotropic virus types 1 and 2 for patients in endemic areas
5. Imaging, if indicated based on history or examination
6. Lymph node biopsy, if enlarged

It is suggested to biopsy 2 or more papules that are inflammatory but have not yet undergone necrosis.

Treatment

The management of LyP depends on the clinical severity and symptoms. Indications to treat include cases that are diffuse or progressive, are physically symptomatic, or lead to disfigurement from significant scarring or pigmentary change. With limited disease burden, active nontreatment may be appropriate and considered first line. To date, treatment has not been reported to alter the natural course of LyP or the risk of developing a secondary malignancy.[34]

If active treatment is required, a therapeutic ladder for treating LyP is outlined in **Table 8**. As with any therapy, and of particular importance in the setting of a recurrent, self-resolving disorder, the benefits of the treatment must outweigh the associated risks. The goal of treatment is to prevent new outbreaks, accelerate resolution of lesions, and prevent secondary scarring and pigmentary changes. With all treatments, lesions recur in more than 40% of patients, typically within weeks of discontinuing or decreasing treatment.[34] **Table 8** lists many therapeutic options; however, the majority of patients with few lesions are managed with potent topical steroids at the first sign of a new papule; those with more diffuse disease respond to low-dose methotrexate or phototherapy. Additional agents are rarely required and multiagent chemotherapy regimens are not indicated or effective at inducing a prolonged remission in this benign disorder. The use of systemic chemotherapy has been associated with rapid recurrence of LyP either during or after treatment.[35]

Table 8 Treatment of LyP	
First line	Active nontreatment
	Topical corticosteroids
	Class I-III for trunk and extremities; class IV, V for face, genitals and axillae
	Phototherapy
	Methotrexate, 5–25 mg/wk[a]
Second line	Topical tacrolimus
	Topical nitrogen mustard
	Topical retinoids (bexarotene)
	Topical carmustine
Third Line	Radiotherapy[b]
	Imiquimod 5% cream
	Interferon-a, Interferon-g
	Brentuximab vendotin (anti-CD30 monoclonal antibody)[c]
	Antibiotics: tetracyclines, penicillin, erythromycin
	Sulfones
	Surgical excision[b]

[a] Generally accepted regimens include starting doses of 7.5 to 12.5 mg/wk, increasing as tolerated every 8 to 12 weeks until clear up to 25 mg/wk. Once control has been maintained for 8 to 12 weeks with no new lesions, the dose is titrated down in a similar fashion to the lowest dose attainable without flares.
[b] For larger, refractory, and persistent lesions.
[c] For multifocal disease.
Adapted from Klein RS, Singer E, Junkins-Hopkins JM, et al. 141: Lymphomatoid papulosis. In: Lebwohl MG, Heymann W, Berth-Jones J, et al, editors. Treatment of skin disease: Comprehensive therapeutic strategies. 4th edition. Edinburgh (United Kingdom): Saunders; 2014. p. 430–4.

Regardless of treatment plan, patients living with LyP should have life-long follow-up to monitor for the development of a secondary hematologic malignancy. Additionally, any lesion that is persistent and/or greater than 2 cm should be biopsied to rule out concomitant ALCL or other secondary neoplasms.

CUTANEOUS ANAPLASTIC LARGE CELL LYMPHOMA

Cutaneous ALCL can be divided into primary cutaneous ALCL (pcALCL) and secondary cutaneous ALCL (scALCL). In scALCL, a systemic ALCL with skin involvement, the skin is the most common extranodal site.[35] Please see Dai Chihara and Michelle A. Fanale's article "Management of Anaplastic Large Cell Lymphoma," in this issue for a more in-depth discussion of systemic ALCL.

Epidemiology

Patients with pcALCL have an older median age of onset (60 years) than their LyP counterparts, and it affects males more than females at a ratio of 3:1 (see **Table 2**).[20] There is a bimodal age distribution with scALCL that varies with anaplastic lymphoma kinase (ALK) expressivity; patients with ALK-positive scALCL present at a median age of 34 years, whereas those who are ALK negative present at a median age of 58 years.[36]

Prognosis

Similar to LyP, pcALCL has a favorable prognosis with greater than 95% survival at 10 years. With draining lymph node involvement in more than one nodal basin, survival decreases to 76%–96% at 5 years; however, the involvement of lymph nodes in a single draining basin has a prognosis similar to patients with disease isolated to the skin.[20] Conversely, patients with systemic ALCL have a less favorable prognosis; those with ALK-positive disease tend to be younger and have a 5-year survival of 70%, whereas ALK-negative disease tends to occur in older patients and has a 5-year survival of 49%. Extranodal involvement of sALCL, such as cutaneous involvement, is a poor prognostic sign.[37]

Clinical

In contrast to the successive crops of small self-healing papulonodules of LyP, pcALCL most often presents with a solitary or local group of nodules or tumors, larger than 2 cm. Patients describe a rapidly growing, red to violaceous nodule or tumor that may ulcerate (**Fig. 4**).[15] Although alarming, these lesions are generally asymptomatic and patients are systemically well, without fevers, chills, fatigue, night sweats, or weight loss. Such B symptoms should raise suspicion of a systemic lymphoma.

Although the majority of patients present with a solitary lesion, approximately 25% of cases of pcALCL present with a localized group of nodulotumors and up to 22% of cases may have multifocal (usually 2) lesions at different anatomic sites.[20] Regression, either partial or total, is variable and occurs in approximately 28% of cases with a range of 0% to 44%. This feature may highlight indeterminate cases or those that are confused with LyP. The spread of pcALCL to extracutaneous sites is uncommon, but has been reported in approximately 13% of cases with a range of 0% to 24%, depending on the series.[37]

Importantly, systemic ALCL commonly presents with B symptoms and approximately 20% of cases of sALCL will develop skin lesions (**Fig. 5**).[38] The lesions tend to be multifocal or generalized in contrast with pcALCL.

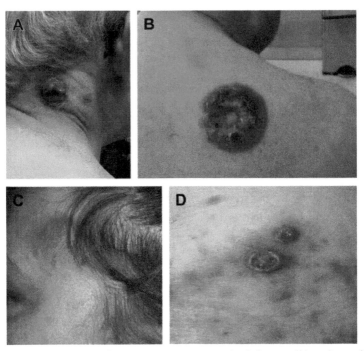

Fig. 4. Clinical presentations of primary cutaneous anaplastic large cell lymphoma (pcALCL). (*A*) Typical pcALCL tumor: Red, friable, 2.5-cm tumor, well-defined with central crusting. (*B*) A pcALCL tumor measuring 5.5 × 7.2 cm with central clearing and hemorrhagic crust. (*C*) Early pink plaque of pcALCL. (*D*) Multifocal, localized, and ulcerative pcALCL.

Pathology

In the majority of cases, routine histopathology of pcALCL demonstrates a dense dermal nodular infiltrate with sheets of atypical large anaplastic lymphocytes. The epidermis is generally uninvolved, unless there is ulceration present. Anaplastic cells refer to cells with irregular nuclei that are often horseshoe shaped, have eosinophilic nucleoli and abundant cytoplasm.[14] Importantly, the sheets of anaplastic lymphocytes cannot be distinguished from LyP type C histologically and differentiation of the 2 entities is made based on the clinical presentation. In 20% to 25% of cases, pcALCL presents with a nonanaplastic pleomorphic or immunoblastic histopathology. In these cases, which show a heterogeneous inflammatory infiltrate including neutrophils and eosinophils, differentiation from LyP type A is made based on the clinical presentation. Interestingly and sometimes complicating the clinicopathologic correlation, cases of pcALCL with LyP-like histopathology are more likely to completely regress.[20]

By definition, at least 75% of the tumor cells must express CD30.[39] In pcALCL, ALK is almost always negative. Importantly, in scALCL, ALK is positive in only 50% of cases[40] and, therefore, ALK negativity does not rule out scALCL. Additionally, cutaneous lymphocyte antigen is generally positive in pcALCL whereas epithelial membrane antigen is typically negative.[20] In contrast, the expression of cutaneous lymphocyte antigen is usually negative and the epithelial membrane antigen is positive in scALCL (see **Table 6**). Please see Dai Chihara and Michelle A. Fanale's article "Management of Anaplastic Large Cell Lymphoma," in this issue for additional details on the pathology of scALCL.

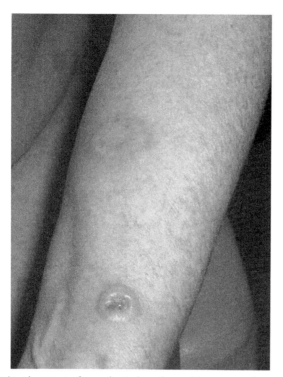

Fig. 5. Cutaneous involvement of anaplastic lymphoma kinase negative systemic anaplastic large cell lymphoma (ALCL), with annular plaques and tumors. Note the evidence of scarring at prior sites on the arm and trunk.

Differential Diagnosis

Again, with histologic evidence of a CD30+ infiltrate, all entities in **Table 1** should be considered. However, the main differential in nodulotumors greater than 2 cm that variably self-resolve are:

1. scALCL
2. LyP
3. Transformed MF
4. Other systemic lymphomas including adult T-cell leukemia–lymphoma or Hodgkin disease with cutaneous involvement
5. Nodular reactive lymphoid hyperplasia owing to arthropod bite, medication, or infection

Workup

The workup for cALCL is more extensive than LyP owing to the greater possibility of extracutaneous involvement. A comprehensive history and physical examination along with a biopsy of suspicious lesions remain the first steps in diagnosis. Similar to LyP, the skin biopsy should be performed and examined for histopathologic appearance, classification of the infiltrate using immunohistochemical, and T-cell gene rearrangement to assess for clonality.

After the establishment of a diagnosis of cALCL based on clinical and pathologic features, systemic involvement must be ruled out. Lack of B-symptoms is supportive

Table 9 Treatment of pcALCL	
Solitary or grouped lesions	Local radiotherapy (first line) Excision
Multifocal	Low-dose methotrexate (5–25 mg/wk) Systemic retinoids Pralatrexate Brentuximab vedotin Monitor for spontaneous resolution
Extracutaneous spread	Nodal radiation, if single basin Brentuximab vedotin Low dose methotrexate (5–25 mg/wk) Pralatrexate Multiagent doxorubicin based chemotherapy

Data from National Comprehensive Cancer Network. Non-Hodgkin lymphomas version 3.2016. Available at: https://www.nccn.org/professionals/physician_gls/PDF/nhl.pdf. Accessed October 24, 2016.

of a diagnosis of pcALCL; however, complete evaluation is recommended to evaluate for extracutaneous disease of all subsets. The following are recommended:

1. Complete blood count with differential
2. Lactate dehydrogenase
3. Contrast-enhanced computed tomography (CT) with PET, which is preferred over computed tomography of the chest, abdomen, and pelvis
4. Biopsy of any avid lymph nodes and those larger than 1.5 cm
5. Bone marrow biopsy is considered in the setting of diffuse or multifocal tumors, abnormal hematologic examination or documented extracutaneous disease.

Treatment

The approach to pcALCL therapy is determined by clinical presentation (**Table 9**). The mainstay of treatment for solitary to a few lesions of pcALCL is radiotherapy or surgical excision. Given the inherent difficulty in determining the margins for cutaneous LPD, radiotherapy is preferred. There are no recommended surgical margins for pcALCL. The optimal dose for radiotherapy also has not been identified but generally 36 to 40 Gy in 2 to 3 fractions are used with a margin of 2 to 3 cm, with complete responses ranging from 86% to 100%.[41]

Historically, treatment for multiple lesions involved multi-agent chemotherapy. Based on the overall prognosis, natural history of pcALCL and high rates of relapse after systemic treatment (40%–70%),[35,38] multiagent chemotherapy is not considered first line; there does not seem to be added benefit beyond less toxic alternatives. Low-dose methotrexate (less than 25 mg/wk) is considered first-line for multifocal pcALCL where radiotherapy is not feasible.[28] Brentuximab vedotin has been used off-label for multifocal, refractory, extracutaneous, or relapsed pcALCL[42] and is increasingly being used early in the treatment course. It is currently approved by the US Food and Drug Administration for the treatment of patients with systemic ALCL after failure of at least 1 prior multiagent chemotherapy regimen.[43] In the case of pcALCL with nodal involvement to a single region, radiotherapy to the primary site and nodal basin may be used.

SUMMARY

CD30+ LPD of the skin are composed of a spectrum of benign and malignant diseases encompassing LyP, pcALCL, and borderline cases. Accurate diagnosis of these conditions requires a thorough history and complete dermatologic and nodal examination, noting the natural course of the lesions and the status of lymph nodes and systemic symptoms. The accurate description of the morphology, distribution, and behavior of lesions is crucial for reaching the correct diagnosis. Although all cases of CD30+ LPD may look malignant histologically, their behavior and knowledge of the natural course of LyP and pcALCL (5-year survival of 100% and >95%, respectively) allows clinicians to avoid aggressive treatment with high recurrence rates. Importantly, ongoing surveillance of these patients is still required to monitor for secondary malignancy with LyP and recurrence or extracutaneous spread of ALCL.

REFERENCES

1. Gilfillan MC, Noel PJ, Podack ER, et al. Expression of the costimulatory receptor CD30 is regulated by both CD28 and cytokines. J Immunol 1998;160(5):2180–7.
2. Smith CA, Gruss HJ, Davis T, et al. CD30 antigen, a marker for Hodgkin's lymphoma, is a receptor whose ligand defines an emerging family of cytokines with homology to TNF. Cell 1993;73(7):1349–60.
3. Bowen MA, Lee RK, Miragliotta G, et al. Structure and expression of murine CD30 and its role in cytokine production. J Immunol 1996;156(2):442–9.
4. Muta H, Podack ER. CD30: from basic research to cancer therapy. Immunol Res 2013;57(1–3):151–8.
5. Younes A, Consoli U, Snell V, et al. CD30 ligand in lymphoma patients with CD30+ tumors. J Clin Oncol 1997;15(11):3355–62.
6. Cerutti A, Schaffer A, Goodwin RG, et al. Engagement of CD153 (CD30 ligand) by CD30+ T cells inhibits class switch DNA recombination and antibody production in human IgD+ IgM+ B cells. J Immunol 2000;165(2):786–94.
7. Song HY, Régnier CH, Kirschning CJ, et al. Tumor necrosis factor (TNF)-mediated kinase cascades: bifurcation of nuclear factor-kappaB and c-jun N-terminal kinase (JNK/SAPK) pathways at TNF receptor-associated factor 2. Proc Natl Acad Sci U S A 1997;94(18):9792–6.
8. Mori M, Manuelli C, Pimpinelli N, et al. CD30-CD30 ligand interaction in primary cutaneous CD30(+) T-cell lymphomas: a clue to the pathophysiology of clinical regression. Blood 1999;94(9):3077–83.
9. Bargou RC, Emmerich F, Krappmann D, et al. Constitutive nuclear factor-kappaB-RelA activation is required for proliferation and survival of Hodgkin's disease tumor cells. J Clin Invest 1997;100(12):2961–9.
10. Muta H, Boise LH, Fang L, et al. CD30 signals integrate expression of cytotoxic effector molecules, lymphocyte trafficking signals, and signals for proliferation and apoptosis. J Immunol 2000;165(9):5105–11.
11. Falini B, Pileri S, Pizzolo G, et al. CD30 (Ki-1) molecule: a new cytokine receptor of the tumor necrosis factor receptor superfamily as a tool for diagnosis and immunotherapy. Blood 1995;85(1):1–14.
12. Bhatt G, Maddocks K, Christian B. CD30 and CD30-targeted therapies in Hodgkin lymphoma and other B cell lymphomas. Curr Hematol Malig Rep 2016;11(6):480–91.
13. Stein H, Mason DY, Gerdes J, et al. The expression of the Hodgkin's disease associated antigen Ki-1 in reactive and neoplastic lymphoid tissue: evidence that Reed-Sternberg cells and histiocytic malignancies are derived from activated lymphoid cells. Blood 1985;66(4):848–58.
14. Willemze R, Jaffe ES, Burg G, et al. WHO-EORTC classification for cutaneous lymphomas. Blood 2005;105(10):3768–85.

15. Stein H, Foss HD, Dürkop H, et al. CD30(+) anaplastic large cell lymphoma: a review of its histopathologic, genetic, and clinical features. Blood 2000;96(12): 3681–95.
16. Macaulay WL. Lymphomatoid papulosis: a continuing self-healing eruption, clinically benign-histologically malignant. Arch Dermatol 1968;97(1):23–30.
17. Wang HH, Lach L, Kadin ME. Epidemiology of lymphomatoid papulosis. Cancer 1992;70(12):2951–7.
18. Willemze R. 120: cutaneous T-cell lymphoma. In: Bolognia J, Jorizzo JL, Schaffer JV, editors. Dermatology, vol. 2, 3rd edition. Philadelphia: Elsevier Saunders; 2012. p. 2029–32. Print.
19. Wang HH, Myers T, Lach LJ, et al. Increased risk of lymphoid and nonlymphoid malignancies in patients with lymphomatoid papulosis. Cancer 1999;86:1240.
20. Bekkenk MW, Geelen FA, van Voorst Vader PC, et al. Primary and secondary cutaneous CD30(+) lymphoproliferative disorders: a report from the Dutch Cutaneous Lymphoma Group on the long-term follow-up data of 219 patients and guidelines for diagnosis and treatment. Blood 2000;95:3653.
21. Gruber R, Sepp NT, Fritsch PO, et al. Prognosis of lymphomatoid papulosis. Oncologist 2006;11(8):955–7 [author reply: 957].
22. de Souza A, el-Azhary RA, Camilleri MJ, et al. In search of prognostic indicators for lymphomatoid papulosis: a retrospective study of 123 patients. J Am Acad Dermatol 2012;66(6):928–37.
23. Kunishige JH, McDonald H, Alvarez G, et al. Lymphomatoid papulosis and associated lymphomas: a retrospective case series of 84 patients. Clin Exp Dermatol 2009;34:576.
24. Wieser I, Oh CW, Talpur R, et al. Lymphomatoid papulosis: treatment response and associated lymphomas in a study of 180 patients. J Am Acad Dermatol 2016;74(1):59–67.
25. Scarisbrick JJ, Evans AV, Woolford AJ, et al. Regional lymphomatoid papulosis: a report of four cases. Br J Dermatol 1999;141(6):1125–8.
26. Chan DV, Staidle J, Tamburro J, et al. Rapid cutaneous dissemination of persistently agminated lymphomatoid papulosis in a 9-year-old boy. Arch Dermatol 2011;147(11):1340–2.
27. Wieser I, Tetzlaff MT, Torres Cabala CA, et al. Primary cutaneous CD30(+) lymphoproliferative disorders. J Dtsch Dermatol Ges 2016;14(8):767–82.
28. LeBoeuf NR, McDermott S, Harris NL. Case records of the Massachusetts General Hospital. Case 5-2015. A 69-year-old woman with recurrent skin lesions after treatment for lymphoma. N Engl J Med 2015;372(7):650–9.
29. Kempf W. Cutaneous CD30-positive lymphoproliferative disorders. Surg Pathol Clin 2014;7(2):203–28.
30. Morimura S, Sugaya M, Tamaki Z, et al. Lymphomatoid papulosis showing γδ T-cell phenotype. Acta Derm Venereol 2011;91:712–3.
31. Karai LJ, Kadin ME, Hsi ED, et al. Chromosomal rearrangements of 6p25.3 define a new subtype of lymphomatoid papulosis. Am J Surg Pathol 2013;37:1173.
32. Rodríguez-Pinilla SM, Ortiz-Romero PL, Monsalvez V, et al. TCR-γ expression in primary cutaneous T-cell lymphomas. Am J Surg Pathol 2013;37(3):375–84.
33. Kadin ME. Current management of primary cutaneous CD30+ T-cell lymphoproliferative disorders. Oncology (Williston Park) 2009;23:1158.
34. Kempf W, Pfaltz K, Vermeer MH, et al. EORTC, ISCL, and USCLC consensus recommendations for the treatment of primary cutaneous CD30-positive lymphoproliferative disorders: lymphomatoid papulosis and primary cutaneous anaplastic large-cell lymphoma. Blood 2011;118:4024.

35. Kadin ME, Carpenter C. Systemic and primary cutaneous anaplastic large cell lymphomas. Semin Hematol 2003;40(3):244–56.
36. Savage KJ, Harris NL, Vose JM, et al. International Peripheral T-Cell Lymphoma Project. ALK- anaplastic large-cell lymphoma is clinically and immunophenotypically different from both ALK+ ALCL and peripheral T-cell lymphoma, not otherwise specified: report from the International Peripheral T-Cell Lymphoma Project. Blood 2008;111(12):5496.
37. Liu HL, Hoppe RT, Kohler S, et al. CD30+ cutaneous lymphoproliferative disorders: the Stanford experience in lymphomatoid papulosis and primary cutaneous anaplastic large cell lymphoma. J Am Acad Dermatol 2003;49:1049.
38. Falini B, Pileri S, Zinzani PL, et al. ALK+ lymphoma: clinico-pathological findings and outcome. Blood 1999;93(8):2697–706.
39. Willemze R, Beljaards RC. Spectrum of primary cutaneous CD30 lymphoproliferative disorders: a proposal for classification and guidelines for management and treatment. J Am Acad Dermatol 1993;28:973–80.
40. Gascoyne RD, Aoun P, Wu D, et al. Prognostic significance of anaplastic lymphoma kinase (ALK) protein expression in adults with anaplastic large cell lymphoma. Blood 1999;93(11):3913–21.
41. Yu JB, McNiff JM, Lund MW, et al. Treatment of primary cutaneous CD30 anaplastic large-cell lymphoma with radiation therapy. Int J Radiat Oncol Biol Phys 2008;70(5):1542–5.
42. Duvic M, Tetzla MT, Gangar P, et al. Results of a phase II trial of brentuximab vedotin for CD30+ cutaneous T-cell lymphoma and lymphomatoid papulosis. J Clin Oncol 2015;33:3759–65.
43. Seattle Genetics Inc. ADCETRIS® full prescribing information including boxed warning – U.S. Bothell (WA): 2016.
44. Yeo W, Chow J, Wong N, et al. Carbamazepine-induced lymphadenopathy mimicking Ki-1 (CD301) T-cell lymphoma. Pathology 1997;29:64.
45. Nathan DL, Belsito DV. Carbamazepine-induced pseudolymphoma with CD-30 positive cells. J Am Acad Dermatol 1998;38:806.
46. Saeed SA, Bazza M, Zaman M, et al. Cefuroxime induced lymphomatoid hypersensitivity reaction. Postgrad Med J 2000;76:577.
47. Marucci G, Sgarbanti E, Maestri A, et al. Gemcitabine-associated CD81 CD301 pseudolymphoma. Br J Dermatol 2001;145:650.
48. Magro CM, Crowson AN, Kovatich AJ, et al. Drug-induced reversible lymphoid dyscrasia: a clonal lymphomatoid dermatitis of memory and activated T cells. Hum Pathol 2003;34(2):119–29.
49. Kim KJ, Lee MW, Choi JH, et al. CD30-positive T-cell-rich pseudolymphoma induced by gold acupuncture. Br J Dermatol 2002;146:882.
50. Cepeda LT, Pieretti M, Chapman SF, et al. CD30- positive atypical lymphoid cells in common non-neoplastic cutaneous infiltrates rich in neutrophils and eosinophils. Am J Surg Pathol 2003;27:912.
51. Gallardo F, Barranco C, Toll A, et al. CD30 antigen expression in cutaneous inflammatory infiltrates of scabies: a dynamic immunophenotypic pattern that should be distinguished from lymphomatoid papulosis. J Cutan Pathol 2002;29(6):368–73.
52. Chai C, White WL, Shea CR, et al. Epstein Barr virus-associated lymphoproliferative-disorders primarily involving the skin. J Cutan Pathol 1999;26:242.
53. Massi D, Trotta M, Franchi A, et al. Atypical CD301 cutaneous lymphoid proliferation in a patient with tuberculosis infection. Am J Dermatopathol 2004;26:234.

54. Smith KJ, Barrett TL, Neafie R, et al. Is CD30 (Ki-1) immunostaining in cutaneous eruptions useful as a marker of Th1 to Th2 cytokine switching and/or as a marker of advanced HIV-1 disease? Br J Dermatol 1998;138:774.

55. Horn T, Lehmkuhle MA, Gore S, et al. Systemic cytokine administration alters the histology of the eruption of lymphocyte recovery. J Cutan Pathol 1996;23:242.

56. Dummer W, Rose C, Bröcker EB. Expression of CD30 on T helper cells in the inflammatory infiltrate of acute atopic dermatitis but not of allergic contact dermatitis. Arch Dermatol Res 1998;290:598.

57. Cordel N, Tressieres B, D'Incan M, et al. Frequency and risk factors for associated lymphomas in patients with lymphomatoid papulosis. Oncologist 2016;21:76.

58. Kempf W, Kazakov DV, Baumgartner H-P, et al. Follicular lymphomatoid papulosis revisited: a study of 11 cases, with new histopathological findings. J Am Acad Dermatol 2013;68(5):809–16.

59. Beyer M, Sterry W. Cutaneous Lymphoma. In: Goldsmith LA, Katz SI, Gilchrest BA, et al, editors. Fitzpatrick's Dermatology in General Medicine, 8th edition. New York: McGraw-Hill; 2012. Available at: http://accessmedicine.mhmedical.com.proxy.bib. uottawa.ca/content.aspx?bookid=392&Sectionid=41138867. Accessed October 24, 2016.

60. Jacobsen E. Primary cutaneous anaplastic large cell lymphoma. 2016. Available at: UpToDate.com. Acceded October 24, 2016.

61. El Shabrawi-Caelen L, Kerl H, Cerroni L. Lymphomatoid papulosis: reappraisal of clinicopathologic presentation and classification into subtypes A, B, and C. Arch Dermatol 2004;140(4):441–7.

62. Burg G, Kempf W, Cozzio A, et al. WHO/EORTC classification of cutaneous lymphomas 2005: histological and molecular aspects. J Cutan Pathol 2005;32(10): 647–74.

63. Droc C, Cualing HD, Kadin ME. Need for an improved molecular/genetic classification for CD30+ lymphomas involving the skin. Cancer Control 2007;14(2): 124–32.

Autologous and Allogeneic Hematopoietic Cell Transplantation in Peripheral T/NK-cell Lymphomas
A Histology-Specific Review

Tejaswini M. Dhawale, MD, Andrei R. Shustov, MD*

KEYWORDS

- Peripheral T-cell lymphoma • Natural killer/T-cell lymphoma
- Hematopoietic stem cell transplantation • Histology • Pathophysiology
- Molecular biology • Treatment

KEY POINTS

- Peripheral T-cell lymphomas and natural killer/T-cell lymphomas (PT/NKCL) comprise a biologically diverse subgroup of rare non-Hodgkin's lymphomas characterized by an aggressive clinical course and dismal outcomes.
- The use of hematopoietic stem cell transplantation in the treatment of PTCL remains controversial owing to the absence of randomized controlled trials.
- Careful consideration of disease biology, history of response to prior therapies, individual patient preferences, and overall treatment goals should guide treatment approaches for every patient.
- Improved understanding of unique biology of each subtype of PTCL and studies incorporating novel agents into treatment regimens may further identify which patients may benefit most from hematopoietic stem cell transplantation.

INTRODUCTION

Peripheral T-cell lymphoma and natural killer (NK)/T-cell lymphomas (PT/NKCL) comprise a diverse subgroup of rare non-Hodgkin's lymphomas that are thought to arise from mature T or NK cells. With a few exceptions, the majority of PT/NKCL are characterized by an aggressive clinical course and historically dismal outcomes. The most common PT/NKCL include peripheral T-cell lymphoma, not otherwise specified (PTCL-NOS), angioimmunoblastic T-cell lymphoma (AITL), anaplastic large cell

Disclosure Statement: The authors have nothing to disclose.
Department of Medicine, University of Washington School of Medicine, SCCA, 825 Eastlake Avenue East, M-Box G3-200, Seattle, WA 98109, USA
* Corresponding author.
E-mail address: ashustov@seattlecca.org

Hematol Oncol Clin N Am 31 (2017) 335–357
http://dx.doi.org/10.1016/j.hoc.2016.11.003
0889-8588/17/© 2016 Elsevier Inc. All rights reserved.

lymphoma (ALCL, ALK-positive and ALK-negative), and extranodal NK/T-cell lymphoma, nasal type.[1] The clinical behavior and prognosis of the different histologic subgroups of PT/NKCL are widely variable and indicative of their individually unique biology. The histology-specific prognosis of the PT/NKCL can be summarized as follows: favorable, 5-year overall survival (OS) of 70% or greater (ALK-positive ALCL, primary cutaneous ALCL); intermediate, 5-year OS of 50% to 70% (ALK-negative ALCL, subcutaneous panniculitis-like TCL [SPTCL]); poor, 5-year OS of 25% to 50% (AITL, PTCL-NOS, nasal NK cell lymphoma); and dismal, 5-year OS of 20% or less (HSTCL, ATL/L, NK/T-cell lymphoma nasal type, aggressive/unclassifiable NK cell leukemia, other extranodal gamma-delta T-cell lymphomas).[2,3] Recent molecular analysis of the PT/NKCL has identified genetic signatures that not only distinguish between specific disease subtypes, but can also inform prognosis.[4] Insights into the biological behavior of these lymphomas has contributed to the development of targeted therapies for these diseases. As appreciation for the molecular fingerprint of PTCL and NKCL increases, it is anticipated that more "personalized" treatment approaches will be available and revolutionize the treatment landscape for these diseases.

Current treatment strategies for the PTCL an NKCL are focused on curative intent and the need to maintain remission given the aggressive nature of these diseases and the frequency with which they relapse. Unfortunately, owing to the absence of any randomized, controlled trials in this setting, there is presently no consensus regarding the optimal therapy for patients with newly diagnosed or relapsed or refractory PT/NKCL. It has been particularly difficult to understand the benefit of hematopoietic stem cell transplantation (HSCT) in these patients as most published studies involving HSCT in the upfront or relapsed setting have been retrospective and/or nonrandomized in nature. Moreover, these studies have often focused on small populations characterized by mixed histologies, varying disease status at transplantation, and treatments with diverse regimens. Selection bias has further limited the interpretation of these results, because many studies have excluded patients with chemorefractory or poor-risk disease who are not eligible for HSCT.

For the purpose of this review, we have focused our attention on the best-available evidence evaluating the role of HSCT in PT/NKCL using a histology-specific approach. We show that certain subtypes of PTCL and NKCL may benefit more from the application of high-dose therapy (HDT) and HSCT than other subtypes and that this benefit is likely a result of their unique clinical characteristics and underlying biology. Ultimately, however, prospective randomized controlled trials are needed to clarify the optimal type and timing of HSCT in patients with PT/NKCL.

PERIPHERAL T-CELL LYMPHOMA, NOT OTHERWISE SPECIFIED

PTCL-NOS is the most common subtype of PTCL, accounting for 25% of all PTCL.[5] The term PTCL-NOS encompasses a heterogeneous group of mature T-cell lymphomas that do not meet criteria for any of the defined T-cell entities in the World Health Organization classification system.[1] PTCL-NOS follows an aggressive clinical course and may present as both nodal and extranodal disease. Most patients with PTCL-NOS have advanced stage disease at diagnosis and in some cases exhibit symptoms of hepatosplenomegaly, pruritus, hemolytic anemia, or hemophagocytic syndrome.[6] The malignant cells in PTCL-NOS are typically characterized by CD4$^+$/CD8$^-$ expression, frequent antigen loss of CD5 and CD7, T-cell receptor (TCR) gene rearrangement and variable cytotoxic granule expression.[5,7] Recent biological insights into PTCL-NOS have identified frequent mutations in the TET2 gene as well as activation of JAK/STAT, mammalian target or rapamycin, and PI3K pathways in varying subsets of

PTCL-NOS tumors cells.[4,8,9] These findings have stimulated interest in the use of single agent therapies such as hypomethylating agents, mammalian target of rapamycin inhibitors, and JAK1 and 2 inhibitors in the treatment of this disease.

At present, however, the optimal treatment of PTCL-NOS remains unknown and participation in clinical trials has been recommended as first line therapy for stages I to IV disease.[10] The prognosis of patients with PTCL-NOS remains poor with a 5-year OS of 25% to 40%.[3,5,6] Relapse is common and the 5-year failure-free survival is only 20%.[3] A small subset of patients can experience long-term survival as evidenced by a 10-year OS of 20%.[6] The strongest predictor for survival is the International Prognostic Index (IPI) score, which can be used to distinguish between high-risk and low-risk individuals. Patients with low-risk IPI of 0 or 1 have an anticipated 5-year OS of 52%, whereas those with a high-risk IPI of 4 or 5 have a 5-year OS of 13% to 16%.[11]

Most patients with PTCL-NOS receive anthracycline-based combination chemotherapy, although there is no clear evidence of superiority to non–anthracycline-containing regimens.[6] Patients with early stage (stages I and II) disease may benefit from the addition of radiation therapy to combination chemotherapy.[5]

The largest prospective phase II trial conducted of autologous stem cell transplantation (ASCT) in first remission, the Nordic study (NLG-T-01 [A Nordic Phase II Study of PTCL Based on Dose-intensive Induction and High-dose Consolidation With ASCT]), evaluated the outcomes of 166 patients, of which 62 were classified as having PTCL-NOS.[12] In this study, patients were treated initially with biweekly chemotherapy with cyclophosphamide, doxorubicin, etoposide, vincristine and prednisone (CHOEP) (or chemotherapy with cyclophosphamide, doxorubicin, vincristine and prednisone [CHOP] for patients age >60). Patients experiencing a complete response (CR) or partial response (72% of enrolled patients) proceeded to consolidation with HDT followed by ASCT. Subtype-specific analysis of patients with PTCL-NOS demonstrated a 5-year OS of 47% and progression-free survival (PFS) of 38%. Reimer and colleagues[13] conducted the second largest prospective study evaluating upfront ASCT in 83 patients with PTCL, 32 of whom carried a diagnosis of PTCL-NOS. In this study, patients with high-risk disease (high or intermediate high IPI) experienced particularly poor outcomes with an OS approaching only 30% at 5 years. Although a head-to-head comparison of ASCT versus chemotherapy alone has not been conducted to date, the German High-Grade Non-Hodgkin Lymphoma Study Group found that for patients with PTCL-NOS, CHOP or CHOP-like therapy (CHOEP) resulted in a 3-year event-free survival (EFS) and OS of 41.1% and 53.9%m respectively. In light of these results, there is little evidence to justify the use of consolidation with HDT/ASCT in patients with PTCL-NOS.

The ideal timing of ASCT in patients with PTCL-NOS remains uncertain. Data from several retrospective studies indicate that ASCT at the time of treatment failure can yield a CR in a fraction of patients with chemosensitive disease. Yang and colleagues[14] performed a multicenter retrospective study with 64 Korean patients treated with HDT/ASCT after primary or salvage chemotherapy. Patients treated with primary chemotherapy mostly received an anthracycline-based regimen, whereas patients with relapsed disease were treated with a variety of salvage regimens include chemotherapy with dexamethasone, high-dose cytarabine, and cisplatin (DHAP), Ifosfamide, carboplatin, and etoposide (ICE), or dose-adjusted etoposide, prednisone, oncovin, cyclophosphamide, and hydroxydaunorubicin (DA-EPOCH). Transplant conditioning regimens varied between institutions. The overall transplant-related mortality cited in the study was 6.2%. An analysis of the posttransplant outcomes demonstrated a cumulative 3-year OS and PFS of 53% and 44.3%, respectively.[14] Importantly, the 3-year OS for patients in first CR/first PR was 60%, whereas the 3-year OS for patients undergoing ASCT in second CR was 70.9%. Taken together, these results suggest that the timing of ASCT in patients with PTCL-NOS is not as critical in determining OS as achieving a CR.

Allogeneic stem cell transplant is a potential curative option for patients with PTCL-NOS, but randomized studies are needed to support this approach. Corradini and co-workers[15] performed the first prospective, phase II, multicenter study evaluating the response of relapsed PTCL after reduced-intensity conditioning (RIC) allogeneic stem cell transplantation (RIC allogeneic HSCT). In this small study, 2 patients with PTCL-NOS developed a response after donor lymphocyte infusion, supporting the notion that a graft-versus-lymphoma effect exists in this setting. A recent retrospective study by Loirat and colleagues[16] of 49 newly diagnosed PTCL patients highlighted the feasibility of upfront allogeneic HSCT by noting a toxicity-related 1-year mortality of only 8.2%. Because patients with high risk disease are infrequently salvaged by ASCT, in our practice we consider the use of allogeneic HSCT in younger patients with high risk PTCL-NOS (IPI of 5) who achieve a first remission.

For patients with chemotherapy-refractory disease or who are not healthy enough to proceed with HDT followed by stem cell transplantation, we consider alternate or novel therapeutic approaches, preferably through a clinical trial. Romidepsin, pralatrexate, and brentuximab vedotin are currently approved in the relapsed/refractory setting.

ANGIOIMMUNOBLASTIC T-CELL LYMPHOMA

AITL is an aggressive T-cell neoplasm that accounts for 15% to 20% of peripheral T-cell lymphomas.[17–19] It is distinguishable from other PTCLs based on unique clinical, morphologic and molecular characteristics. Patients with AITL commonly present with advanced stage disease by Ann Arbor criteria. The majority are elderly with a mean age of 65 years at diagnosis and have signs or symptoms of systemic illness including generalized lymphadenopathy, hepatosplenomegaly, skin rash, hemolytic anemia, and hypergammaglobulinemia. Prognosis is dismal with the 5-year OS, failure-free survival, and PFS after intensive chemotherapy being 33%, 18%, and 13%, respectively (International T-Cell Lymphoma Project, British Columbia Cancer Agency).[3,20] With chemotherapy alone, the median OS is only 15 to 36 months.

AITL is thought to originate from malignant follicular T-helper cells. On morphology, the lymph node architecture is effaced by a complex milieu of neoplastic cells, arborizing blood vessels, follicular dendritic cells and Epstein-Barr virus–positive B-cell blasts.[21] Immunohistochemical studies are often positive for CD4, CD10, CXCL-13, PD1, and BCL-6.[7,22] Recent genome-wide studies have identified recurrent mutations in genes encoding epigenetic regulators such as *TET2*, *DNMT3A*, and *IDH2* in patients with AITL.[19,23,24] Insight into the unique biology of AITL has driven further investigation into novel therapies for this disease. Two different phase II studies found AITL to be particularly responsive to treatment with the histone deacetylase inhibitors belinostat and romidepsin.[25–28] Brentuximab vedotin, a CD30-specific antibody–drug conjugate, has also been found to be active in a subset of patients with CD30-positive AITL.[25–29]

For patients newly diagnosed with AITL, therapeutic options include observation, initiation of steroids, combination chemotherapy, stem cell transplantation, or clinical trial enrollment. At present, there are no randomized, controlled trials that compare these treatment approaches to guide selection of first-line therapy. In patients with AITL who are able to tolerate high-dose chemotherapy, we recommend the use of ASCT for consolidation in first remission. The strongest evidence supporting this approach comes from a prospective single arm study, the Nordic study, which evaluated the use of upfront ASCT in 166 patients with untreated PTCL.[12] In this study, patients received 6 cycles of biweekly CHOEP followed by HDT/ASCT if a CR or partial response was achieved. At a median follow-up of 60.5 months, the 5-year overall and PFS was 51% and 44%, respectively. A subgroup analysis of 30 patients with AITL demonstrated a 5-year OS and PFS of 52% and 49%, respectively. Overall, the treatment-related mortality was 4%. The largest study evaluating patients specifically with AITL was a performed by the European Group for Blood and Marrow Transplantation.[30] In this retrospective, multicenter study consisting of 146 patients with AITL, the 4-year OS and PFS after HDT-ASCT was reported to be 59% and 42%, respectively, after a median follow-up of 31 months. The majority of the patients in this study received carmustine, etoposide, cytarabine, and melphalan (BEAM) conditioning before ASCT. Of note, although the overall response rate to HDT-ASCT was high (77%), the cumulative incidence of relapse at 4 years was 51%. A multivariate analysis found that patients receiving ASCT in CR had significantly lower relapse rates when compared with patients with chemotherapy-sensitive disease without CR at the time of transplant. Importantly, the study did not assess the outcomes of patients in first CR versus second CR or later at the time of transplant. Thus, although not curative, ASCT seems to extend disease-free survival in patients with AITL with outcomes optimized when transplantation occurs in CR.

For patients who do not undergo upfront ASCT and relapse after standard chemotherapy, salvage HDT-ASCT remains an option. Several studies have reported long-term overall and event-free survival is possible even when patients are transplanted after relapse.[31,32] These studies, however, are limited by selection bias, small sample sizes, and their retrospective nature. Ideally, a prospective randomized controlled trial would be needed to determine the optimal first-line strategy for patients with AITL and the best timing for consolidation with HDT-ASCT. As our understanding of the biology of AITL improves, it has also become apparent that monotherapy with brentuximab vedotin, pralatrexate, and romidepsin are of benefit in the relapsed refractory setting.[29] The role of these novel agents in conjunction with HDT-ASCT is an area of active investigation.

Given the frequency of relapse after ASCT, additional treatment modalities are needed for patients with AITL. Allogeneic transplantation has been shown to result in long-term survival, but at the cost of significant treatment-related toxicities.[33,34] A retrospective analysis of 45 patients with AITL treated with allogeneic HSCT between 1998 and 2005 demonstrated a 3-year OS and PFS of 64% and 53%, respectively.[34] Twenty-five patients in the study received a myeloablative conditioning regimen and 20 patients underwent a RIC allogeneic HSCT with a corresponding 3-year OS of 58% and 71%, respectively. The combined 1-year non-relapse mortality (NRM) was 25% and did not differ between the 2 conditioning groups. The relapse rate was low (20% at 3 years) and seemed to be lower in patients with chronic GVHD. Although this study supports the notion that a clinically potent graft-versus-lymphoma effect exists with allogeneic HSCT in AITL, the concurrent risk of treatment-related mortality limits the widespread use of allogeneic HSCT.

Future randomized or prospective trials in this setting are necessary to confirm the benefit and optimal timing of both ASCT and allogeneic HSCT in patients with newly diagnosed and relapsed/refractory AITL.

ANAPLASTIC LARGE CELL LYMPHOMA

ALCL is the third most common subtype of PTCL and comprises approximately 3% of all non-Hodgkin's lymphomas.[3,35] The neoplastic cells in ALCL have universally strong expression of CD30 and are characterized by pleomorphic horseshoe or kidney-shaped nuclei along with abundant cytoplasm (so-called hallmark cells).[36] In addition to CD30, ALCL typically exhibits a EMA[+], PAX5[-], and CD45[-] (in one-third of cases) immunophenotype with a clonal TCR gene rearrangement.[7,37] A rearranged *ALK* gene is present in 65% of ALCL and defines a subtype of ALCL with unique clinical and genetic characteristics.[1,3] Patients with ALK-positive ALCL tend to present at a younger age (median, 34 years) whereas those with ALK-negative disease tend to be older (median, 58 years). Both subtypes seem to have a male predominance and present with advanced stage disease at diagnosis.[3,11,38,39]

The prognosis of ALK-positive ALCL is generally more favorable than ALK-negative ALC with a 5-year OS of 70% (vs 49%) and failure-free survival of 60% (vs 36%).[3] The IPI can be used to stratify disease risk in patients with ALCL. Patients with high-risk ALK-positive ALCL (an IPI of 4 or 5) have a 5-year OS of 33% and 5-year failure-free survival of 25% whereas the outcome of patients with low-risk ALK-negative (an IPI of 0 or 1) is favorable (5-year OS of 74% and 5-year failure-free survival of 62%).[3] Age (>40 years) and high beta2-microglobulin have also been found to be predictors of adverse outcomes in ALK-negative ALCL.[40]

Recently published gene expression studies have found that ALK-negative ALCL is itself a genetically diverse subgroup with specific gene rearrangements that impact prognosis. Rearrangements involving *DUSP22* and *IRF4* in chromosome 6p25 (*DUSP22* rearrangement) are associated with superior prognosis similar to that of patients with ALK-positive ALCL.[41] In contrast, patients with *TP63* rearrangements tend to have a poor prognosis and an estimated 5-year OS of 17%.[41]

The optimal treatment for all patients with ALCL remains unknown because the disease is relatively rare and no randomized controlled trials have been completed in this setting. Published outcomes of ALCL from prospective and retrospective studies are limited by small sample sizes and a heterogeneous sample population in which ALK rearrangement status is not always identified.

For patients presenting with early stage disease, there is general agreement that these patients should receive a truncated course of combination chemotherapy followed by targeted radiation therapy. The largest study supporting this approach retrospectively evaluated the outcomes of 46 patients with stage I or II ALCL after short-course doxorubicin-based chemotherapy and radiotherapy.[42] After a median follow-up of 55 months, the 5-year OS and PFS was found to be 84.4% and 63.6%, respectively.

Unfortunately, the majority of patients with ALCL present with advanced stage disease at diagnosis and require more long-term and intensive therapy. The role of autologous or allogeneic stem cell transplantation in the upfront setting remains unclear because neither treatment strategy has been compared directly with patients with ALCL receiving chemotherapy alone in a prospective, randomized study.

A subset of patients with ALCL, namely, those with low-risk (IPI < 2) ALK-positive disease, may be cured with chemotherapy alone.[39] Although chemotherapy with CHOP is the standard regimen for aggressive lymphomas, the German High-grade Non-Hodgkin Lymphoma Study Group found that patients younger than 40 with ALK-positive ALCL seem to benefit from the addition of etoposide (3-year EFS 57.1% without vs 91.2% with etoposide; *P* = .012) to the standard CHOP backbone.[43,44] In general, upfront CHOP or CHOP-like chemotherapy for ALK-positive ALCL is associated with an overall response rate of approximately 90%, a 5-year relapse-free survival of approximately 60%, and a 5-year OS of 70%.[39,45]

Published outcomes of HDT/ASCT in first remission demonstrate superior outcomes for patients with ALK-positive ALCL compared with other PTCLs.[45,46] Corradini and colleagues[46] conducted a prospective phase II study evaluating upfront ASCT in 62 patients with PTCL with mixed histologies (30% of which had ALK-positive ALC).

After a mean follow-up period of 76 months, patients with ALK-positive ALCL were found to have significantly improved OS (62% vs 21%; P = .005) and EFS (54% vs 18%; P = .006) compared with non–ALK-positive histologies. More impressive, however, are the results of a recent phase II trial using DA-EPOCH in the frontline treatment of ALK-positive and ALK-negative ALCL.[47] At a median follow-up of 14 years, the authors of this study found the EFS and OS in ALK-positive ALCL to be a remarkable 72% and 78%, respectively. Although a head-to-head comparison between standard chemotherapy and HDT-ASCT in first CR for patients with ALCL has not been performed, these recent data make the benefit of ASCT more doubtful.

With the current evidence, we cannot recommend ASCT for every patient with ALK-positive ALCL, but selected patients may benefit. We consider a risk-stratified approach to upfront therapy based on age and disease risk. For patients with low-risk ALK-positive ALCL or age less than 40 years, we recommend upfront chemotherapy without ASCT in first remission given the excellent prognosis anticipated with chemotherapy alone. For selected high-risk patients (IPI > 3) with an age of greater than 40 years, we conduct a careful assessment of the individual's risks and benefits of HDT/ASCT and discuss these with each patient, noting that, although feasible, the benefit of this approach is not clear from available data.

Patients with ALK-negative ALCL may potentially benefit from upfront HDT-ASCT, although randomized studies are needed to be certain. The largest prospective phase II study evaluating this approach was the Nordic study, which evaluated the benefit of ASCT for PTCL in first remission.[12] In this study, patients received induction chemotherapy consisting of 6 cycles of CHOP14 (if age > 60 years) or CHOEP (age < 60 years). Responders proceeded to conditioning with BEAM followed by ASCT. Of the 166 total patients, 31 had ALK-negative ALCL. Importantly, this subgroup was noted to have the highest OS and PFS (5-year OS, 70%; 5-year PFS, 61%) with a median follow-up of almost 4 years. The second largest prospective study addressing this approach assessed the outcomes of 83 patients with PTCL treated with upfront ASCT after CHOP.[13] After a median follow-up of 33 months, the study demonstrated a 3-year OS and PFS of 48% and 36% respectively. Unlike the Nordic study, histology-specific subgroup analysis in this study population did not reveal superior outcomes for ALK-negative ALCL over non-ALCL PTCLs.[13] Moreover, a recent report by Schmitz and colleagues[44] found that the 5-year EFS in ALK-negative patients after frontline CHOEP chemotherapy was 60.7%, which is similar to outcomes quoted by the Nordic study. These results are very similar to those a recently published phase II study in which DA-EPOCH resulted in an EFS and OS of 62.5% and 87.5%, respectively, in patients with ALK-negative ALCL.[47] Taken together, these data suggest that upfront ASCT is feasible and may result in long-term remissions in patients with ALK-negative ALCL, but that no clear comparison to chemotherapy alone can be made in the absence of a randomized study. Future studies that examine these results in light of the presence or absence of *DUSP22* or *TP63* rearrangements may help to clarify the discordant conclusions seen regarding the superior outcomes of ALK-negative ALCL. In addition, results of ongoing clinical trials such as the ECHELON-2 study (A Comparison of brentuximab vedotin and CHP with standard-of-care CHOP in the treatment of patients with CD30-positive mature T-cell lymphomas) evaluating the benefit and safety of novel agents such as brentuximab vedotin, an anti-CD30 antibody–drug conjugate, added to CHOP in the frontline setting may alter the future treatment approach to ALCL.[48]

In our assessment, the currently available data do not support the use of ASCT in all patients with ALCL. At our institution, we consider the use of upfront ASCT in patients with high-risk ALK-negative ALCL achieving CR with frontline therapy.

For patients with chemosensitive relapsed but not refractory ALCL, HDT followed by ASCT remains the standard of care. This approach is an abstraction of the insights from the PARMA trial and the treatment of relapsed refractory B-cell lymphomas.[49] Unfortunately, there are no similar prospective randomized control trials conducted in patients with relapsed refractory ALCL that assess the relative benefit of ASCT or allogeneic HSCT to guide treatment decisions. There are, however, numerous retrospective studies that have been conducted.[50–54] Although the interpretation of these studies is limited inherently by their retrospective nature and the heterogeneity of the sample population with regard to prognostic factors and ALK status, these data largely support the notion that good salvage rates can be accomplished by ASCT, although this finding is not consistent across all studies.

A registry analysis of data from the Center for International Blood and Marrow Transplant Research consisting of 241 patients (112 of which had ALCL) undergoing ASCT or allogeneic HSCT recently reported a histology specific 3-year OS and PFS of 65% and 50%, respectively, in patients with ALCL undergoing ASCT beyond first CR.[51] Likewise, Fanin and colleagues[50] published an European Group for Blood and Marrow Transplantation registry analysis of 64 adult and pediatric patients with relapsed T-cell and null-cell ALCL undergoing HDT/ASCT. The median age of the participants was 25 years and at the time of transplant, 47% were in CR. Although the study reported an excellent 5-year OS and PFS of 70% and 56%, respectively, these results are biased by the young age, transplant status, and absence of ALK status of the study population.[50] In comparison, Zamkoff and colleagues[52] published a retrospective analysis of 16 patients with recurrent, chemosensitive, ALK-negative ALCL treated with ASCT at the time of first relapse. The median age of the 16 patients was 51 years. The study found a strikingly low OS and PFS of 72 and 12 weeks, respectively, and concluded that ASCT did not offer a survival benefit to patients in this setting. In the absence of randomized studies, these data can only suggest that ASCT is feasible and that the benefit is likely restricted to patients with chemosensitive disease at the time of first relapse.

Because the relapse rate after transplantation remains high, alternative treatment strategies involving clinical trial enrollment, treatment with novel agents such as brentuximab vedotin or consideration of allogeneic stem cell transplantation for transplant eligible patients with available donors is our preferred approach.

Brentuximab vedotin, an anti-CD30 monoclonal antibody–drug conjugate has been approved for relapsed ALCL (regardless of ALK status) and seems to be far more effective than prior regimens used for first salvage. A recent phase II study of 58 patients with relapsed ALCL found that treatment with brentuximab vedotin yielded an overall objective response of 86% and a CR in more than one-half of the patients evaluated.[55] The median duration of overall response and CR were 12.6 and 13.2 months, respectively. A second novel agent, crizotinib, has been demonstrated to have activity in patients with relapsed ALK-positive ALCL. Crizotinib is an oral ALK inhibitor currently approved by the US Food and Drug Administration for therapeutic use in ALK-positive nonsmall cell lung cancer. In a phase I study of crizotinib in pediatric patients with refractory solid tumors and ALCL, 7 of 9 patients (78%) with ALK-positive ALCL experienced a CR.[56] Similar remarkable results have been reported as case reports by other groups.[57] These agents, along with other novel agents approved for relapsed/refractory ALCL may serve as an alternative salvage therapy before HSCT. At present, their role in induction and maintenance in the setting of salvage therapy and HSCT is being investigated.

The role of allogeneic HSCT in patients with ALCL remains controversial. The theoretic benefit of allogeneic transplantation lies in the potential for inducing a powerful graft-versus-lymphoma effect. However, there have been no studies performed to date specific to patients with ALCL to guide management decisions for those who may be transplant eligible. Most studies evaluating allogeneic HSCT have been small retrospective studies that collectively analyze multiple histologies of PTCLs. Recently, the Center for International Blood and Marrow Transplant Research retrospectively evaluated the outcomes of 115 autologous transplants and 126 allogeneic transplants in patients with ALCL, PTCL-NOS, and AITL. Not surprisingly, nonrelapse mortality relative risk was higher for allogeneic HSCT (3.543 vs 1.000; $P < .01$); however, no difference in relapse rates was found between the 2 treatment modalities.[51] Interestingly, the authors found that patients with ALCL undergoing ASCT experienced superior outcomes in comparison with those patients undergoing allogeneic HSCT. The largest single institution study evaluated the outcomes of 76 patients undergoing ASCT or allogeneic HSCT for relapsed T-cell lymphoma, 18 of whom had ALK-negative ALCL. The 4-year OS for all patients with relapsed disease treated with ASCT and allogeneic HSCT were 50% and 36%, respectively. The OS seen in patients receiving allogeneic HSCT seemed to be largely limited by NRM as the 4-year NRM for autologous HSCT and allogeneic HSCT was 17% and 40%, respectively. More favorable results for allogeneic HSCT were published by a French group evaluating 77 patients, including 27 patients with ALCL. This study demonstrated a 5-year OS and EFS of 55% and 48%, respectively, in patients receiving allogeneic HSCT, but a fair comparison with other studies is limited given that patients receiving transplant in the upfront setting were included in this analysis.[33] A few investigators have evaluated RIC and allogeneic HSCT (RIC allogeneic HSCT). Corradini and colleagues[15] published results of a small prospective phase II study of 17 patients (4 of whom had ALK-negative ALCL) with relapsed/refractory PTCL treated with RIC allogeneic HSCT. The study demonstrated a remarkable 3-year OS and PFS of 81% and 64%, respectively. These studies demonstrate that, although allogeneic stem cell transplantation may be potentially curative in patients with ALCL, OS is limited by high treatment-related mortality, predominantly from graft-versus-host disease, infections, and organ toxicities. A fair comparison between allogeneic and autologous transplantation is severely limited without randomized studies. The studies performed to date are, moreover, influenced by selection bias wherein those patients proceeding to allogeneic HSCT inevitably have more advanced disease, are chemorefractory, and have seen a greater number of prior therapies. RIC protocols offer a promising approach that may minimize treatment-related mortality and are especially attractive in the largely elderly population affected by this disease.

Because this treatment modality remains investigational, these authors favor the use of allogeneic stem cell transplantation in patients with multiply relapsed and refractory ALCL who are transplant eligible, have an HLA-matched donor, and can be treated in the context of a clinical trial. Novel therapies are likely to alter dramatically the treatment recommendations in the near future given their very high activity in ALCL.

EXTRANODAL NATURAL KILLER/T-CELL LYMPHOMA

Extranodal NK/TCL (ENKTL) is a unique clinical entity characterized by an aggressive clinical course. The disease is more prevalent in Asian and Hispanic populations, with the majority of cases presenting in the upper aerodigestive tract (nasal NK/TCL).[58] On histologic examination, ENKTL generally exhibits necrosis, local angioinvasion, and Epstein-Barr virus infection of the neoplastic cells. Malignant cells typically express phenotypic markers of NK cells, including CD2, CD56, and cytoplasmic CD3. Although surface expression of CD3 is absent, a small minority of cases do exhibit clonal rearrangement of TCR genes.[59] The overall prognosis of ENKTL is poor, with an expected 5-year OS of less than 20%.[2] The NK/T cell Lymphoma Prognostic Index can be used to identify high-risk patients based on the presence of B symptoms, nodal spread, increased lactate dehydrogenase level, and Ann Arbor stage IV disease.[60] Both treatment strategy and outcome depend on disease stage. For patients presenting with limited (stage I/II) disease, combined chemotherapy and radiation therapy is recommended and associated with a 5-year OS rate ranging from 42% to 83%.[61] In contrast, patients presenting with advanced disease (stages III or IV) have not been shown to benefit from the addition of radiotherapy and generally receive systemic chemotherapy. L-Asparaginase–based regimens have been found to have particularly high activity in patients with advanced NK cell lymphoma.[62] However, given the significant toxicity of these regimens and that a significant number of ENKTL patients still relapse after primary therapy, there remains substantial interest in alternate treatment strategies.[62–64] A potential consideration has been the use of HDT followed by HSCT; however, at present, no prospective randomized trials evaluating the benefit of upfront HSCT in ENKTL have been conducted. Most reports of HDT followed by HSCT are limited by small sample sizes and are composed of a heterogeneous patient population that limits comparison. The largest study to date retrospectively evaluated the feasibility and efficacy of upfront ASCT in 62 patients with newly diagnosed ENKTL.[65] The majority (80%) of patients were treated with non–anthracycline-based chemotherapy (dexamethasone, methotrexate, fosfamide, L-asparaginase, and etoposide [SMILE], etoposide, fosfamide, dexamethasone, and L-asparaginase [VIDL], fosfamide, methotrexate, etoposide, and prednisolone [IMEP] plus L-asp, and etoposide,[19] fosfamide, cisplatin, and dexamethasone [VIPD]), resulting in a complete remission in 61.3% of patients before transplantation. Upfront ASCT yielded a complete remission in 78.3% of patients with a 3-year PFS of 52.4% and a 3-year OS of 60.0%. Of note, both the PFS and the OS were significantly better for patients in the limited disease group when compared with the advanced disease group (PFS, 64.5% vs 40.1% [P = .017]; OS, 67.6% vs 52.3% [P = .048]). The survival outcomes seen in the limited disease group were similar to those seen previously in patients treated with chemotherapy or chemoradiotherapy alone. A second study examined the benefit of upfront ASCT after non–anthracycline-based chemotherapy (SMILE) in 27 patients with advanced-stage ENKTL. Induction with SMILE resulted in a 59% response rate (16 of 27), but was associated with significant toxicity with 5 deaths resulting from neutropenic fever. Of the remaining patients, 11 proceeded to ASCT. Although the study demonstrated improved OS and PFS in patients undergoing ASCT over those patients who did not (P < .003), the total number of patients was small and 4 patients ultimately relapsed. Multiple studies have shown that the benefit of ASCT in patients with ENKTL seems to depend on obtaining a CR at the time of transplantation. A retrospective study compared the outcomes of 47 patients after ASCT with a historical control group of 107 patients matched to the ASCT group by NK/T cell lymphoma International Prognostic Index risk group and disease status at transplantation.[61] Although no survival difference was found between patients in the ASCT and non-ASCT groups, a subgroup analysis showed that the benefit of ASCT was greater in patients who achieved CR with primary therapy and had a high-risk NK/T cell lymphoma International Prognostic Index. Importantly, most patients in this subgroup had limited stage (stage I and II disease) and would likely have experienced prolonged remission in the absence of ASCT. Multiple additional studies now corroborate these data and support the notion that upfront ASCT is of little value in patients with limited disease, but may be considered in patients with advanced or relapsed disease.[66,67] It remains unclear whether patients with refractory disease may benefit from ASCT over L-asparaginase containing chemotherapy. Given that the use of L-asparaginase–based chemotherapy (SMILE, L-asparaginase with methotrexate and dexamethasone) is highly efficacious in this setting,[62–64] these authors recommend considering treatment with ASCT after primary therapy with such regimens if CR is achieved. Prospective studies are clearly needed to further clarify the benefit of ASCT in this setting.

Because relapse is common after ASCT, several groups have investigated the benefit of allogeneic stem cell transplantation and its putative graft-versus-lymphoma effect in patients with newly diagnosed, and relapsed or refractory disease.[68–71] Although multiple studies have proven the feasibility of allogeneic stem cell transplantation in the setting of ENKTL, high treatment-related mortality limits its widespread use. In a combined analysis of 28 patients with NK cell neoplasms, 22 of which were ENKTL, treatment-related mortality was higher in patients receiving a conventional myeloablative stem cell transplantation (30% vs 20%) in comparison with those receiving a reduced-intensity stem cell transplantation (RIC) with no observed difference in overall response rate (60% vs 52%).[71] A retrospective study of 120 patients with NKTL compared the benefit of ASCT to allogeneic stem cell transplantation and found that ASCT yielded a better OS (60% vs 45% at 2 years; $P = .002$).[72] The allogeneic stem cell transplantation cohort, however, contained a greater number of patients with advanced stage and high IPI risk disease. Furthermore, on multivariate analysis, the type of HSCT was not found to be prognostic but advanced stage, lack of CR, and performance status were. A more recent multicenter study of 18 patients with mostly advanced, high-risk ENKTL found that the use of SMILE as induction or salvage therapy before allogeneic HSCT resulted in improved OS and EFS compared with those treated with non-SMILE regimens.[69] Most important, patients transplanted in first CR and second CR were found to have similar survival outcomes. These data suggest that upfront allogeneic HSCT for patients achieving first CR is not necessary and that its value in patients with advanced stage or relapsed or refractory ENKTL should be evaluated in the context of known treatment toxicities. At present, we consider allogeneic HSCT only in patients with multiply relapsed disease or refractory disease. Because circulating Epstein-Barr virus DNA and posttreatment PET with computed tomography scans have been found to be predictive of disease recurrence, future studies should focus on developing a risk-stratified approach to the use of allogeneic HSCT in advanced stage or high-risk ENKTL.[73]

ADULT T-CELL LEUKEMIA/LYMPHOMA

Adult T-cell leukemia/lymphoma (ATL) is a malignancy of peripheral T lymphocytes associated with chronic infection by the human T-cell lymphotropic virus type I retrovirus. There are between 5 and 20 million individuals infected with virus worldwide. The vast majority of those individuals are geographically clustered in southwestern Japan, the Caribbean, Western Africa, the Middle East, South America, and Papua New Guinea.[74,75] ATL develops in approximately 3% to 5% of individuals infected with T-cell lymphotropic virus type I after a long period of latency.[74,76] The clinical presentation can be greatly variable and ranges from asymptomatic disease, to systemic illness characterized by circulating neoplastic cells, lymphadenopathy, hepatosplenomegaly, rashes, infections, and hypercalcemia. The Japanese Clinical Oncology Group has proposed a classification system, the Shimoyama classification system, that highlights 4 distinct clinical subtypes of ATL (acute, lymphoma, chronic, and smoldering) on the basis of adverse prognostic factors including organ involvement, leukemic manifestations, and biochemical paramenters.[77] Acute, lymphoma, and chronic type with unfavorable prognostic factors are characteristically aggressive ATLs. The median survival time (MST) for patients with aggressive ATL is 6 to 10 months despite chemotherapy.[78–80] In contrast, smoldering and chronic ATL are typically indolent diseases with a MST of between 31 and 55 months and may not require upfront treatment if individuals are asymptomatic.[78]

The intrinsic difficulty in treating aggressive ATL is a result of their unique biological features. ATL leukemic cells overexpress multidrug resistance proteins such as P-glycoprotein and lung resistance-related protein, which may explain the poor response of ATL to chemotherapy.[81,82] ATL is also genetically complex with 30% to 50% of cases harboring mutations in tumor suppressor genes such as *p53* or *p13*[INK4B]/*p16*[INK4A] and multiple clones can present. The severe immunosuppression and high relapse rates are additional factors that affect long-term survival.[83]

Given the difficulty of treating aggressive ATL, newly diagnosed patients are encouraged to enroll in clinical trials whenever possible. At present, no standard of care has been established for relapsed or resistant ATL. For newly diagnosed patients with aggressive ATL who do not have access to clinical trial enrollment, published guidelines recommend first-line treatment with combination chemotherapy (eg, vindesine, cyclophosphamide, adriblastine, and prednisone [VCAP], doxorubicin, ranimustine, and prednisone [AMP], vindesine, etoposide, carboplatin, and prednisone [VCEP]) and consideration of subsequent allogeneic HSCT.[83] For patients with acute and unfavorable chronic type ATL, more recent evidence suggest that antiviral therapy with interferon-alpha and zidovudine may also be used as first-line therapy.[84] In addition, combined azidothymidine, interferon-alpha, and chemotherapy seems to be particularly effective in patients with ATL lymphoma.[85]

Although the use of chemotherapy and antiretroviral agents has been shown to achieve CR rates of 40% to 54%, the OS remains poor.[86] High-dose chemotherapy followed by HSCT has been considered as a possible way of improving outcomes. ASCT has not been found to be beneficial, owing to the high risk of infection and relapse within 1 year of transplantation.[87] Multiple studies and case reports, however, have shown that patients undergoing allogeneic HSCT may experience longer survival, but this benefit comes at the cost of high treatment-related mortality ranging between 30% to 40%.[88–90] No prospective randomized controlled clinical trials have directly compared allogeneic HSCT over combination chemotherapy alone, so the benefit of allogeneic HSCT remains unknown. That said, several retrospective studies support the notion that a powerful graft-versus-lymphoma effect yields durable remissions in ATL in patients who are transplanted early in first CR.[78,89,91] The largest retrospective study conducted to date analyzed the outcomes of 1186 Japanese patients with acute and lymphoma type ATL. The most commonly used chemotherapy regimen was CHOP21. No patients with acute or lymphoma type ATL received interferon/azidothymidine because the agent was not approved for the treatment of ATL in Japan. In this study, patients with aggressive ATL who did not undergo allogeneic HSCT experienced a MST and 4-year OS of 6.7 to 9.7 months and 6.8% to 13.7%, respectively. For patients with aggressive ATL who received allogeneic HSCT (n = 214), the MST and 4-year OS were 5.9 months and 26%, respectively. Importantly, those transplanted in first CR experienced a significantly longer MST of 22 months compared with those transplanted with active disease who experienced an MST of 3 months. Although an obvious selection bias limits the interpretation of retrospective data, these data do indicate that, for patients with aggressive ATL who respond to initial combination chemotherapy, transplantation in the first CR can yield durable survival. For patients who relapse after allogeneic HSCT, additional studies have found that withdrawal of immunosuppression and donor lymphocyte infusion with or without chemotherapy can be effective, suggesting that a graft-versus-lymphoma effect is essential to maintaining durable remissions.[89,92] At present, it remains unclear which donor source is ideal for allogeneic HSCT, although data from clinical trials investigating this question are forthcoming.

Although allogeneic HSCT may yield prolonged survival in patients with ATL, its widespread use is limited as the majority of patients presenting with ATL are elderly and have multiple comorbidities at the time of disease onset. For this reason, alternative treatment strategies for aggressive ATL remains an area of tremendous interest and active investigation. Recently, mogamulizumab, an anti-CCR4 monoclonal antibody, was approved in Japan for the treatment of ATL. In addition to mogamulizumab, there are ongoing phase I and II studies evaluating the role of novel agents such as brentuximab vedotin, bortezomib, lenalidomide, panobinostat, forodesine, pralatrexate, and denileukin diftitox in the treatment of ATL.[93] Although progress in our understanding of the biology of ATL will likely lead to the development of novel agents, the epidemiology and geographic distribution of the disease necessitate that future treatment strategies be both tolerated by and affordable to elderly patients in resource limited-settings to achieve a significant impact on the global burden of disease.

ENTEROPATHY-ASSOCIATED T-CELL LYMPHOMA

Enteropathy-associated TCL (EATCL) is a rare intestinal lymphoma arising from intraepithelial T lymphocytes. It is rare in the general population with an incidence of 0.5 in 1 million people in Western countries. Although there is a well-known association with celiac disease, EATCL can present in patients with no prior history of celiac disease.[94,95]

There are 2 subtypes of EATCL that are distinguishable on the basis of their clinical, morphologic, and genetic characteristics.[58] EATCL, formerly known as EATCL type I, is associated with celiac disease, the HLA-DQ2 haplotype as well as genetic alterations in chromosomes 9 and 16 (9q31.3 gain, 16q12.1 deletion).[96] Histologically, these lymphomas are composed of $CD30^+$ large pleomorphic cells with negative CD56 expression.[95] In contrast, monomorphic epitheliotropic intestinal TCL (formerly known as EATCL type II), is characterized by the monomorphic accumulation of small-to medium-sized $CD8^+$, $CD56^+$, $MATK^+$, and CD30-cells. The most common genetic alterations seen in monomorphic epitheliotropic intestinal TCL include chromosome 8q24 gain (involving *MYC*) and 1q or 5q gains.[96] In comparison to EATCL, monomorphic epitheliotropic intestinal TCL is less frequently associated with an antecedent history of celiac disease.[95,97–99]

EATCL commonly involves the small bowel and can result in malabsorption syndrome, ulcerations, perforations, obstruction, or intestinal bleeding.[96,100] At diagnosis, most patients with EATCL are in the sixth or seventh decade of their life and present with abdominal pain, fatigue, anorexia, and advanced stage disease.[95,96]

Unfortunately, EATCL portends one of the worst prognoses for any subtype of PTCL. The mean survival of patients with EATCL in the International Peripheral T-Cell Lymphoma Project was only 10 months.[96] The estimated 5-year OS and PFS for EATCL are 20% and 4%, respectively.[3]

The dismal outcomes seen for EATCL is not only a result of the severity and chemotherapy-refractory nature of the lymphoma, but also to the poor functional and nutritional status of most patients on presentation.[101] There is no standard treatment for EATCL because prospective studies evaluating therapeutic options are uncommon and retrospective studies involving patients with EATCL have been limited by small sample sizes and a heterogeneous study population.

Treatment strategies that have been used with variable success for patients with newly diagnosed EATCL include surgery, standard dose chemotherapy, HDT/ASCT, allogeneic stem cell transplantation, radiotherapy, and novel agents. Surgery performed to alleviate intestinal obstructions or perforations may aid diagnosis and is commonly followed by chemotherapy after 2 to 5 weeks.[100,101] Anthracycline-based regimens have been the most commonly used regimens used in this setting, but outcomes have remained poor.[102,103] Only 35% to 40% of patients undergoing combination chemotherapy attain a complete remission with the median duration of CR being only 6 months.[95,97,102,104,105] Radiotherapy has been used rarely and the outcome with allogeneic transplantation has been dismal.[100,101,103]

For newly diagnosed and medically fit patients with EATCL, we recommend high-dose chemotherapy followed by ASCT in first remission. The most robust evidence supporting this approach comes from 2 prospective studies, which demonstrate that upfront HDT/ASCT results in improved OS and PFS when compared with standard chemotherapy or surgery alone. Sieniawski and colleagues[106] prospectively evaluated 26 patients with EATCL treated with the Newcastle regimen of CHOP plus 6 cycles of alternating IVE (ifosfamide, epirubicin, etoposide) and MTX (intermediate-dose methotrexate) followed by ASCT. The 5-year OS and PFS were 60% and 52%, respectively, and significantly higher when compared with a historical group treated primarily with anthracycline-based chemotherapy (where the OS and PFS were 22% and 22%, respectively). A second study, the Nordic study, prospectively evaluated the benefit of upfront ASCT in 160 patients with confirmed PTCL after an induction regimen of 6 cycles of biweekly CHOEP (etoposide was omitted for patients >60 years of age). In this study, a subtype-specific analysis of 21 patients with EATCL showed that upfront ASCT resulted in a 5-year OS and PFS of 48% and 38%, respectively.[12] Although these studies were not randomized and limited by a selection bias favoring patients fit enough to tolerate ASCT, they nonetheless support the notion that ASCT is not only feasible, but can result in long-term remissions when performed as first-line therapy.

Patients with EATCL who fail first-line therapy respond poorly to second-line conventional chemotherapy.[97] One of the largest retrospective studies to date evaluating the outcomes of patients with EATCL suggests that ASCT may be an effective salvage therapy for EATCL. This analysis included 44 patients with EATCL undergoing ASCT, of which 19 (46%) received second-line or beyond chemotherapy before ASCT. At the time of transplantation, 31 patients (70%) were in first complete or partial remission. Although survival based on treatment line was not analyzed separately, the cumulative 4-year OS and PFS was 59% and 54%, respectively, with a trend toward better survival in patients transplanted in first CR or partial response.[107] Because of the retrospective nature of the study and the lack of additional prospective randomized trials, the true role of ASCT in relapsed or refractory EATCL remains unknown at this time.

It has been suggested that allogeneic HSCT may be the only curative strategy for EATCL. Unfortunately, results have been frankly disappointing owing to high mortality and early relapse.[101,103] Given that more than 50% of patients presenting with EATCL are unable to tolerate this intensive therapy, alternative strategies with novel agents are a key area interest.[95] As noted, a subset of EATCL is characterized by CD30 expression and may benefit from targeted therapy with brentuximab vedotin, an anti-CD30 drug conjugate with evidence of efficacy in relapsed lymphoma, systemic anaplastic lymphoma, and primary cutaneous T-cell non-Hodgkin lymphoma.[108] Additional agents that have been or are being actively investigated include alemtuzumab, cladribine, and romidepsin.[95,97] In the future, randomized prospective trials will be needed to ascertain whether novel agents may either replace or be used in conjunction with ASCT to improve the poor prognosis of patients with EATCL.

OTHER RARE PERIPHERAL T-CELL LYMPHOMAS

The role of stem cell transplantation in the treatment of extremely rare subtypes of PTCLs including hepatosplenic T-cell lymphoma (HSTL), primary cutaneous γδ TCL (PCGD-TCL), subcutaneous SPTCL, T-cell prolymphocytic leukemia, and aggressive NK cell leukemia is unknown; the optimal therapeutic approach for these disorders remains undefined. These uncommon PTCLs together comprise less than 3% of all PTCLs and have widely diverse clinical, immunophenotypic, and histopathologic features.[1] The rarity of these disorders limits the best available evidence evaluating treatment strategies to small, retrospective, and nonrandomized studies. As such, the use of HSCT in the treatment of these disorders remains largely investigational.

Retrospective data suggest that early stem cell transplantation may improve the otherwise poor outcomes seen in patients with HSTL who tend to present with rapidly progressive disease. The International Peripheral T-Cell/NK Cell Lymphoma Study estimated the 5-year OS and PFS of patients with HSTL to be only 7% and 0%, respectively[3] and anthracycline-based induction regimens have consistently shown low rates of durable remissions.[109,110] In comparison, non-CHOP induction regimens (ICE, IVAC) have shown improved survival when followed by stem cell transplantation (allogeneic HSCT or autologous HSCT) but this approach has only been studied retrospectively in a small cohort of patients.[111] The European Group for Blood and Marrow Transplantation Lymphoma Working Party recently published a registry-based retrospective review of 18 patients undergoing allogeneic HSCT for HSTL and demonstrated a 3-year OS and PFS of 54% and 48%, respectively.[112] NRM was high, however, at 40%. Of note, of the 7 patients in this study who underwent autologous HSCT, there remained only 1 long-term survivor who was alive and progression free at 58 months after transplantation. A retrospective review of 42 patients with HSTL from The North American Peripheral T-Cell Lymphoma Consortium similarly found that all but 1 long-term survivor had undergone allogeneic HSCT.[113] Collectively, these data suggest, that in transplant-eligible patients with HSTL, non-CHOP induction followed by allogeneic stem cell transplantation in first CR may yield improved survival but additional studies are needed to confirm benefit.

In comparison, it seems that patients with SPTCL may not require upfront stem cell transplantation. Patients with SPTCL classically present with lymphocytic panniculitis that may be associated with constitutional symptoms and is distinguished from the more aggressive PCGD-TCL on the basis of TCR phenotype.[114] SPTCL expresses a αβ TCR and follows a more indolent clinical course as opposed to PCGD-TCL which expresses the γδ TCR and is associated with poorer prognosis.[1,114] Although retrospective studies and case reports have show that stem cell transplantation is feasible and may result in long-term remission both in patients with SPTCL and PCGD-TCL, milder approaches in the upfront setting are generally favored.[115] A small study of 11 patients with SPTCL or PCGD-TCL treated with single agent bexarotene (a retinoid X receptor agonist) alone had an overall response rate of 82% (9 of 11) with CR in 55% (6 of 11).[116] Alternative agents that have also been tried with variable success in this setting include corticosteroids, interferon-alpha, zidovudine, cyclosporine, oral methotrexate, and, more recently, romidepsin.[115,117]

Treatment experience using HSCT for T-cell prolymphocytic leukemia and aggressive NK cell leukemia is likewise severely limited by the rarity of these diseases. Both subtypes are frequently resistant to conventional chemotherapy, in part owing to the production of P-glycoproteins. Two recently published registry-based studies from the European Group for Blood and Marrow Transplantation and French Society for Stem Cell Transplantation suggest that allogeneic HSCT may result in long-term survival; however, in both studies relapse after HSCT was high (41%–47%), as was 3-year transplant-related mortality (31%–41%).[118,119] ASCT has been demonstrated to be feasible after initial treatment with alemtuzumab, but this approach has not been evaluated in larger studies.[120] Although the optimal treatment of aggressive NK cell leukemia is not presently known, L-asparaginase–based regimens followed by allogeneic HSCT may improve upon dismal historical outcomes.[121]

Ultimately, it is anticipated that an improved understanding of the biologic underpinnings of all rare subtypes of PTCL will expand treatment options for these diseases in the future and likely include the use of single agent therapies with reduced toxicities. Until then, the use of stem cell transplantation in this setting remains investigational and must be balanced with the substantial risks of treatment related mortality.

SUMMARY

The use of HSCT in the treatment of PTCL remains controversial owing to the absence of randomized, controlled trials. Careful consideration of disease biology, history of response to prior therapies, individual patient preferences and overall treatment goals should guide treatment approaches for every patient. Participation in clinical trials is particularly encouraged for all subtypes of PTCL. Based on the available data, HDT followed by ASCT may be considered in first remission for patients with AITL or EATCL and in first or second remission for patients with ALK-negative ALCL. For the remainder of PTCL histologies, the benefit of ASCT and allogeneic HSCT is difficult to assess given the limitations of available data and future studies are needed. An improved understanding of unique biology of each subtype of PTCL and studies incorporating novel agents into treatment regimens may help to further identify which patients may benefit the most from HSCT.

REFERENCES

1. Swerdlow S. World Health Organization classification of tumours. 4th edition. Geneva, Switzerland: World Health Organization; 2008.
2. Shustov A. Controversies in autologous and allogeneic hematopoietic cell transplantation in peripheral T/NK-cell lymphomas. Best Pract Res Clin Haematol 2013;26(1):89–99.
3. Vose J, Armitage J, Weisenburger D. International T-Cell Lymphoma Project. International peripheral T-cell and natural killer/T-cell lymphoma study: pathology findings and clinical outcomes. J Clin Oncol 2008;26(25):4124–30.
4. Iqbal J, Wilcox R, Naushad H, et al. Genomic signatures in T-cell lymphoma: how can these improve precision in diagnosis and inform prognosis? Blood Rev 2016;30(2):89–100.
5. Savage KJ, Ferreri AJM, Zinzani PL, et al. Peripheral T-cell lymphoma–not otherwise specified. Crit Rev Oncol Hematol 2011;79(3):321–9.
6. Weisenburger DD, Savage KJ, Harris NL, et al. Peripheral T-cell lymphoma, not otherwise specified: a report of 340 cases from the International Peripheral T-cell Lymphoma Project. Blood 2011;117(12):3402–8.
7. d'Amore F, Gaulard P, Trümper L, et al. Peripheral T-cell lymphomas: ESMO Clinical Practice Guidelines for diagnosis, treatment and follow-up. Ann Oncol 2015; 26(Suppl 5):v108–15.

8. Lemonnier F, Couronné L, Parrens M, et al. Recurrent TET2 mutations in peripheral T-cell lymphomas correlate with TFH-like features and adverse clinical parameters. Blood 2012;120(7):1466–9.

9. Horwitz SM, Porcu P, Flinn I, et al. Duvelisib (IPI-145), a Phosphoinositide-3-Kinase-δ,γ Inhibitor, Shows Activity in Patients with Relapsed/Refractory T-Cell Lymphoma. Blood 2014;124(21):803.

10. NCCN Clinical Practice Guidelines in Oncology. Available at: http://www.nccn.org/professionals/physician_gls/f_guidelines.asp. Accessed September 6, 2015.

11. Savage KJ, Harris NL, Vose JM, et al. ALK- anaplastic large-cell lymphoma is clinically and immunophenotypically different from both ALK+ ALCL and peripheral T-cell lymphoma, not otherwise specified: report from the International Peripheral T-Cell Lymphoma Project. Blood 2008;111(12):5496–504.

12. d'Amore F, Relander T, Lauritzsen GF, et al. Up-front autologous stem-cell transplantation in peripheral T-cell lymphoma: NLG-T-01. J Clin Oncol 2012;30(25): 3093–9.

13. Reimer P, Rüdiger T, Geissinger E, et al. Autologous stem-cell transplantation as first-line therapy in peripheral T-cell lymphomas: results of a prospective multicenter study. J Clin Oncol 2009;27(1):106–13.

14. Yang D-H, Kim WS, Kim SJ, et al. Prognostic factors and clinical outcomes of high-dose chemotherapy followed by autologous stem cell transplantation in patients with peripheral T cell lymphoma, unspecified: complete remission at transplantation and the prognostic index of peripheral T cell lymphoma are the major factors predictive of outcome. Biol Blood Marrow Transplant 2009;15(1):118–25.

15. Corradini P, Dodero A, Zallio F, et al. Graft-versus-lymphoma effect in relapsed peripheral T-cell non-Hodgkin's lymphomas after reduced-intensity conditioning followed by allogeneic transplantation of hematopoietic cells. J Clin Oncol 2004; 22(11):2172–6.

16. Loirat M, Chevallier P, Leux C, et al. Upfront allogeneic stem-cell transplantation for patients with nonlocalized untreated peripheral T-cell lymphoma: an intention-to-treat analysis from a single center. Ann Oncol 2015;26(2):386–92.

17. Federico M, Rudiger T, Bellei M, et al. Clinicopathologic characteristics of angioimmunoblastic T-cell lymphoma: analysis of the international peripheral T-cell lymphoma project. J Clin Oncol 2013;31(2):240–6.

18. Rüdiger T, Weisenburger DD, Anderson JR, et al. Peripheral T-cell lymphoma (excluding anaplastic large-cell lymphoma): results from the Non-Hodgkin's Lymphoma Classification Project. Ann Oncol 2002;13(1):140–9.

19. Cortés JR, Palomero T. The curious origins of angioimmunoblastic T-cell lymphoma. Curr Opin Hematol 2016;23(4):434–43.

20. Mourad N, Mounier N, Brière J, et al. Clinical, biologic, and pathologic features in 157 patients with angioimmunoblastic T-cell lymphoma treated within the Groupe d'Etude des Lymphomes de l'Adulte (GELA) trials. Blood 2008;111(9):4463–70.

21. Foss FM, Zinzani PL, Vose JM, et al. Peripheral T-cell lymphoma. Blood 2011; 117(25):6756–67.

22. Gaulard P, de Leval L. Pathology of peripheral T-cell lymphomas: where do we stand? Semin Hematol 2014;51(1):5–16.

23. Couronné L, Bastard C, Bernard OA. TET2 and DNMT3A mutations in human T-Cell lymphoma. N Engl J Med 2012;366(1):95–6.

24. Cairns RA, Iqbal J, Lemonnier F, et al. IDH2 mutations are frequent in angioimmunoblastic T-cell lymphoma. Blood 2012;119(8):1901–3.

25. Piekarz RL, Frye R, Prince HM, et al. Phase 2 trial of romidepsin in patients with peripheral T-cell lymphoma. Blood 2011;117(22):5827–34.

26. O'Connor OA, Horwitz S, Masszi T, et al. Belinostat in patients with relapsed or refractory peripheral T-Cell lymphoma: results of the pivotal phase II BELIEF (CLN-19) Study. J Clin Oncol 2015;33(23):2492–9.

27. Horwitz SM, Advani RH, Bartlett NL, et al. Objective responses in relapsed T-cell lymphomas with single-agent brentuximab vedotin. Blood 2014;123(20): 3095–100.

28. Lunning MA, Horwitz S. Treatment of peripheral T-cell lymphoma: are we data driven or driving the data? Curr Treat Options Oncol 2013;14(2):212–23.

29. Moskowitz AJ, Lunning MA, Horwitz SM. How I treat the peripheral T-cell lymphomas. Blood 2014;123(17):2636–44.

30. Kyriakou C, Canals C, Goldstone A, et al. High-dose therapy and autologous stem-cell transplantation in angioimmunoblastic lymphoma: complete remission at transplantation is the major determinant of Outcome-Lymphoma Working Party of the European Group for Blood and Marrow Transplantation. J Clin Oncol 2008;26(2):218–24.

31. Schetelig J, Fetscher S, Reichle A, et al. Long-term disease-free survival in patients with angioimmunoblastic T-cell lymphoma after high-dose chemotherapy and autologous stem cell transplantation. Haematologica 2003;88(11):1272–8.

32. Rodríguez J, Conde E, Gutiérrez A, et al. Prolonged survival of patients with angioimmunoblastic T-cell lymphoma after high-dose chemotherapy and autologous stem cell transplantation: the GELTAMO experience. Eur J Haematol 2007;78(4):290–6.

33. Le Gouill S, Milpied N, Buzyn A, et al. Graft-versus-lymphoma effect for aggressive T-cell lymphomas in adults: a study by the Société Francaise de Greffe de Moëlle et de Thérapie Cellulaire. J Clin Oncol 2008;26(14):2264–71.

34. Kyriakou C, Canals C, Finke J, et al. Allogeneic stem cell transplantation is able to induce long-term remissions in angioimmunoblastic T-cell lymphoma: a retrospective study from the lymphoma working party of the European group for blood and marrow transplantation. J Clin Oncol 2009;27(24):3951–8.

35. Project TN-HLC. A clinical evaluation of the International Lymphoma Study Group Classification of Non-Hodgkin's Lymphoma. The Non-Hodgkin's Lymphoma Classification Project. Blood 1997;89(11):3909–18.

36. Harris NL, Jaffe ES, Stein H, et al. A revised European-American classification of lymphoid neoplasms: a proposal from the International Lymphoma Study Group [see comments]. Blood 1994;84(5):1361–92.

37. Hapgood G, Savage KJ. The biology and management of systemic anaplastic large cell lymphoma. Blood 2015;126(1):17–25.

38. Beaven AW, Diehl LF. Peripheral T-cell lymphoma, NOS, and anaplastic large cell lymphoma. Hematology Am Soc Hematol Educ Program 2015;2015(1): 550–8.

39. Ferreri AJM, Govi S, Pileri SA, et al. Anaplastic large cell lymphoma, ALK-positive. Crit Rev Oncol Hematol 2012;83(2):293–302.

40. Sibon D, Fournier M, Brière J, et al. Long-term outcome of adults with systemic anaplastic large-cell lymphoma treated within the Groupe d'Etude des Lymphomes de l'Adulte trials. J Clin Oncol 2012;30(32):3939–46.

41. Parrilla Castellar ER, Jaffe ES, Said JW, et al. ALK-negative anaplastic large cell lymphoma is a genetically heterogeneous disease with widely disparate clinical outcomes. Blood 2014;124(9):1473–80.

42. Zhang X-M, Li Y-X, Wang W-H, et al. Favorable outcome with doxorubicin-based chemotherapy and radiotherapy for adult patients with early stage primary systemic anaplastic large-cell lymphoma. Eur J Haematol 2013;90(3):195–201.

43. Fisher RI, Gaynor ER, Dahlberg S, et al. Comparison of a standard regimen (CHOP) with three intensive chemotherapy regimens for advanced non-Hodgkin's lymphoma. N Engl J Med 1993;328(14):1002–6.

44. Schmitz N, Trümper L, Ziepert M, et al. Treatment and prognosis of mature T-cell and NK-cell lymphoma: an analysis of patients with T-cell lymphoma treated in studies of the German High-Grade Non-Hodgkin Lymphoma Study Group. Blood 2010;116(18):3418–25.

45. Jagasia M, Morgan D, Goodman S, et al. Histology impacts the outcome of peripheral T-cell lymphomas after high dose chemotherapy and stem cell transplant. Leuk Lymphoma 2004;45(11):2261–7.

46. Corradini P, Tarella C, Zallio F, et al. Long-term follow-up of patients with peripheral T-cell lymphomas treated up-front with high-dose chemotherapy followed by autologous stem cell transplantation. Leukemia 2006;20(9):1533–8.

47. Dunleavy K, Pittaluga S, Shovlin M, et al. Phase II trial of dose-adjusted EPOCH in untreated systemic anaplastic large cell lymphoma. Haematologica 2016; 101(1):e27–9.

48. ECHELON-2: A Comparison of brentuximab vedotin and CHP with standard-of-care CHOP in the treatment of patients with CD30-positive mature T-cell lymphomas - Full Text View - ClinicalTrials.gov. Available at: https://clinicaltrials.gov/ct2/show/NCT01777152. Accessed August 5, 2016.

49. Philip T, Chauvin F, Bron D, et al. PARMA international protocol: pilot study on 50 patients and preliminary analysis of the ongoing randomized study (62 patients). Ann Oncol 1991;2(Suppl 1):57–64.

50. Fanin R, Ruiz de Elvira MC, Sperotto A, et al. Autologous stem cell transplantation for T and null cell CD30-positive anaplastic large cell lymphoma: analysis of 64 adult and paediatric cases reported to the European Group for Blood and Marrow Transplantation (EBMT). Bone Marrow Transplant 1999;23(5):437–42.

51. Smith SM, Burns LJ, van Besien K, et al. Hematopoietic cell transplantation for systemic mature T-cell non-Hodgkin lymphoma. J Clin Oncol 2013;31(25): 3100–9.

52. Zamkoff KW, Matulis MD, Mehta AC, et al. High-dose therapy and autologous stem cell transplant does not result in long-term disease-free survival in patients with recurrent chemotherapy-sensitive ALK-negative anaplastic large-cell lymphoma. Bone Marrow Transplant 2004;33(6):635–8.

53. Song KW, Mollee P, Keating A, et al. Autologous stem cell transplant for relapsed and refractory peripheral T-cell lymphoma: variable outcome according to pathological subtype. Br J Haematol 2003;120(6):978–85.

54. Jantunen E, Wiklund T, Juvonen E, et al. Autologous stem cell transplantation in adult patients with peripheral T-cell lymphoma: a nation-wide survey. Bone Marrow Transplant 2004;33(4):405–10.

55. Pro B, Advani R, Brice P, et al. Brentuximab vedotin (SGN-35) in patients with relapsed or refractory systemic anaplastic large-cell lymphoma: results of a phase II study. J Clin Oncol 2012;30(18):2190–6.

56. Mossé YP, Lim MS, Voss SD, et al. Safety and activity of crizotinib for paediatric patients with refractory solid tumours or anaplastic large-cell lymphoma: a Children's Oncology Group phase 1 consortium study. Lancet Oncol 2013;14(6): 472–80.

57. Gambacorti-Passerini C, Messa C, Pogliani EM. Crizotinib in anaplastic large-cell lymphoma. N Engl J Med 2011;364(8):775–6.

58. Swerdlow SH, Campo E, Pileri SA, et al. The 2016 revision of the World Health Organization classification of lymphoid neoplasms. Blood 2016;127(20):2375–90.

59. Jaffe ES, Nicolae A, Pittaluga S. Peripheral T-cell and NK-cell lymphomas in the WHO classification: pearls and pitfalls. Mod Pathol 2013;26(S1):S71–87.

60. Lee J, Suh C, Park YH, et al. Extranodal natural killer T-Cell lymphoma, nasal-type: a prognostic model from a retrospective multicenter study. J Clin Oncol 2006;24(4):612–8.

61. Lee J, Au W-Y, Park MJ, et al. Autologous hematopoietic stem cell transplantation in extranodal natural killer/T cell lymphoma: a multinational, multicenter, matched controlled study. Biol Blood Marrow Transplant 2008;14(12):1356–64.

62. Yamaguchi M, Kwong Y-L, Kim WS, et al. Phase II study of SMILE chemotherapy for newly diagnosed stage IV, relapsed, or refractory extranodal natural killer (NK)/T-cell lymphoma, nasal type: the NK-Cell Tumor Study Group study. J Clin Oncol 2011;29(33):4410–6.

63. Jaccard A, Gachard N, Marin B, et al. Efficacy of L-asparaginase with methotrexate and dexamethasone (AspaMetDex regimen) in patients with refractory or relapsing extranodal NK/T-cell lymphoma, a phase 2 study. Blood 2011; 117(6):1834–9.

64. Kwong Y-L, Kim WS, Lim ST, et al. SMILE for natural killer/T-cell lymphoma: analysis of safety and efficacy from the Asia Lymphoma Study Group. Blood 2012; 120(15):2973–80.

65. Yhim H-Y, Kim JS, Mun Y-C, et al. Clinical outcomes and prognostic factors of up-front autologous stem cell transplantation in patients with extranodal natural killer/T Cell Lymphoma. Biol Blood Marrow Transplant 2015;21(9):1597–604.

66. Yamaguchi M, Tobinai K, Oguchi M, et al. Phase I/II study of concurrent chemoradiotherapy for localized nasal natural killer/T-cell lymphoma: Japan Clinical Oncology Group Study JCOG0211. J Clin Oncol 2009;27(33):5594–600.

67. Kim SJ, Kim K, Kim BS, et al. Phase II trial of concurrent radiation and weekly cisplatin followed by VIPD chemotherapy in newly diagnosed, stage IE to IIE, nasal, extranodal NK/T-Cell Lymphoma: consortium for Improving Survival of Lymphoma study. J Clin Oncol 2009;27(35):6027–32.

68. Yokoyama H, Yamamoto J, Tohmiya Y, et al. Allogeneic hematopoietic stem cell transplant following chemotherapy containing l-asparaginase as a promising treatment for patients with relapsed or refractory extranodal natural killer/T cell lymphoma, nasal type. Leuk Lymphoma 2010;51(8):1509–12.

69. Tse E, Chan TSY, Koh L-P, et al. Allogeneic haematopoietic SCT for natural killer/T-cell lymphoma: a multicentre analysis from the Asia Lymphoma Study Group. Bone Marrow Transplant 2014;49(7):902–6.

70. Ennishi D, Maeda Y, Fujii N, et al. Allogeneic hematopoietic stem cell transplantation for advanced extranodal natural killer/T-cell lymphoma, nasal type. Leuk Lymphoma 2011;52(7):1255–61.

71. Murashige N, Kami M, Kishi Y, et al. Allogeneic haematopoietic stem cell transplantation as a promising treatment for natural killer-cell neoplasms. Br J Haematol 2005;130(4):561–7.

72. Paper: comparison of autologous and allogeneic hematopoietic stem cell transplantation for extranodal NK/T-Cell lymphoma, nasal type: analysis of the Japan Society for Hematopoietic Cell Transplantation (JSHCT) Lymphoma Working Group. Available at: https://ash.confex.com/ash/2011/webprogram/Paper43317.html. Accessed July 14, 2016.

73. Kwong Y-L, Pang AW, Leung AY, et al. Quantification of circulating Epstein-Barr virus DNA in NK/T-cell lymphoma treated with the SMILE protocol: diagnostic and prognostic significance. Leukemia 2014;28(4):865–70.

74. de Thé G, Bomford R. An HTLV-I vaccine: why, how, for whom? AIDS Res Hum Retroviruses 1993;9(5):381–6.
75. Gessain A, Cassar O. Epidemiological Aspects and World Distribution of HTLV-1 Infection. Front Microbiol 2012;3:388.
76. Iwanaga M, Watanabe T, Yamaguchi K. Adult T-cell leukemia: a review of epidemiological evidence. Front Microbiol 2012;3:322.
77. Shimoyama M. Diagnostic criteria and classification of clinical subtypes of adult T-cell leukaemia-lymphoma. A report from the Lymphoma Study Group (1984-87). Br J Haematol 1991;79(3):428–37.
78. Katsuya H, Ishitsuka K, Utsunomiya A, et al. Treatment and survival among 1594 patients with ATL. Blood 2015;126(24):2570–7.
79. Yamada Y, Tomonaga M, Fukuda H, et al. A new G-CSF-supported combination chemotherapy, LSG15, for adult T-cell leukaemia-lymphoma: Japan Clinical Oncology Group Study 9303. Br J Haematol 2001;113(2):375–82.
80. Tsukasaki K, Utsunomiya A, Fukuda H, et al. VCAP-AMP-VECP Compared With Biweekly CHOP for Adult T-Cell Leukemia-Lymphoma: Japan Clinical Oncology Group Study JCOG9801. J Clin Oncol 2007;25(34):5458–64.
81. Yasunami T, Wang Y, Tsuji K, et al. Multidrug resistance protein expression of adult T-cell leukemia/lymphoma. Leuk Res 2007;31(4):465–70.
82. Kuwazuru Y, Hanada S, Furukawa T, et al. Expression of P-glycoprotein in adult T-cell leukemia cells. Blood 1990;76(10):2065–71.
83. Tsukasaki K, Hermine O, Bazarbachi A, et al. Definition, prognostic factors, treatment, and response criteria of adult T-cell leukemia-lymphoma: a proposal from an international consensus meeting. J Clin Oncol 2009;27(3):453–9.
84. Bazarbachi A, Suarez F, Fields P, et al. How I treat adult T-cell leukemia/lymphoma. Blood 2011;118(7):1736–45.
85. Paper: addition of anti-viral therapy to chemotherapy improves overall survival in acute and lymphomatous Adult T-Cell Leukaemia/Lymphoma (ATLL). Available at: https://ash.confex.com/ash/2010/webprogram/Paper33893.html. Accessed July 25, 2016.
86. Ishitsuka K, Tamura K. Human T-cell leukaemia virus type I and adult T-cell leukaemia-lymphoma. Lancet Oncol 2014;15(11):e517–26.
87. Tsukasaki K, Maeda T, Arimura K, et al. Poor outcome of autologous stem cell transplantation for adult T cell leukemia/lymphoma: a case report and review of the literature. Bone Marrow Transplant 1999;23(1):87–9.
88. Fukushima T, Miyazaki Y, Honda S, et al. Allogeneic hematopoietic stem cell transplantation provides sustained long-term survival for patients with adult T-cell leukemia/lymphoma. Leukemia 2005;19(5):829–34.
89. Kanda J, Hishizawa M, Utsunomiya A, et al. Impact of graft-versus-host disease on outcomes after allogeneic hematopoietic cell transplantation for adult T-cell leukemia: a retrospective cohort study. Blood 2012;119(9):2141–8.
90. Ishida T, Hishizawa M, Kato K, et al. Impact of graft-versus-host disease on allogeneic hematopoietic cell transplantation for adult T cell leukemia-lymphoma focusing on preconditioning regimens: nationwide retrospective study. Biol Blood Marrow Transplant 2013;19(12):1731–9.
91. Fuji S, Fujiwara H, Nakano N, et al. Early application of related SCT might improve clinical outcome in adult T-cell leukemia/lymphoma. Bone Marrow Transplant 2016;51(2):205–11.
92. Itonaga H, Tsushima H, Taguchi J, et al. Treatment of relapsed adult T-cell leukemia/lymphoma after allogeneic hematopoietic stem cell transplantation: the Nagasaki Transplant Group experience. Blood 2013;121(1):219–25.

93. Kato K, Akashi K. Recent advances in therapeutic approaches for adult T-cell Leukemia/Lymphoma. Viruses 2015;7(12):6604–12.

94. Catassi C, Bearzi I, Holmes GK. Association of celiac disease and intestinal lymphomas and other cancers. Gastroenterology 2005;128(4 Suppl 1):S79–86.

95. Chandesris M-O, Malamut G, Verkarre V, et al. Enteropathy-associated T-cell lymphoma: a review on clinical presentation, diagnosis, therapeutic strategies and perspectives. Gastroenterol Clin Biol 2010;34(11):590–605.

96. Delabie J, Holte H, Vose JM, et al. Enteropathy-associated T-cell lymphoma: clinical and histological findings from the international peripheral T-cell lymphoma project. Blood 2011;118(1):148–55.

97. Di Sabatino A, Biagi F, Gobbi PG, et al. How I treat enteropathy-associated T-cell lymphoma. Blood 2012;119(11):2458–68.

98. Chott A, Haedicke W, Mosberger I, et al. Most CD56+ intestinal lymphomas are CD8+CD5-T-cell lymphomas of monomorphic small to medium size histology. Am J Pathol 1998;153(5):1483–90.

99. Chott A, Dragosics B, Radaszkiewicz T. Peripheral T-cell lymphomas of the intestine. Am J Pathol 1992;141(6):1361–71.

100. Malamut G, Chandesris O, Verkarre V, et al. Enteropathy associated T cell lymphoma in celiac disease: a large retrospective study. Dig Liver Dis 2013;45(5): 377–84.

101. Nijeboer P, Malamut G, Mulder CJ, et al. Enteropathy-associated T-cell lymphoma: improving treatment strategies. Dig Dis 2015;33(2):231–5.

102. Gale J, Simmonds PD, Mead GM, et al. Enteropathy-type intestinal T-cell lymphoma: clinical features and treatment of 31 patients in a single center. J Clin Oncol 2000;18(4):795–803.

103. Nijeboer P, de Baaij LR, Visser O, et al. Treatment response in enteropathy associated T-cell lymphoma; survival in a large multicenter cohort. Am J Hematol 2015;90(6):493–8.

104. Daum S, Ullrich R, Heise W, et al. Intestinal non-Hodgkin's lymphoma: a multicenter prospective clinical study from the German Study Group on Intestinal non-Hodgkin's Lymphoma. J Clin Oncol 2003;21(14):2740–6.

105. Egan LJ, Walsh SV, Stevens FM, et al. Celiac-associated lymphoma. A single institution experience of 30 cases in the combination chemotherapy era. J Clin Gastroenterol 1995;21(2):123–9.

106. Sieniawski M, Angamuthu N, Boyd K, et al. Evaluation of enteropathy-associated T-cell lymphoma comparing standard therapies with a novel regimen including autologous stem cell transplantation. Blood 2010;115(18):3664–70.

107. Jantunen E, Boumendil A, Finel H, et al. Autologous stem cell transplantation for enteropathy-associated T-cell lymphoma: a retrospective study by the EBMT. Blood 2013;121(13):2529–32.

108. Thomas A, Teicher BA, Hassan R. Antibody–drug conjugates for cancer therapy. Lancet Oncol 2016;17(6):e254–62.

109. Belhadj K, Reyes F, Farcet J-P, et al. Hepatosplenic gammadelta T-cell lymphoma is a rare clinicopathologic entity with poor outcome: report on a series of 21 patients. Blood 2003;102(13):4261–9.

110. Falchook GS, Vega F, Dang NH, et al. Hepatosplenic gamma-delta T-cell lymphoma: clinicopathological features and treatment. Ann Oncol 2009;20(6): 1080–5.

111. Voss MH, Lunning MA, Maragulia JC, et al. Intensive induction chemotherapy followed by early high-dose therapy and hematopoietic stem cell transplantation

results in improved outcome for patients with hepatosplenic T-cell lymphoma: a single institution experience. Clin Lymphoma Myeloma Leuk 2013;13(1):8–14.

112. Tanase A, Schmitz N, Stein H, et al. Allogeneic and autologous stem cell transplantation for hepatosplenic T-cell lymphoma: a retrospective study of the EBMT Lymphoma Working Party. Leukemia 2015;29(3):686–8.

113. Shustov AS, Wilson WH, Beaven AW, et al. Hepatosplenic T-Cell Lymphoma: clinicopathological features and treatment outcomes: report from the North American Peripheral T-Cell Lymphoma Consortium. Blood 2013;122(21):3032.

114. Willemze R, Jansen PM, Cerroni L, et al. Subcutaneous panniculitis-like T-cell lymphoma: definition, classification, and prognostic factors: an EORTC Cutaneous Lymphoma Group Study of 83 cases. Blood 2008;111(2):838–45.

115. Go RS, Wester SM. Immunophenotypic and molecular features, clinical outcomes, treatments, and prognostic factors associated with subcutaneous panniculitis-like T-cell lymphoma: a systematic analysis of 156 patients reported in the literature. Cancer 2004;101(6):1404–13.

116. Mehta N, Wayne AS, Kim YH, et al. Bexarotene is active against subcutaneous panniculitis-like T-cell lymphoma in adult and pediatric populations. Clin Lymphoma Myeloma Leuk 2012;12(1):20–5.

117. Bashey S, Krathen M, Abdulla F, et al. Romidepsin is effective in subcutaneous panniculitis-like T-cell lymphoma. J Clin Oncol 2012;30(24):e221–5.

118. Guillaume T, Beguin Y, Tabrizi R, et al. Allogeneic hematopoietic stem cell transplantation for T-prolymphocytic leukemia: a report from the French society for stem cell transplantation (SFGM-TC). Eur J Haematol 2015;94(3):265–9.

119. Wiktor-Jedrzejczak W, Dearden C, de Wreede L, et al. Hematopoietic stem cell transplantation in T-prolymphocytic leukemia: a retrospective study from the European Group for Blood and Marrow Transplantation and the Royal Marsden Consortium. Leukemia 2012;26(5):972–6.

120. Dearden CE, Matutes E, Cazin B, et al. High remission rate in T-cell prolymphocytic leukemia with CAMPATH-1H. Blood 2001;98(6):1721–6.

121. Jung KS, Cho S-H, Kim SJ, et al. L-asparaginase-based regimens followed by allogeneic hematopoietic stem cell transplantation improve outcomes in aggressive natural killer cell leukemia. J Hematol Oncol 2016;9:41.

Novel Agents in the Treatment of Relapsed or Refractory Peripheral T-Cell Lymphoma

Enrica Marchi, MD, PhD, Alexander G. Raufi, MD,
Owen A. O'Connor, MD, PhD*

KEYWORDS

- Peripheral T-cell lymphoma (PTCL) • Histone deacetylase (HDAC) inhibitors
- Pralatrexate • Epigenetic • Antibody drug conjugates

KEY POINTS

- Peripheral T-cell lymphomas (PTCLs) are rare disease and the best was to clarify the biology of these entities and improve treatment outcome is to enroll patients in clinical trials with novel agents and novel combination treatments based on the recent insight into the pathophysiology of these disease.
- The available data suggest that there is a benefit to incorporating newer agents in earlier line of therapy, but clinical trials are needed to assess the safety and the efficacy of such approaches.
- In the relapsed and refractory settings, encouraging results are seen with novel agents, and some of these drugs (eg, pralatrexate and romidepsin) can achieve high rate of response and result in durable remission.

INTRODUCTION

Malignancies derived from postthymic (mature) T cells and natural killer cells, collectively referred to as peripheral T-cell lymphomas (PTCL), encompass a variety of rare and often therapeutically challenging diseases.[1] PTCL represents 10% to 15% of all non-Hodgkin lymphoma (NHL) cases worldwide, accounting for 6000 to 10,000 cases annually in the United States.[1] The global prevalence of T-cell lymphoma (TCL) on the

Disclosure: Dr O.A. O'Connor has received research funding from Mundipharm, Seattle genetics, Celgene, DSMC, TGTR, ADCT and Edo Mundi.

Columbia University Medical Center, Center for Lymphoid Malignancies, 51 West 51st Street, Suite 200, New York, NY 10019, USA

* Corresponding author. Department of Medicine, Columbia University Medical Center, College of Physicians and Surgeons, The New York Presbyterian Hospital, 51 West 51st Street, Suite 200, New York, NY.

E-mail address: owenoconnor@columbia.edu

other hand is less well characterized and varies considerably with regards to geography. In East Asia, for example, particularly high rates of PTCL have been observed, possibly due to the high prevalence of eliciting viruses such as Epstein-Barr virus and human T-cell leukemia virus-1.[1,2] Nevertheless, the incidence of TCL appears to be on the increase in both Western and Asian countries, perhaps as a consequence of aging populations and/or improved diagnostic tests. In general PTCLs tend to be more common in men and are typically diagnosed after 50 years of age, although the median age of diagnosis can vary between the different subtypes which are shown in order of prevalence in **Fig. 1**. In between the non Hodgkin lymphomas, PTCL is among the worst in terms of 5-years survival (36%–56%).[3]

With the exception of the ALK-positive anaplastic large cell lymphoma (ALCL) subtype, PTCLs are associated with a poor prognosis. CHOP (cyclophosphamide, doxorubicin, vincristine, and prednisone) and CHOP-like chemotherapy programs are still the most commonly used regimens despite suboptimal outcomes. CHOP-based chemotherapies achieve overall response rates (ORRs) of 30% to 60%, but overall survival (OS) rates at 5 years are approximately 15% to 25%. Although autologous stem cell transplant (SCT) may improve long-term outcomes, most patients are ineligible due to refractory disease and/or poor performance status.[4]

Efforts to improve on these approaches with more dose-intense combination chemotherapy regimens have failed to show a benefit.[5,6] Given the dismal outcomes that patients with PTCL are facing, there is an urgent need to identify new agents with activity in these diseases. Fortunately, several promising new drugs with marked single-agent activity in TCLs are recently emerging.

Since 2009, 4 novel agents have been approved by the US Food and Drug Administration (FDA) in patients with relapsed or refractory PTCL. Initial trials aimed to

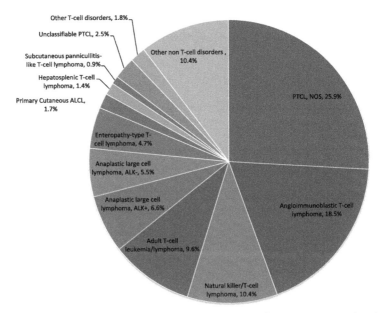

Fig. 1. PTCL subtypes. (*Data from* Vose J, Armitage J, Weisenburger D. International peripheral T-cell and natural killer/T-cell lymphoma study: pathology findings and clinical outcomes. J Clin Oncol 2008;26:4124–30.)

incorporate these agents into conventional treatment backbones (alemtuzumab-CHOP, bexarotene–CHOP, Denileukin diftitox-CHOP) have been disappointing. Another approach has been to identify novel doublets with promising preclinical activity, which could then be used to form the basis for innovative treatment platforms. In the authors' experience, many of these regimens exhibited profound synergy in both the preclinical setting and early clinical studies.

In this review, the authors discuss unique agents presently available to treat PTCL and future changes to the treatment paradigm brought about by new insight into the pathogenesis of PTCL.

US FOOD AND DRUG ADMINISTRATION–APPROVED AGENTS IN RELAPSED/REFRACTORY PERIPHERAL T-CELL LYMPHOMAS
Pralatrexate

Pralatrexate was the first drug approved for patients with relapsed/refractory PTCL. Like other antifolates, pralatrexate inhibits dihydrofolate reductase, thereby limiting intracellular synthesis of thymidylate, the rate-limiting nucleotide required for uninterrupted DNA synthesis. Pralatrexate was rationally designed to have a high affinity for both the reduced folate receptor (RFC) and folylpolyglutamate synthetase, enabling enhanced internalization specifically into tumor cells.[7–9] Although it is significantly more cytotoxic when compared with first-generation antifolates, its precise mechanism of action and T-cell specificity are not completely understood.[10] Gene expression array analyses performed following exposure to pralatrexate and methotrexate have demonstrated radically different genetic profiles. Gene Set Enrichment Analysis studies have demonstrated that many of the genes perturbed by pralatrexate exposure are associated with immunomodulatory pathways, while genes most widely affected by methotrexate involve, as one might expect, nucleotide biosynthesis. Future investigation is necessary to elucidate the physiologic mechanisms of pralatrexate because this may lead to additional biomarkers, beyond merely RFC-1, capable of predicting activity in patients with PTCL.

The PROPEL (Pralatrexate in Relapsed or Refractory Peripheral T-cell Lymphoma) study, published in 2011, was the largest prospective phase 2 trial designed to evaluate the efficacy and safety profile of pralatrexate.[11] A total of 115 patients with PTCL who had evidence of progression despite prior treatment with at least one line of prior therapy were enrolled. This population was very heavily pretreated with a median of 3 prior treatment regimens. Eighteen patients had previously undergone autologous transplant and 20% of patients had received more than 5 lines of prior therapy. Fifty-three percent of the patients were refractory to their last regimen, and 25% of patients had primary refractory disease that had not responded to any prior treatment. A total of 111 patients received pralatrexate, administered at 30 mg/m^2 weekly for 6 weeks followed by 1 week of rest on 7-week cycles, in addition to prior supplementation with folic acid and vitamin B12. Based on an independent review, the ORR was 29% with 12% of patients achieving complete remission. Strikingly, 69% of the responses occurred after the first cycle of therapy and the median duration of response (DOR) was 12.4 months. The PROPEL trial led to the FDA approval of pralatrexate for the treatment of relapsed and refractory TCL in October 2009.

Several subset analyses have been performed on the PROPEL dataset after its publication. Shustov and colleagues[9] analyzed the impact of prior therapy on response in 15 patients who had previously received CHOP-based therapy. Eleven of these patients achieved a response to pralatrexate (including 7 complete response [CR] and 4 partial response [PR]), 2 remained on treatment at the time of data cutoff

(12.9 and 18.5 months), and 2 patients proceeded to SCT (and thus were censored at 2.3 and 3.3 months). Interestingly, the ORR, CR, DOR, and progression-free survival (PFS) were 47%, 20%, not reached, and 8.4 months, respectively, based on the Independent Central Review. The investigator-assessed ORR, CR, DOR, and PFS were 40, 34%, 12.5 months, and 7.4 months, respectively. These data, albeit based on a small number of patients, confirm that earlier treatment with pralatrexate could produce better results.

A second similar analysis of the PROPEL study performed by Goy and colleagues[12] examined 20 patients who had received 2 lines of prior therapy: CHOP followed by ifosfamide, carboplatin, and etoposide (ICE). The ORR in this patient population was 40%. Two of the 20 patients achieved a CR on pralatrexate and proceeded to SCT. The PROPEL study also collected information on response to therapies administered before study entry. In the 20 patients included in the analysis, the ORR to prior ICE-based regimens was 25%, with 3 patients achieving CR (15%) and 2 patients achieving PR (10%). An additional 3 patients had stable disease (SD) (15%), 7 had progression of disease (PD) (35%), and 5 patients had nonassessable response.[11] These data further support the notion that earlier use of pralatrexate (eg, first line) would produce comparable ORR to combination chemotherapy.

Although pralatrexate is generally well tolerated, it is associated with mucositis. In the PROPEL study, mucosal inflammation was noted in more than 70% of patients, although grade 3 and 4 toxicity was seen in only 21% of patients. More recent data suggest that leucovorin may markedly reduce this risk. Hematologic toxicities consisted of grade 3 and 4 thrombocytopenia, noted to affect 14% and 19% of cases, respectively. A grade 3 anemia was seen in 16% of cases. Other adverse effects to treatment with pralatrexate included mild fatigue, nausea, dyspnea, and mild abnormalities of transaminases and serum electrolytes. Febrile neutropenia was noted in only 5% of cases.[11]

The results of the PROPEL study were compelling and led to the accelerated FDA approval of pralatrexate for patients with relapsed or refractory PTCL in 2009. Since then, South America, Asia, and Europe have approved its use in this population.

Histone Deacetylases Inhibitors

Over the last several decades, it has become clear that epigenetics likely plays a more significant role in cancer pathophysiology than previously thought. Posttranslational modifications of histones modulate gene transcription, chromatin remodeling, and nuclear architecture. Acetylation of the histone proteins is controlled by the activities of histone acetyltransferases and histone deacetylases (HDACs). By removing acetyl groups, HDACs reverse chromatin acetylation and alter transcription of oncogenes and tumor suppressor genes. In addition, HDACs deacetylate numerous nonhistone cellular substrates that govern a wide array of biologic and pathologic processes. More recently, it has been shown that epigenetic regulation plays a central role in the pathogenesis of specific types of PTCL. Although the precise mechanism of action still remains unclear, epigenetic therapies using the HDAC inhibitors have shown significant activity in these diseases. The recent approval of belinostat adds to the list of HDAC inhibitors that have been approved for TCL that includes romidepsin for cutaneous T-cell lymphoma (CTCL) and PTCLs, and vorinostat for CTCL.[13,14]

Romidepsin

Romidepsin is a macrolide small molecule belonging to a family of bicyclic peptides, which selectively inhibit class I and to a lesser extent class II HDACs. Romidepsin was approved by the FDA in 2009 for treatment of CTCL and in 2011 for the treatment of relapsed and refractory PTCL. The results of 2 separate phase 2 clinical trials formed the basis of this approval in Relapsed/Refractory PTCL. In the first study, Piekarz and colleagues[15] enrolled 47 patients with various subtypes of PTCL, including PTCL-NOS (not otherwise specified), angioimmunoblastic, ALK-negative ALCL, and enteropathy-associated TCL. All of these patients had received prior therapy with a median of 3 prior treatments (range 1–11) and 18 (38%) patients had previously undergone autologous SCT. The ORR was 38%, with CRs in 8 of the 45 patients. Responses were seen across the spectrum of subtypes enrolled, and the median DOR was 8.9 months (range 2–74). Patients with angioimmunoblastic T-cell lymphoma (AITL), of which there were 6 cases enrolled, were noted to have a lower response rate, and only one patient achieved a response, albeit a sustained PR for 23 months. It is unclear why this aggressive subtype of PTCL responded less to romidepsin; however, the sample size was small, and responses were more robust in future trials. Common toxicities included nausea, fatigue, transient thrombocytopenia, and neutropenia.[15]

In the second study, a larger registration-directed trial, 130 patients whose disease had failed to respond to at least one prior systemic therapy with PTCL were enrolled.[16] An independent review revealed an ORR of 25%, including 15% of patients who achieved a CR or complete response unconfirmed (CRu). Similar response rates were seen across a variety of subset analyses, including number of prior therapies, presence of a prior SCT, and refractoriness to the most recent therapy. The median DOR was 17 months, and of the 19 patients who achieved CR/CRu, 17 (89%) continued to remain progression-free at a median follow-up of 13.4 months. Although the study population was not as diverse or as heavily treated as the one accrued in the PROPEL study, responses were seen in many of the subtypes, including PTCL-NOS (29%), AITL (33%), and ALK-negative ALCL (24%). A recent update published longer durations of response on the order of 22.3 months and median PFS and OS times of 4 and 11.3 months, respectively.[17] The median DOR for all responders measured at 28 months was not reached for those who achieved a CR or CRu. Remarkably, even patients with a lack of response or a transient response to prior therapy achieved durable responses. None of the baseline characteristics examined in the subgroup analysis, including heavy pretreatment, response to prior therapy, and advanced disease, barred long-term responses to romidepsin.

Belinostat

Belinostat, N-hydroxy-3-[3-(phenylsulfamoyl) phenyl] prop-2-enamide, is a low-molecular-weight HDAC inhibitor with a sulfonamide-hydroxamide structure. Similar to vorinostat, the hydroxamate region of belinostat chelates zinc, a necessary element for the HDAC family of enzymes to properly function. Belinostat is a pan-HDAC inhibitor, inhibiting class I, II, and IV HDAC isoforms with nanomolar potency. In July 2014, the FDA granted accelerated approval to belinostat for the treatment of patients with relapsed and/or refractory PTCL, making it the latest HDAC inhibitor to be approved.

In March 2015, Foss and colleagues[18] published the results of an open-label, multi-center phase 2 study of belinostat in 53 patients with relapsed and refractory PTCL or CTCL who failed at least one prior systemic therapy. Patients were treated with belinostat given as 1000 mg/m^2 intravenously for 5 days on a 21-day cycle. Twenty-four patients with PTCL, 40% of whom had stage IV disease at the time of enrollment, had already received a median of 3 prior systemic therapies. Twenty-nine patients with CTCL had received a median of one prior skin-directed therapy (range 0–4) and 4 prior systemic therapies (range 1–9); 55% had stage IV disease. The ORRs were 25% (PTCL) and 14% (CTCL). Treatment-related adverse events (AEs) occurred in 77% of patients and primarily included nausea (43%), vomiting (21%), infusion site pain (13%), and dizziness (11%). Treatment-related serious AEs included one grade 5 ventricular fibrillation; grade 4 thrombocytopenia; grade 3 peripheral edema, apraxia, paralytic ileus, and pneumonitis; and grade 2 jugular vein thrombosis.

Recently, O'Connor and colleagues[19] published the results of the pivotal phase 2 BELIEF trial. In this study, 129 patients with relaxed or refractory PTCL who relapsed after or were refractory to at least one prior systemic therapy received treatment with belinostat 1000 mg/m^2 daily on days 1 to 5 on a 21-day cycle. The ORR in the 120 evaluable patients was 25.8%, including 13 (10.8%) patients with CR and 18 (15%) patients with PR. The median DOR was 13.6 months, with the longest ongoing response currently reaching more than 36 months. Median PFS and OS were 1.6 and 7.9 months, respectively. Twelve of the enrolled patients underwent stem-cell transplantation after belinostat monotherapy. Similar to other HDAC inhibitors, the most common grade 3/4 AEs involved anemia (10.8%), thrombocytopenia (7%), dyspnea (6.2%), and neutropenia (6.2%). Subjects with AITL did surprisingly well with 46% of these patients showing response to treatment. It is important to recognize, however, that the subset analysis of this heterogeneous population was not designed to explore the effectiveness of belinostat in this specific subpopulation of patients. These data further emphasize the need for future disease focused investigation with HDAC inhibitors.

Brentuximab Vedotin

Brentuximab vedotin (SGN-35) is a novel anti-CD30 antibody linked via a protease-cleavable linker to monomethyl auristatin E (MMAE), a potent antimicrotubule agent.[20] MMAE is a mitotic spindle poison that induces G2-M cell-cycle arrest and apoptosis. Brentuximab vedotin was approved for relapsed Hodgkin lymphoma and relapsed, refractory systemic ALCL, but not for patients with other subtypes of PTCL.[21–24]

A multicenter, phase 2, open-label study evaluating the efficacy and safety of brentuximab vedotin was conducted in 35 patients with relapsed/refractory CD30(+) NHL. Brentuximab vedotin was dosed at 1.8 mg/kg and given every 3 weeks until progression or unacceptable toxicity. The subset analysis included patients only with AITL and PTCL-NOS of whom 63% were refractory to most recent therapy. The ORR was 41% with 24% complete remissions, and the PFS was 6.7 months. Importantly, the duration of the benefit of brentuximab vedotin was shorter than that noted in other studies with romidepsin and pralatrexate. The safety data were consistent with the side-effect profile of brentuximab vedotin. Grade 3 events included neutropenia (14%), peripheral sensory neuropathy (9%), and hyperkalemia (9%).[25] Overall, this study population was not as heavily treated as those discussed above. **Table 1** summarizes the novel FDA agents approved for PTCLs.

EMERGING DRUGS
Alisertib

Alisertib (MLN8237) is an oral Aurora A kinase (AAK) inhibitor. AAK functions as a serine/threonine kinase regulating G2-M transition and centrosome separation during mitosis. AAK has been found to be upregulated in PTCL most strongly in ALK-positive ALCL, followed by ALK-negative ACLC and PTCL-NOS. An initial phase 2 trial evaluated alisertib efficacy against a variety of NHL. In this trial, patients received 50 mg twice daily for 7 days every 21-day cycle, until PD or unacceptable toxicities. The ORR in the 48 patients enrolled was 27% and 50% among the 8 patients with aggressive TCL.[26] Alisertib was also recently evaluated by the Southwest Oncology in a

Table 1
Novel therapies approved for relapsed/refractory peripheral T-cell lymphomas

Approved Single-Agent Therapies	Indications	Mechanism of Action	Outcomes (ORR, CR, DOR)	Pivotal Trials
Belinostat	PTCL	HDAC inhibitor	26%, 11%, 13.6 mo	O'Connor et al,[19] 2015
Chidamine (approved only in China)	PTCL	HDAC inhibitor	28%, 14%, 9.9 mo	Shi et al,[59] 2015
Brentuximab vedotin	ALCL	α-CD30 linked to auristatin (antitubulin agent)	86%, 57%, 13.2 mo	Pro et al,[21] 2012
Pralatrexate	PTCL	DHFR/thymidylate synthase inhibitor	29%, 11%, 10.1 mo	O'Connor et al,[11] 2011
Romidepsin	PTCL	HDAC inhibitor	25%, 15%, 28 mo	Coiffier et al,[16] 2014
			38%, 18%, 8.9 mo	Piekarz et al,[15] 2011

phase II trial in patients with relapsed, refractory PTCL and transformed mycosis fungoides. In 37 patients with relapsed and refractory PTCL, Barr and colleagues[27] reported 2 CRs and 7 PRs, with an ORR of 24%; the ORR was 33% for the most common subtypes (PTCL-NOS, AITL, and ALCL) when mycosis fungoides was excluded. These data with single-agent alisertib in relapsed and refractory PTLC suggested promising antitumor activity.

The LUMIERE trial was a phase 3, randomized, 2-arm, Open-Label, Multicenter, International Trial of Alisertib versus Investigator's Choice in Patients with Relapsed or Refractory Peripheral T-Cell Lymphoma. O'Connor and colleagues[28] presented the results of this recently closed study at the American Society of Hematology meeting in 2015. Patients taking alisertib were followed for a median of 9.5 months, whereas those in the comparator regimens were followed for a median of 9.2 months. The ORR was 33% for the alisertib arm, and 43% for the investigators choice arm. Interestingly, the ORR was lower among those taking alisertib, with an odds ratio of 0.65 (95% confidence interval [CI] 0.34–1.23), and the median OS was shorter among patients receiving alisertib compared with the investigator's choice of treatment: 9.2 months versus 12.2 months (hazard ratio = 0.901; 95% CI 0.607–1.337). Likewise, the median PFS was similar among both groups: 3.7 months for the alisertib cohort versus 3.4 months for the comparator cohort. One interesting of the LUMIERE study was the individual ORR for patients receiving pralatrexate and romidepsin, which was 40% and 59%, respectively. Although the study population was not as heavily treated as in the PROPEL study, these data confirm a relatively higher ORR for these agents in a relapsed or refractory PTCL population. This discrepancy in the number of treatments received may have accounted for the negative results of the study given that the study was powered on data from the respective registration directed study data.

Treatment duration was longer in patients receiving alisertib than with the other cohorts (12 weeks vs 10 weeks, respectively), with 15% and 5% of patients remaining on treatment after 2 years. Grade 3 or higher AEs occurring in the alisertib versus comparator cohorts included neutropenia (44% vs 27%), thrombocytopenia (29% vs 27%), and anemia (30% vs 11%, respectively). Although alisertib showed activity in relapsed/refractory PTCL, there was no significant efficacy benefit versus the comparator (pralatrexate, romidepsin, and gemcitabine).

Bendamustine

Bendamustine is an alkylating agent that exhibits activity in several hematologic malignancies and solid tumors. The BENTLY trial[29] explored the activity of bendamustine in patients with CTCL and PTCL (mainly AITL and PTCL-NOS). In this trial, 60 patients were treated with bendamustine infused at a dose of 120 mg/m^2 on days 1 and 2 every 3 weeks, for 6 cycles. Twenty patients (33%) received fewer than 3 cycles of bendamustine, mostly because of disease progression. The ORR was 50%, including a CR in 17 patients (28%) and a PR in 13 patients (22%). The median DOR was 3.5 months, with 30% of responses lasting greater than 6 months. The median PFS and OS were 3.6 and 6.2 months, respectively. The most frequent ($\geq$5%) grade 3/4 AEs were neutropenia (30%), thrombocytopenia (24%), and infections (20%). Infections and hematological AEs led to discontinuation in 5 patients (8%). Because bendamustine showed an encouraging response rate and acceptable toxicity, the National Comprehensive Cancer Network has recommended it as a second-line and subsequent therapy, regardless of high-dose therapy and SCT.

Crizotinib and Sorafenib

In patients with ALK-positive ALCL, there are efforts to study the use of crizotinib that is an oral small-molecule tyrosine kinase inhibitor of ALK that has been FDA approved for the treatment of lung cancer harboring a translocation in the ALK gene. In a small study consisting of 11 patients with refractory ALK-positive lymphoma, 9 had ALCL histology. Patients received crizotinib at a dose of 250 mg twice daily as monotherapy until disease progression. There was an ORR of 91% of patients. The OS was 72.7%, and the PFS was 63.7% at 2 years; in addition, 3 patients experienced a CR for greater than 30 months under continuous crizotinib administration. All toxicities were grade 1/2, including ocular flashes, peripheral edema, and neutropenia.[30,31] More recently, 2 cases of abrupt relapse in patients with *ALK*-positive anaplastic large-cell lymphoma after discontinuation of crizotinib have been described, suggesting that residual neoplastic cells can persist for up to 3 years during crizotinib treatment.[32]

Likewise, sorafenib is a multikinase inhibitor that modulates multiple intracellular pathways, including platelet-derived growth factor receptor/vascular endothelial growth factor receptor and MAPK signaling and has shown cytotoxic in vitro activity in NHL including TCL.[33] A small pilot study recently evaluated sorafenib in 12 patients with TCL (3 with PTCL and 9 with CTCL). The median number of prior therapies for the patients with PTCL was 2. Of the patients with PTCL, 3 achieved a CR and 1 received an allogeneic SCT. The median event-free survival for the entire cohort was 3.5 months. At a median follow-up of 11.2 months, 10 patients were alive (83%), and SD and PR were noted in 75% of patients.[34]

Duvelisib

Duvelisib (IPI-145) is an oral inhibitor of phosphoinositide 3-kinase (PI3K)-δ and PI3K-γ. PI3K has been found to play key regulatory roles in many cellular processes, including cell survival, proliferation, and differentiation.[35] PI3K-δ and-PI3K-γ isoforms are preferentially expressed in leukocytes and do play a central role in proliferation and survival in specific T-cell malignancies. Horwitz and colleagues[36] explored the safety of duvelisib in a phase 1 trial with a disease-specific expansion cohort. Thirty-three patients including 17 with CTCL and 16 patients with PTCL were enrolled in the study and received duvelisib at the maximum tolerated dose (MTD) of 75 mg twice daily. Thirty-one patients were evaluable for efficacy, with an ORR of 42% (13/31). The ORR in PTCL was 47% (7/15, 2 CRs, 5 PRs), and in CTCL 38% (6/16, 6 PR). The median time to response was 1.9 months (range: 1.5–3.8). Median OS was 36.4 weeks (95% CI: 18.6, –) for patients with PTCL. The median number of treatment cycles was 3.1 (range: 0.5–12.5), with 14 (42%) on treatment of 4 or more cycles (16 weeks). The median number of prior therapies was 4 (range: 1–11).

Plitidepsin

Plitidepsin is a cyclic depsipeptide originally isolated from the tunicate *Aplidium albicans* that is commercially produced by chemical synthesis. It displays a broad spectrum of anticancer activities, including induction of apoptosis and G1/G2 cell-cycle arrest. Plitidepsin has shown activity against several human malignant cell lines, including lymphoma cell lines.[37] A phase 2 trial evaluated plitidepsin in 67 patients and included 34 patients with relapsed/refractory PTCL. Of the 29 evaluable patients with PTCL, 6 demonstrated an objective response to plitidepsin (2 CRs and 4 PRs; ORR, 20.7%), with a median PFS and a median DOR of 1.6 and 2.2 months, respectively.[38]

Mogamulizumab

Mogamulizumab is a monoclonal antibody targeting CC chemokine receptor 4 (CCR4). Regulatory T cells (Tregs) that overexpress CCR4 in aggressive PTCL impair host antitumor immunity and provide an environment for the tumor to grow. Mogamulizumab depletes CCR4-positive Tregs, potentially evoking antitumor activity.[39] A phase 2 study of weekly administered mogamulizumab infusions at a dose of 1.0 mg/kg in 27 patients with relapsed, aggressive CCR4-positive TCL showed an ORR of 50%, including 31% with a CR. The median PFS was 5.2 months, and the median OS was 13.7 months. The most common ($\geq$15%) grade 3/4 AEs were lymphopenia (74%), leukocytopenia (30%), thrombocytopenia (19%), neutropenia (19%), and rash (19%).[40,41]

COMBINATION THERAPIES

The TCLs remain one of the more challenging areas in lymphoma research, where progress has been slow and conventional chemotherapy has not been able to significantly improve patient outcomes. One of the major research goals in PTCL has been to develop novel treatment platforms based on biological observation, preclinical data, and clinical efficacy, to challenge the front-line conventional chemotherapy.

Although TCLs have been classified on the basis of gene expression profiling (GEP),[42] insights into driving mutations and pathogenically dysregulated pathways are still largely unknown. There is growing evidence that epigenetic changes play an important role in the cause of TCL, and recurrent mutations in epigenetic factors, including *TET2*, *DNMT3A*, *IDH2*, impaired DNA damage response, and escape from immune surveillance, have been identified as major mechanisms contributing to the pathogenesis of PTCLs.[43,44] Frequent mutations affecting RHOA, TET2, DNMT3A, and isocitrate dehydrogenase 2 (IDH2) have been demonstrated specifically in AITL and PTCL-NOS.[45,46] Although IDH2 mutations are largely confined to AITL,[47] mutations of *RHOA*, *TET2*, and *DNMT3* can be found in other types of PTCL, with lower frequencies. In addition, the observation of recurring mutations in genes involved in genome methylation seems to be highly clustered, at least in some subtypes of PTCL, including AILT[46] and PTCL-NOS.[42] These biological observations, coupled with the efficacy of HDAC inhibitors and immunomodulatory drugs including proteasome inhibitors[48,49] in the treatment of PTCLs, suggests that rationally designed treatment platforms targeting these pathways could be a valuable therapeutic approach. Our group has focused on the development of "doublet combination treatments" that were explored initially in the preclinical setting and produced promising data that supported the development of early clinical trials that are currently ongoing. The FDA approval of several new agents for the treatment of PTCLs has facilitated the development of new combinations. The results of the principal preclinical and early clinical study in the field of PTCLs are addressed in later discussion.

Decitabine and Romidepsin

Based on the recent evidence of epigenetic mutations in PTCLs and well-known synergistic interaction between hypomethylating agents (HMA) and HDAC inhibitors in B-cell NHL,[50] the authors' group systematically explored the merits of combining HMA and HDAC inhibitors using in vitro and in vivo models of TCL. The authors demonstrated profound in vitro synergistic activity when combining the HMA decitabine with multiple HDAC inhibitors, including romidepsin, belinostat, vorinostatat, and panobinostat. Specifically, the authors demonstrated a synergy coefficient less than 0.0007 when using romidepsin in combination with decitabine. These findings were validated in a severe combined immunodeficiency beige mouse model of TCL. The molecular basis for the synergistic effect of HDAC inhibitors and DNMT inhibitors was explored by GEP and methylation array. A significant downregulation of genes involved in biosynthetic pathways, including protein and lipid synthesis, and a significant upregulation of genes responsible for cell-cycle arrest were seen. Of the genes modulated by single agents, 92% were similarly modulated by the combination, but the combination induced a further significant change in the transcriptome that affected an additional 390 genes. Decitabine in combination with romidepsin decreased the number of demethylated gene regions, and when GEP and methylation data were compared, a significant inverse relationship ($R^2 = 0.657$) was found, with genes differentially expressed in the GEP and methylation analyses.[51] Based on these data, a phase 1/2a dose escalation study (NCT01998035) is currently ongoing in patients with NHL, including TCL, to evaluate the combination of oral 5-azacytidine and the HDAC inhibitor, romidepsin.

Pralatrexate and Romidepsin

Based on the clinical observation that pralatrexate and romidepsin are active single-agent drugs in PTCLs, Jain and colleagues[52] explored the in vitro and in vivo activity of the combination using a high-throughput screening approach and multimodality in vivo imaging of surface bioluminescence and 3-dimensional ultrasound xenograft murine model of TCL. In vitro, the combination of pralatrexate and romidepsin exhibited concentration-dependent synergy against a panel of TCL cell lines. In a murine model of TCL, the group of mice treated with pralatrexate plus romidepsin demonstrated a statistically significant reduction in bioluminescent intensity compared with the romidepsin-alone, pralatrexate-alone, and control groups after 21 days. A CR was observed by day 18 only in the combination cohort, in which all 6 mice exhibited a CR. In addition, the fraction of actively proliferating cells was lower in the combination-treated mice (20%), and these mice demonstrated a statistically significant reduction in 3-dimensional tumor volumes compared with the other 3 mouse cohorts. Furthermore, the median OS time was statistically superior to that observed in the other cohorts. Based on these preclinical findings, a phase 1/2 study of the combination was performed in patients with relapsed/refractory TCL (NCT01947140).[53] Final results of this study are pending.

Alisertib and Romidepsin

Preclinical studies by Zullo and colleagues[54] supported the combination of alisertib with romidepsin. High-throughput screening has shown alisertib to be synergistic with romidepsin, although not with pralatrexate or ixazomib. During simultaneous exposure to alisertib and romidepsin at their IC10, IC20, and IC30 values, marked synergy was observed only in TCL cell lines, and not in the B-cell lymphoma cell lines. Induction of apoptosis was demonstrated by increased expression of p53 upregulated modulator of apoptosis (PUMA), caspase 3–mediated cleavage of poly(ADP-ribose) polymerase, and decreased expression of BCL-xL and BCL-2. Alisertib was induced a G2-M arrest, whereas the combination of the 2 agents seemed to induce polyploidy and a failure of cytokinesis. In vivo in a xenograft mouse model, alisertib and romidepsin synergistically induced inhibition of tumor growth. Based on the synergist effect of alisertib and romidepsin demonstrated in both in vitro and in vivo models of TCL, a phase 1 trial exploring the combination of alisertib and romidepsin in relapsed/refractory NHL was initiated. Nine patients were enrolled in the study at the time of data presentation, 3 at each of 3 dose levels. Nine patients were enrolled and 8 were evaluable for response at the time of presentation of the data. Patient's histology included 3 patients with PTCL. The median number of prior therapies was 4 (2–7), and no patients underwent prior transplant given refractory disease. The observed toxicities included grade 3/4 neutropenia, thrombocytopenia, and anemia in 45%, 45%, and 20% of the cycles, respectively. The responses included a CR (PTCL, dose level 1), SD (PTCL, dose level 3), PD (3 DHL, 1 HG DLBCL, 1 DLBCL with c-Myc, 1 PTCL). The CR patient received 7 prior lines of treatment and remained in remission at 5 months.[55]

Bortezomib and Panobinostat

Another interesting and promising drug combination that was explored in patients with relapsed and refractory PTCL included the combination of panobinostat and bortezomib. Upregulation of the nuclear factor kB pathway is a key feature in PTCL, and bortezomib, a known inhibitor of the pathway, induces apoptosis in PTCL cell lines in vitro.[56] Bortezomib showed some clinical efficacy in CTCL but has never been broadly used in PTCL as single agent.[48] In vitro data for the combination of bortezomib and HDAC inhibitors suggested a synergy between the 2 drugs by targeting the proteasome with bortezomib and the aggresome pathway via HDAC 6 inhibition.[57] Tan and colleagues[58] described a series of 25 patients treated with relapsed PTCL treated with bortezomib and the pan-deacetylase inhibitor panobinostat. The ORR was 43% with 10 of 23 patients achieving a response, including 5 patients that demonstrated a CR, and the responses to treatment were observed across all histology subtypes. The toxicities recorded included 68% of patients with grade 3/4 thrombocytopenia, 40% with peripheral neuropathy, including 8% of patients with grade 3/4 leading to drug discontinuation. Although the ORR suggested significant activity of the combination, the median PFS was 2.59 months and median DOR was 5.6 months.

   Table 2 summarizes the single agents and combination treatment currently under investigation for the treatment of PTCLs.

Table 2
Novel therapies under investigation for relapsed/refractory peripheral T-cell lymphomas

Single-Agent Trials	Mechanism of Action	Phase	ClinicalTrial.gov ID
Endostar	Angiogenesis inhibitor	II	NCT02520219
E7777	Diphtheria Toxin Fragment-Interleukin-2 Fusion protein	II	NCT02676778
Selinexor	Selective inhibitor of nuclear export	II	NCT0231247
Tipifarnib	Farnesyltransferase inhibitor	II	NCT02464228
Darinaparsin	Organic arsenic compound	II	NCT02653976
Ixazomib	Proteasome inhibitor	II	NCT02158975
Forodesine	PNP inhibitor	I/II	NCT01776411
Ruxolitinib	JAK inhibitor	II	NCT01431209
Temsirolimus	mTOR inhibitor	I	NCT01614197
Carfilzomib	Proteasome inhibitor	I	NCT01336920
Panobinostat	Pan-deacetylase inhibitor	II	NCT01261247
Clofarabine (completed)	DNA synthesis inhibitor	I/II	NCT00644189
MK2006 (completed)	AKT inhibitor	II	NCT01258998
Sorafenib (completed)	Multikinase inhibitor	II	NCT00131937
Alefacept	Immunosuppressive dimeric fusion protein	I	NCT00438802
Pembrolizumab	PD-1 antibody	II	NCT02535247
Fenretinide	Synthetic retinoid derivative	II	NCT02495415
MEDI-570	Anti-ICOS monoclonal antibody	I	NCT02520791
EDO-S101	Alkylating HDAC inhibitor	I	NCT02576496
ALRN-6924	MDM2/MDMX antagonist	I/II	NCT02264613
MLN9708	Proteasome inhibitor	II	NCT02158975

Combination Trials	Mechanism of Action	Phase	ClinicalTrial.gov ID
Chidamide + CHOP	HDAC inhibitor	I	NCT02809573
Pralatrexate + CHOP	DHFR/thymidylate synthase inhibitor	I	NCT02594267
Chidamide + Cyclophosphamide + Thalidomide	HDAC inhibitor	II	NCT02879526
Romidepsin + CHOEP	HDAC inhibitor	I/II	NCT02223208
Romidepsin + CHOP	HDAC inhibitor	III	NCT01796002
Romidepsin + ICE	HDAC inhibitor	I	NCT01590732
Romidepson + Lenalidomide	HDAC inhibitor	II	NCT02232516
		I/II	NCT01742793
Chidamide + ICE	HDAC inhibitor	II	NCT02856997
CPI-613 + Bendamustine	Antimitochondrial metabolism agent	I	NCT02168140
Belinostat + Carfilzomib	HDAC inhibitor + proteasome inhibitor	I	NCT02142530
Brentuximab vedotin + Rituximan	α-CD30 linked to auristatin (antitubulin agent)	I/II	NCT01805037
Brentuximab vedotin + CHP	α-CD30 linked to auristatin (antitubulin agent)	III	NCT01777152
Brentuximab vedotin + Bendamustine	α-CD30 linked to auristatin (antitubulin agent)	II	NCT02499627
Pralatrexate + Romidepson	DHFR/thymidylate synthase inhibitor + HDAC inhibitor	I/II	NCT01947140
Romidepsin + 5-Azacitadine	HDAC inhibitor	I/II	NCT01998035

SUMMARY

The authors believe that the use of rational combination treatment with novel agents should be further implemented based on improved understanding of the pathogenetic mechanism of PTCL and the results of preclinical studies. The best way to further understand the biology of and to improve treatment for PTCLs is to enroll as many patients as possible in clinical trials with novel agents and novel combination treatment. The available data suggest that there is a benefit to incorporating newer agents in earlier lines of therapy, but clinical trials are needed to assess the safety and efficacy of such approaches. In the relapsed and refractory setting, encouraging results are seen mostly with novel agents, and some of these drugs (eg, pralatrexate and romidepsin) can achieve a comparatively high rate of response and result in durable remissions. It is clear that to have a real chance of improving outcomes and potentially cure these diseases, novel agents are required and further investigation of these agents as first-line therapy is needed. The ability to identify more mechanistically based combination therapies will lead to more tailored therapy and, it is hoped, better survival for patients with PTCLs.

REFERENCES

1. Vose J, Armitage J, Weisenburger D. International peripheral T-cell and natural killer/T-cell lymphoma study: pathology findings and clinical outcomes. J Clin Oncol 2008;26:4124–30.
2. Foss FM, Zinzani PL, Vose JM, et al. Peripheral T-cell lymphoma. Blood 2011;117: 6756–67.
3. Teras LR, DeSantis CE, Cerhan JR, et al. 2016 US lymphoid malignancy statistics by World Health Organization subtypes. CA Cancer J Clin 2016;66:443–59.
4. Mak V, Hamm J, Chhanabhai M, et al. Survival of patients with peripheral T-cell lymphoma after first relapse or progression: spectrum of disease and rare long-term survivors. J Clin Oncol 2013;31:1970–6.
5. Simon A, Peoch M, Casassus P, et al. Upfront VIP-reinforced-ABVD (VIP-rABVD) is not superior to CHOP/21 in newly diagnosed peripheral T cell lymphoma. Results of the randomized phase III trial GOELAMS-LTP95. Br J Haematol 2010;151:159–66.
6. Escalon MP, Liu NS, Yang Y, et al. Prognostic factors and treatment of patients with T-cell non-Hodgkin lymphoma: the M. D. Anderson Cancer Center experience. Cancer 2005;103:2091–8.
7. Sirotnak FM, DeGraw JI, Moccio DM, et al. New folate analogs of the 10-deaza-aminopterin series. Basis for structural design and biochemical and pharmacologic properties. Cancer Chemother Pharmacol 1984;12:18–25.
8. Sirotnak FM, DeGraw JI, Schmid FA, et al. New folate analogs of the 10-deaza-aminopterin series. Further evidence for markedly increased antitumor efficacy compared with methotrexate in ascitic and solid murine tumor models. Cancer Chemother Pharmacol 1984;12:26–30.
9. Shustov A, Pro B, Gisselbrecht C, et al. Pralatrexate is effective as second-line treatment following cyclophosphamide/doxorubicin/vincristine/prednisone (CHOP) failure in patients with relapsed or refractory peripheral T-Cell lymphoma (PTCL). Blood 2010;116:4882.
10. Wang ES, O'Connor O, She Y, et al. Activity of a novel anti-folate (PDX, 10-propargyl 10-deazaaminopterin) against human lymphoma is superior to methotrexate and correlates with tumor RFC-1 gene expression. Leuk Lymphoma 2003;44: 1027–35.

11. O'Connor OA, Pro B, Pinter-Brown L, et al. Pralatrexate in patients with relapsed or refractory peripheral T-cell lymphoma: results from the pivotal PROPEL study. J Clin Oncol 2011;29:1182–9.

12. Goy A, Pro B, Savage KJ, et al. Pralatrexate is effective in patients with relapsed or refractory peripheral T-Cell lymphoma (PTCL) with prior ifosfamide, carboplatin, and etoposide (ICE)-based regimens. Blood 2010;116:1753.

13. Duvic M, Talpur R, Ni X, et al. Phase 2 trial of oral vorinostat (suberoylanilide hydroxamic acid, SAHA) for refractory cutaneous T-cell lymphoma (CTCL). Blood 2007;109:31–9.

14. Olsen EA, Kim YH, Kuzel TM, et al. Phase IIb multicenter trial of vorinostat in patients with persistent, progressive, or treatment refractory cutaneous T-cell lymphoma. J Clin Oncol 2007;25:3109–15.

15. Piekarz RL, Frye R, Prince HM, et al. Phase 2 trial of romidepsin in patients with peripheral T-cell lymphoma. Blood 2011;117:5827–34.

16. Coiffier B, Pro B, Prince HM, et al. Romidepsin for the treatment of relapsed/refractory peripheral T-cell lymphoma: pivotal study update demonstrates durable responses. J Hematol Oncol 2014;7:11.

17. Pro B, Horwitz SM, Prince HM, et al. Romidepsin induces durable responses in patients with relapsed or refractory angioimmunoblastic T-cell lymphoma. Hematol Oncol 2016. [Epub ahead of print].

18. Foss F, Advani R, Duvic M, et al. A Phase II trial of Belinostat (PXD101) in patients with relapsed or refractory peripheral or cutaneous T-cell lymphoma. Br J Haematol 2015;168:811–9.

19. O'Connor OA, Horwitz S, Masszi T, et al. Belinostat in patients with relapsed or refractory peripheral T-cell lymphoma: results of the pivotal phase II BELIEF (CLN-19) Study. J Clin Oncol 2015;33:2492–9.

20. Francisco JA, Cerveny CG, Meyer DL, et al. cAC10-vcMMAE, an anti-CD30-monomethyl auristatin E conjugate with potent and selective antitumor activity. Blood 2003;102:1458–65.

21. Pro B, Advani R, Brice P, et al. Brentuximab vedotin (SGN-35) in patients with relapsed or refractory systemic anaplastic large-cell lymphoma: results of a phase II study. J Clin Oncol 2012;30:2190–6.

22. Younes A, Gopal AK, Smith SE, et al. Results of a pivotal phase II study of brentuximab vedotin for patients with relapsed or refractory Hodgkin's lymphoma. J Clin Oncol 2012;30:2183–9.

23. Fanale MA, Horwitz SM, Forero-Torres A, et al. Brentuximab vedotin in the frontline treatment of patients with CD30+ peripheral T-cell lymphomas: results of a phase I study. J Clin Oncol 2014;32:3137–43.

24. Perini GF, Pro B. Brentuximab vedotin in CD30+ lymphomas. Biol Ther 2013;3:15–23.

25. Horwitz SM, Advani RH, Bartlett NL, et al. Objective responses in relapsed T-cell lymphomas with single-agent brentuximab vedotin. Blood 2014;123:3095–100.

26. Friedberg JW, Mahadevan D, Cebula E, et al. Phase II study of alisertib, a selective Aurora A kinase inhibitor, in relapsed and refractory aggressive B- and T-cell non-Hodgkin lymphomas. J Clin Oncol 2014;32:44–50.

27. Barr PM, Li H, Spier C, et al. Phase II intergroup trial of alisertib in relapsed and refractory peripheral T-cell lymphoma and transformed mycosis fungoides: SWOG 1108. J Clin Oncol 2015;33:2399–404.

28. O'Connor OE, Leonard J, Benaim E. Phase III study of investigational MLN8237 (alisertib) versus investigator"s choice in patients (pts) with relapsed/refractory (rel/ref) peripheral T-cell lymphoma (PTCL). J Clin Oncol 2012;30(suppl; abstr TPS8110).

29. Damaj G, Gressin R, Bouabdallah K, et al. Results from a prospective, open-label, phase II trial of bendamustine in refractory or relapsed T-cell lymphomas: the BENTLY trial. J Clin Oncol 2013;31:104–10.

30. Gambacorti Passerini C, Farina F, Stasia A, et al. Crizotinib in advanced, chemo-resistant anaplastic lymphoma kinase-positive lymphoma patients. J Natl Cancer Inst 2014;106:djt378.

31. Gambacorti-Passerini C, Messa C, Pogliani EM. Crizotinib in anaplastic large-cell lymphoma. N Engl J Med 2011;364:775–6.

32. Gambacorti-Passerini C, Mussolin L, Brugieres L. Abrupt relapse of ALK-positive lymphoma after discontinuation of crizotinib. N Engl J Med 2016;374:95–6.

33. Chapuy B, Schuelper N, Panse M, et al. Multikinase inhibitor sorafenib exerts cy-tocidal efficacy against Non-Hodgkin lymphomas associated with inhibition of MAPK14 and AKT phosphorylation. Br J Haematol 2011;152:401–12.

34. Gibson JF, Foss F, Cooper D, et al. Pilot study of sorafenib in relapsed or refrac-tory peripheral and cutaneous T-cell lymphoma. Br J Haematol 2014;167:141–4.

35. Engelman JA, Luo J, Cantley LC. The evolution of phosphatidylinositol 3-kinases as regulators of growth and metabolism. Nat Rev Genet 2006;7:606–19.

36. Horwitz SM, Porcu P, Flinn I, et al. Duvelisib (IPI-145), a phosphoinositide-3-ki-nase-δ,γ inhibitor, shows activity in patients with relapsed/refractory T-cell lym-phoma. Blood 2014;124:803.

37. Depenbrock H, Peter R, Faircloth GT, et al. In vitro activity of aplidine, a new marine-derived anti-cancer compound, on freshly explanted clonogenic human tumour cells and haematopoietic precursor cells. Br J Cancer 1998;78:739–44.

38. Ribrag V, Caballero D, Fermé C, et al. Multicenter phase II study of plitidepsin in patients with relapsed/refractory non-Hodgkin's lymphoma. Haematologica 2013; 98:357–63.

39. Remer M, Al-Shamkhani A, Glennie M, et al. Mogamulizumab and the treatment of CCR4-positive T-cell lymphomas. Immunotherapy 2014;6:1187–206.

40. Ishida T, Joh T, Uike N, et al. Defucosylated anti-CCR4 monoclonal antibody (KW-0761) for relapsed adult T-cell leukemia-lymphoma: a multicenter phase II study. J Clin Oncol 2012;30:837–42.

41. Ogura M, Ishida T, Hatake K, et al. Multicenter phase II study of mogamulizumab (KW-0761), a defucosylated anti-cc chemokine receptor 4 antibody, in patients with relapsed peripheral T-cell lymphoma and cutaneous T-cell lymphoma. J Clin Oncol 2014;32:1157–63.

42. Iqbal J, Wright G, Wang C, et al. Gene expression signatures delineate biological and prognostic subgroups in peripheral T-cell lymphoma. Blood 2014;123: 2915–23.

43. Couronne L, Bastard C, Bernard OA. TET2 and DNMT3A mutations in human T-cell lymphoma. N Engl J Med 2012;366:95–6.

44. Palomero T, Couronné L, Khiabanian H, et al. Recurrent mutations in epigenetic regulators, RHOA and FYN kinase in Peripheral T cell lymphomas. Nat Genet 2014;46:166–70.

45. Odejide O, Weigert O, Lane AA, et al. A targeted mutational landscape of an-gioimmunoblastic T-cell lymphoma. Blood 2014;123:1293–6.

46. Wang C, McKeithan TW, Gong Q, et al. IDH2R172 mutations define a unique sub-group of patients with angioimmunoblastic T-cell lymphoma. Blood 2015;126: 1741–52.

47. Cairns RA, Iqbal J, Lemonnier F, et al. IDH2 mutations are frequent in angioimmu-noblastic T-cell lymphoma. Blood 2012;119:1901–3.

48. Zinzani PL, Musuraca G, Tani M, et al. Phase II trial of proteasome inhibitor bortezomib in patients with relapsed or refractory cutaneous T-cell lymphoma. J Clin Oncol 2007;25:4293–7.

49. Marchi E, Paoluzzi L, Scotto L, et al. Pralatrexate is synergistic with the proteasome inhibitor bortezomib in in vitro and in vivo models of T-cell lymphoid malignancies. Clin Cancer Res 2010;16:3648–58.

50. Kalac M, Scotto L, Marchi E, et al. HDAC inhibitors and decitabine are highly synergistic and associated with unique gene-expression and epigenetic profiles in models of DLBCL. Blood 2011;118:5506–16.

51. Marchi E, Zullo KM, Amengual JE, et al. The combination of hypomethylating agents and histone deacetylase inhibitors produce marked synergy in preclinical models of T-cell lymphoma. Br J Haematol 2015;171:215–26.

52. Jain S, Jirau-Serrano X, Zullo KM, et al. Preclinical pharmacologic evaluation of pralatrexate and romidepsin confirms potent synergy of the combination in a murine model of human T-cell lymphoma. Clin Cancer Res 2015;21:2096–106.

53. Amengual JE, Lichtenstein R, Rojas C, et al. Development of novel backbones for the treatment of peripheral T-cell lymphoma (PTCL): the pralatrexate/romidepsin doublet. ASCO Meeting Abstracts 2016;34:2552.

54. Zullo KM, Guo Y, Cooke L, et al. Aurora A kinase inhibition selectively synergizes with histone deacetylase inhibitor through cytokinesis failure in T-cell lymphoma. Clin Cancer Res 2015;21:4097–109.

55. Fanale MA, Hagemeister FB, Fayad L, et al. A Phase I trial of alisertib plus romidepsin for relapsed/refractory aggressive B- and T-cell lymphomas. Blood 2014; 124:1744.

56. Nasr R, El-Sabban ME, Karam JA, et al. Efficacy and mechanism of action of the proteasome inhibitor PS-341 in T-cell lymphomas and HTLV-I associated adult T-cell leukemia/lymphoma. Oncogene 2005;24:419–30.

57. Hideshima T, Bradner JE, Wong J, et al. Small-molecule inhibition of proteasome and aggresome function induces synergistic antitumor activity in multiple myeloma. Proc Natl Acad Sci U S A 2005;102:8567–72.

58. Tan D, Phipps C, Hwang WY, et al. Panobinostat in combination with bortezomib in patients with relapsed or refractory peripheral T-cell lymphoma: an open-label, multicentre phase 2 trial. Lancet Haematol 2015;2:e326–33.

59. Shi Y, Dong M, Hong X, et al. Results from a multicenter, open-label, pivotal phase II study of chidamide in relapsed or refractory peripheral T-cell lymphoma. Ann Oncol 2015;26(8):1766–71.

Index

Note: Page numbers of article titles are in **boldface** type.

Hematol Oncol Clin N Am 31 (2017) 377–387
http://dx.doi.org/10.1016/S0889-8588(17)30020-5
0889-8588/17

Z

Moving?

Make sure your subscription moves with you!

To notify us of your new address, find your **Clinics Account Number** (located on your mailing label above your name), and contact customer service at:

Email: **journalscustomerservice-usa@elsevier.com**

800-654-2452 (subscribers in the U.S. & Canada)
314-447-8871 (subscribers outside of the U.S. & Canada)

Fax number: **314-447-8029**

Elsevier Health Sciences Division
Subscription Customer Service
3251 Riverport Lane
Maryland Heights, MO 63043

Printed and bound by CPI Group (UK) Ltd, Croydon, CR0 4YY

03/10/2024

01040392-0001